The Ultimate Conspiracy
The Biomedical Paradigm

James McCumiskey

Literally PUBLISHING

Literally Publishing Limited

The Ultimate Conspiracy
The Biomedical Paradigm

By James McCumiskey

Published by Literally Publishing Limited (www.literallypublishing.com)

ISBN 978-0-9557161-0-2

Literally Publishing Limited
Oxfordshire
United Kingdom

Legal Disclaimer

It is quite evident from reading this book the author's trenchant opinion of Modern Medicine and Medical Doctors. The author believes that 95% of Modern Medicine is scientifically and medically wrong. As an example, the author mostly accepts the diagnosis of a Medical Doctor (MD) such as "you have prostate cancer" but would strongly reject any of the MD's therapies for prostate cancer, which is clearly explained in the book.

It is also quite clear that the author is certain that the five Biological Laws of Nature are natural biological laws and are therefore 100% correct in each and every case of any cancer or disease. These five Biological laws are the central discovery of what is called New Medicine or German New Medicine, which is the life-work of Dr Ryke Geerd Hamer. The author's fervent desire is that we discard Modern Medicine as quickly as possible and replace it with German New Medicine, which is 100% scientific and 100% medically correct .

However despite these sincerely held convictions, this book cannot be relied upon by the reader for medical advice and the author is forced solely for legal reasons to state that if the reader has a medical problem you should seek appropriate medical advice, which currently means taking the advice of a medically qualified doctor, an MD.

Table of Contents

Introduction

When my father died from liver cancer in October 2002, just a few weeks before his 65th birthday, I knew nothing about the Ultimate Conspiracy. My voyage of discovery into the Ultimate Conspiracy began with his dying, death and my observations of the various doctors attending to him. The doctors knew that he was going to die very soon because of liver cancer. But none of the doctors expressed an interest in the origin of liver cancer; none of them questioned why he got liver cancer. They only explained the various tests and procedures which indicated full-blown liver cancer. They were only interested in describing the symptoms of liver cancer. They had no cure. There was only one certainty; painful and premature death.

Modern Medicine is based on a pattern of thinking called the "Biomedical Paradigm", which is fundamentally flawed. The fact that all the doctors believe in it and promote it to the wider general public, and that fact that most of us, more than 99% of us, believe it to be true, is the Ultimate Conspiracy. A conspiracy is normally the work of a few people with a specific clandestine goal. In contrast, the Ultimate Conspiracy is the work of the entire medical profession, with a declared objective of improving health. However they cannot achieve this goal because they are operating according to the Biomedical Paradigm.

What if 95% of Modern Medicine could be discarded because it is unscientific, medically wrong and is therefore killing and injuring far more people than it cures? This is what is meant by the Ultimate Conspiracy - the Biomedical Paradigm.

When enough of us understand the full nature of the Biomedical Paradigm, we will recoil in horror and demand a complete change of course in approach to medicine. This will firstly require a revolution in thinking among the general public. It will involve discarding the current Biomedical Paradigm and accepting a new paradigm for our health. The Turning Point in our understanding of medicine will only be reached after a far-reaching scientific debate about the Germ Theory of Disease medical myth in particular. The Turning Point will have been completed when most of us understand the New Medicine, which gives a scientific explanation for the origin and mechanism of all cancers and most other diseases.

I want to bring you on this incredible voyage of discovery to understand the true nature of the Biomedical Paradigm and the absolute perfection of God or Mother Nature. The human body is not a bag full of chemical formulas to be administered by increasing quantities and varieties of pharmaceuticals.[1] We do not get cancer for an unknown reason or because Mother Nature has made a mistake. Apart from diseases caused by poisoning such as from radiation and other toxins, diseases caused by malnutrition, vitamin deficiency or polluted water, and injuries caused by trauma such as a car crash, all cancers and other diseases are caused by events that have occurred in our lives prior to the onset of the cancer or disease. This sounds absurd and simplistic but is absolutely true and has been proven scientifically on thousands of occasions.

"The real voyage of discovery lies not in seeking new lands, but in seeing with new eyes."[2] All I ask is that you suspend your natural scepticism and read what follows with an open mind. I do not expect you nor do I want you to believe anything written in this book. All I ask you to do is to think about and reflect on what is written because information is only relevant when it is understood.

Once you do this you will have made the greatest voyage of discovery of your entire life. What you will see and learn will change your life for ever as it did mine.

Bon voyage![3]

The Ultimate Conspiracy
The Biomedical Paradigm

1

The Biomedical Paradigm

Cast a cold Eye
On Life, on Death.
Horseman, pass by!
Epitaph of William Butler Yeats (Irish poet, 1865–1939)

For this is the great error of our day in the treatment of the human body, that physicians separate the soul from the body.
Plato (Greek philosopher, 427–347 BC)

Through the millennia, humanity has more or less consciously known that all diseases ultimately have a psychic origin. This understanding became a "scientific" asset, firmly anchored in the inheritance of universal knowledge. It is only 'Orthodox Medicine' that has turned our animated beings into a bag full of chemical formulas.
Ryke Geerd Hamer (German physician, 1935–)

Even when all the experts agree, they may well be mistaken.
Bertrand Russell (British philosopher, 1872–1970)

Everybody gets so much information all day long that they lose their common sense.
Gertrude Stein (American writer, 1874–1946)

We don't see things as they are, we see them as we are.
Anaïs Nin (American writer, 1903–1977)

The real voyage of discovery lies not in seeking new lands, but in seeing with new eyes.
Marcel Proust (French writer, 1871–1922)

CHAPTER 1

The Ultimate Conspiracy

By Tuesday 19th October 2005, I understood the Ultimate Conspiracy. I call it the "Ultimate Conspiracy", because it involves all of us and most of us believe in it and accept it as plain common sense and scientific fact.

More than 99% of us are not even aware that we are part of the Ultimate Conspiracy. This conspiracy can be best illustrated by examining the medical stories for one day. I picked a Tuesday, because the *Irish Times* (an Irish daily newspaper) has a medical supplement that day. I noted all the medical stories for that day, Tuesday 19th October 2005.

I live in Belfast, Ireland. While eating breakfast with my family, the radio news was on in the background. The latest bird flu story was being reported on the radio[4]. I was eating, chatting with my wife and sons, and not paying much attention to the radio. However, I was very much aware that the bird flu story was on the radio and had been running in the media for the last few weeks.

That day I visited two clients for a particular assignment. While driving I listened intently to a morning talk show[5]. The guest was the Northern Ireland Health Minister, Shaun Woodward. He was interviewed about the proposed smoking ban in the workplace and all enclosed public places in Northern Ireland in April 2007. The minister is an ex-smoker; he smoked 20 cigarettes a day for ten years and gave them up with great difficulty about six months previously. He was positively evangelistic about the ban, claiming that thousands of people will be alive because they won't die from passive smoking after the ban is introduced. Some people phoned in and questioned the alleged statistics about passive smoking and lung cancer and other diseases. The Minister dismissed their queries with his absolute belief that he will be saving thousands of lives.

I read the Irish Times that night and noted all the medical-related stories for that day:

1. The bird flu pandemic was on the front page. The bird flu pandemic story was the most important current medical story at the end of October 2005. The avian flu that the experts are all worried about is the H5N1 strain, which can be transmitted from birds to humans. The Asian bird flu has killed more than 60 people (at the time of the article) since 2003. Scientists fear that the virus could mutate, enabling it to pass between people creating an influenza pandemic. The last great flu pandemic was in 1918, killing up to 50 million people. There were smaller pandemics in 1957 and 1968, killing up to a million people each. Apparently it is only a matter of time before we get another pandemic as big as the 1918 outbreak.
2. The proposed smoking ban in Northern Ireland was briefly mentioned on page seven. The Cancer Research Northern Ireland Director, Professor Alex Mark, said the smoking ban would cause "the most significant health improvement that Northern Ireland has seen in decades".
3. There were two articles on page eight about stem cell research. The first article was about two teams of scientists in Massachusetts, USA, who have provided definitive evidence that embryonic stem cells can be grown in laboratory conditions without harming human embryos.
4. The second article on stem cell research is an opinion piece by the science editor of the Irish Times. It tells us that the researchers around the world agree that the ability to manipulate stem cells would quickly lead to remarkable new cures for diseases such as multiple sclerosis (MS), diabetes and Parkinson's disease.
5. The business section had an article on page 19 about General Motors (GM) wanting to slash its health care costs by three billion dollars per year. GM Chairman and CEO, Rick Wagoner, warned that health care costs remained a major obstacle to the competitiveness of US manufacturing and called for a reform of the US health care system.
6. Page 18 of the business section had a story about Elan Corporation, plc, an Irish pharmaceutical company. Its share price rose 3% the previous day because the company said that Tysabri®, its then suspended MS treatment had passed another safety hurdle in its bid to return to market.

The Irish Times' medical supplement had two interesting front page stories:

1. One story concerned the low take up of measles, mumps, and rubella (MMR) vaccinations in the Republic of Ireland. The World Health Organization (WHO) target is 95% of the population. Ireland along with a number of other European countries has a vaccination rate below 85%. The Irish Minister of Health, Ms Mary Harney, stated that immunization is one of the most effective ways of preventing disease. A WHO doctor, Dr Nedret Emiroglu, stated that 1.4 million children under five die from vaccine-preventable diseases each year.
2. The other story concerned a 75-year-old man, Patrick Joseph Walsh, who died in a small local hospital in county Monaghan from a bleeding ulcer. The doctors weren't allowed to operate in Monaghan Hospital, but there were no beds in the other nearby hospitals for this man to be operated on. He died unnecessarily and painfully from a bleeding ulcer. There is an ongoing investigation into this tragic death.

What if the only factually correct medical stories on Tuesday 19th October 2005 were about Patrick Joseph Walsh dying unnecessarily from a bleeding ulcer, and the escalating costs of medical care in the US? What if all the other medical stories were wrong?

What if most of us have been deceived and had our sensibilities dulled, and would agree in the interests of Modern Medicine and scientific progress to stem cell research, with the laudable aim of curing diseases like MS, diabetes and Parkinson's disease, despite the fact that it would involve the destruction of human embryos? But what if stem cell research is a scientific dead-end and cannot cure any disease?

What if there is no miracle drug for curing MS, nor any other disease?

What if the bird flu/H5N1 virus does not exist?

What if the HIV virus that allegedly causes AIDS does not exist? What if AIDS is simply a collection of different diseases lumped together under this name?

What if all these so-called disease-inducing and infectious viruses like measles, mumps, and rubella (that we vaccinate our children against) have never been scientifically isolated according to established scientific criteria, and do not in fact exist?

What if the figures produced by the WHO doctor about 1.4 million children under five dying from vaccine-preventable diseases are bogus? What if vaccinations are totally unnecessary and have instead killed millions of children? What if vaccines are responsible only for creating new diseases like autism, attention deficit disorders, sudden infant death syndrome (SIDS), or shaken baby syndrome (SBS)?

What if smoking does not cause lung cancer?

What if 95% of the procedures carried out by Modern Medicine are completely unnecessary? What if Modern Medicine is inherently wrong because it is based on a pattern of thinking called the Biomedical Paradigm?

What has happened is a horror that affects us all: It is the Ultimate Conspiracy.

CHAPTER 2

How I Discovered the Ultimate Conspiracy

In August 2002, I knew nothing about the Ultimate Conspiracy. I knew nothing until my father was diagnosed with liver cancer.

My father, Bill McCumiskey, died on October 24th 2002 from acute liver failure caused by liver cancer. He was almost 65 years old. He had been diagnosed nearly three months earlier in August.

My father wasn't the type of man to go to a medical doctor (MD[6]) too often. He had never been hospitalised since his birth. If he went to the MD he would have had a real problem.

He visited his local MD in May 2002, saying that he was losing weight, couldn't sleep, had a persistent itch, and generally felt bad. He had not visited that MD before. The only reason he would have had an MD was because my mother is a regular visitor. The MD gave him the requisite five minutes and then prescribed him tranquillisers. My father had never taken tranquillisers in his life. He simply wasn't the type of man to have "bad nerves". But the MD didn't know him as a person. I found out later that the itch was significant in that it can be indicative of liver problems.

Bill attended his MD again in mid-August 2002. At this stage he looked awful and felt absolutely miserable. The MD examined his abdomen and discovered that he had an enlarged liver. His liver had expanded by at least four finger lengths[7] from its normal position. He referred him to a general surgeon for a more detailed examination.

The examination a few days later confirmed what the MD had belatedly discovered. A computed tomography (CT) scan showed multiple lesions of a low attenuation throughout an enlarged liver. This was consistent with extensive multiple hepatic metastases. This meant that his liver was riddled with cancer and they suspected that it had originated somewhere else,[8] probably in the colon, which is the large intestine.

The general surgeon in Wexford said that whilst chemotherapy could be used, there was no firm evidence that it would prolong life by a significant period. He had considered the possibility of a needle biopsy, but in view of my father's already weakened state, and the extensive nature of the abnormality on the CT scan, he had wondered if it was advisable. The biopsy wasn't going to tell him anything he didn't know.

In Wexford, being a provincial town in Ireland, it was considered normal to go to Dublin for a second opinion. The Dublin opinion merely confirmed the opinion given in Wexford. The oncologist (cancer specialist) in Dublin wanted my father to have chemotherapy for "palliative" purposes or to relieve pain and prolong life. One session of chemotherapy was enough for my father. It took an enormous toll on him.

He had gone down the conventional route; he had the first opinion and the second opinion. There was nothing more that Modern Medicine could do for him. We had to try some alternatives.

In relation to any future treatment for Bill, I deferred to one of my sisters because she had had a cancer scare a few months earlier. Having gone down the conventional medical route as we had with our father, she now seemed to rely on two alternative approaches: Dr Hamer and food.

I read some books on the food angle: on eating organic food, drinking vegetable juices and taking coffee enemas. The idea behind these books was that by eating these foods one prevented the cancer from growing or spreading and therefore one lived longer. They simply didn't ring true to me although I did not doubt the sincerity of the people who wrote them.[9]

I read a Canadian web-site[10] and understood the basics of Dr Hamer's approach to cancer. It seemed plausible. It was certainly worth a go.

Dr Hamer is a German physician. His full name is Dr Ryke Geerd Hamer. Dr Hamer had discovered a unifying explanation for all cancers and diseases. His body of work is now called German New Medicine.

My sister arranged a number of appointments for my father with a German New Medicine physician in Brussels, Belgium. The Belgian German New Medicine therapist was a conventionally trained MD who had converted to Dr Hamer's German New Medicine. He had the results of my father's liver biopsy and his liver CT scans. He did an anamnesis[11] with Bill. Anamnesis is a Greek word meaning to recall and basically it is the patient recalling his past, major events in his life such as the birth of siblings, birth of children or marriage date. The anamnesis is done so that the German New Medicine therapist can understand the psyche of the person, and his previous medical history, and then determine the cause of the cancer. Basically, in two separate hour-long sessions, the German New Medicine therapist got to know my father as a person. At this time I didn't fully understand what the German New Medicine therapist was doing, but in essence he was trying to understand my father as a person, in order to ascertain what events in my father's life had caused his liver cancer.

But Bill wanted to return home. German New Medicine isn't a magic bullet. My sister had arranged more sessions, but he still wanted to go home. He was weak. He was tired, he knew he was dying, and he had obtained the first and second opinions from Modern Medicine; he had tried the alternative approach; he had done all we had asked him to do, but he was exhausted mentally and physically. Now he just wanted to die in peace at home with his wife and family.

Modern Medicine had nothing to offer. He was too weak to continue with the alternative German New Medicine. The only thing left to do was to pray and pray hard. But there was to be no miracle. The tumour kept growing.

I reflected upon my father's death and was struck by the fact that not one MD could say why my father had liver cancer. Why was the tumour growing in his liver? Why his liver? Why not the bowel? Why him? They knew that it was inoperable: They knew the tumour was growing rapidly, but they didn't know why it had happened. Just one of those things!

Bill told me in one conversation, a month or so before he died, to get a full medical check-up every year or so. He felt if he had done so, they might have caught the liver cancer in time. He didn't go on about it; he mentioned it once. I perfunctorily nodded and said I'd do it, but I didn't dwell on it, after all he was dying. But in the year leading up to his first anniversary mass,[12] I thought about it on and off. I had already purchased Dr Hamer's book *Summary of the New Medicine* in early 2003 and had read bits of it intermittently. It's a difficult read, especially for a non-medic. In the weeks coming up to my father's anniversary mass, I realised I had to do something. I arranged an appointment with our local MD. It was for a few weeks before the 24th of October 2003, the first anniversary of my father's death.

I went to the MD's clinic and was called in to the nurse's office. She weighed me, measured my height, measured my blood pressure, and took some blood and urine samples.

I was then ushered into the MD's office. He reviewed the information given to date, told me that my body mass index (BMI) was 26, which isn't great. BMI is your weight in kilograms divided by the square of your height in metres. I weighed about 99 kg (235 pounds) and am 1.95 m (6 feet, four inches). The BMI range for ideal weight is 20–25. A BMI of 26 means that I need to lose about 7 kg (or about 15 pounds).

He then asked me to take my trousers down. The look on my face gave it away. He joked and was reassuring. He was checking for prostate cancer. For a 39-year-old male to be "intimately" examined, no matter that the person is an MD, is a traumatic experience. Well traumatic is probably overdoing it. Having said that, though, I'll never forget it. It is not nice.

I consented rather wryly to this examination. I knew that he thought he was doing the right thing. Prostate cancer, statistically speaking, does seem to be the cancer that hits men of my age. But at this stage I had gleaned enough from Dr Hamer's book *Summary of the New Medicine* to know that I was not in danger.

This would be my last consultation with an MD – a conventional medical doctor practicing Modern Medicine.

I resolved to have a good understanding of the German New Medicine in the next year, by the time of the second anniversary of my father's death. Every anniversary of his death is a milestone for me. I think of him almost every day, but his anniversary is a reminder to me that I must continue to make progress in my understanding of the German New Medicine. I don't make a New Year's resolution in January. My resolutions are determined by what I have achieved by every 24th October in relation to the New Medicine and what I must achieve the following year.

Nobody else should have their life cut short by cancer like my father.

I had no interest in medicine until my father died unnecessarily from liver cancer. I am an accountant. I am not an MD. I have no formal medical training whatsoever. But I desperately wanted to understand why people get cancers and other diseases, and how these deadly diseases could be effectively cured using Dr Hamer's German New Medicine.

By 24th October 2004, the second anniversary of my father's death, I had thoroughly studied Dr Hamer's book[13] and I understood the causes of cancer. I had an understanding of how the New Medicine explained the mechanism of other diseases, but it was a vague understanding. I desperately needed to go on a course and develop my knowledge further.

I e-mailed a Canadian lady[14] via her web-site about a course in Europe. She referred me to a Swiss man, Harald Baumann. I made contact with him in January 2005 and he told me there would be a course in Ireland in April 2005. Fantastic! It was a six-day course in Limerick city, Ireland. My wife, Donna, gave her blessing for me to go on this course; I was so excited about finally going on a course about the German New Medicine.

The course was excellent. Harald gave many examples of patients with specific cancers and other diseases, and how they were cured using German New Medicine, or how sadly they died because of their treatment by Modern Medicine. It was the case studies, the stories about real human beings that interested me. I wasn't particularly interested in the symptoms of a particular cancer or disease (unlike Modern Medicine), but I was interested in the stories of how people got a particular disease and how they cured it or unfortunately died from it.

At this time I thought that German New Medicine applied only to cancers and major diseases. I didn't realise it also applied to so-called "infectious" diseases like measles, mumps and rubella. Harald mentioned in passing the work of another German, Dr Stefan Lanka, who alleged that viruses did not exist! This seemed incredible! This surely couldn't be true? Other people on the course were confirmed vaccine-sceptics and were not at all surprised. I was astonished at the lack of reaction by the course participants to the incredible claim that viruses simply didn't exist! But every single day on that course we were told new things that completely contradicted our previous understanding of medicine.

Harald explained Dr Lanka's work over coffee one day: If the viruses didn't exist, this meant that vaccinations were therefore unnecessary, at the very least, for viral diseases. In fact vaccinations were positively dangerous because the vaccines contained poisons, and caused diseases like autism, SIDS, and attention deficit disorders. There was so much more to this German New Medicine.

I had a lot in common with Harald Baumann. He too was not an MD and, like me, had no medical training whatsoever. His journey into the New Medicine began with a book by Dr Hamer called, in English, "Legacy of a New Medicine"[15]. Harald read it on and off for a few years in the late 80s and early 90s. In the summer of 1994, his partner, Arlette Büchel, had a number of friends who had been diagnosed with breast cancer. She was naturally very upset about this. Harald had been talking to her about Dr Hamer's book and read her a few passages about breast cancer which resonated with her, because she was familiar with the life-story of her friends with breast cancer. Both Arlette and Harald were now intrigued by the possibility that Dr Hamer had discovered the true cause of all cancers. In early 1995, Harald found by chance an advertisement announcing a talk by Dr Hamer in Lindau at Lake Constance, Germany. Within a few minutes of that talk, both Harald and Arlette were hooked. They attended their first seminar on the New Medicine within a week and have been working with the New Medicine ever since. They both worked very closely with Dr Hamer for five years and got to know him very well.

I was intrigued from the moment I read about the German New Medicine on Ilsedora Laker's web-site (www.newmedicine.ca). It struck a chord with me. It just made sense. I had *Summary of the New Medicine* as my bedside reading for over a year. This book hooked me in and I too had to learn more about German New Medicine and to attend a course on it.

Evangelical Christians believe that you must be "born again"[16] in order to enter Heaven. That course had the same effect on me: after six days I knew more valuable information about medicine than any conventionally trained MD! I certainly knew a whole lot more about cancer than any oncologist or cancer MD. I clearly didn't complete a six-year medical degree in six days. Modern Medicine is only concerned with the symptoms of a disease: the oncologist will not know why the person got the cancer in the first place, and has no interest in the cause. However I understood the cause of various cancers and other diseases in only six days. This was absolutely astounding and exhilarating for me.

I felt born again. I was renewed. I felt obliged to evangelise, to spread the word about German New Medicine. Harald's course energised and empowered me. I had to continue reading, studying, thinking about and understanding German New Medicine.

With the exception of diseases caused by malnutrition, lack of clean water, vitamin deficiency, poisoning, and trauma caused by a car crash or accident, German New Medicine explains the mechanism of every cancer and every single disease known to mankind.

In April 2005, (while I was on the German New Medicine course in Limerick), Dr Hamer was in jail in France. At this time I didn't understand why the medical and scientific world wouldn't honour Dr Hamer for his tremendous discoveries.

Over the rest of 2005, I gradually became aware of the nature and full extent of the Ultimate Conspiracy. It will later become apparent that my absolute lack of medical knowledge from the outset has been in fact a help, not a hindrance, in uncovering the Ultimate Conspiracy.

CHAPTER 3

The Death of Dirk Hamer

Dr Ryke Geerd Hamer

Dr Ryke Geerd Hamer was born on 17th May 1935 in Frisia, Germany. He studied medicine and theology at the University of Tübingen. He met his wife Sigrid Oldenburg (a medical student) there and married her in 1956. At the age of 22, in 1957, he completed his degree in theology and then, four years later in 1961, he qualified as an MD.[17]

In the following years he practiced at different university clinics in Germany. In 1972 Dr Hamer completed his specialization in internal medicine and began to work at the University Clinic in Tübingen as an internist in charge of cancer patients. At the same time, he ran a private practice with his wife Dr Sigrid Hamer.[18]

Dr Hamer also showed an extraordinary talent for inventing medical devices, one of which was the Hamer-scalpel. The Hamer-scalpel is used for plastic surgery and cuts 20 times more sharply than a razor. His intention was to treat the sick in Rome free of charge, from the money obtained from his patents.[19]

Dr Hamer and his wife Sigrid had four children, two boys and two girls. They were born roughly two years apart. Birgit was the eldest, then Dirk born in March 1959, then Gunhild and finally Bernd.[20]

Prior to the tragic death of his son, Dr Hamer was, however inadvertently, a key player in the Biomedical Paradigm. He was a 43-year-old specialist in internal medicine: an extremely successful MD.

Dr Hamer discovered what is now called German New Medicine because of the effect the tragic death of his son Dirk had on him: A few months after Dirk died, Dr Hamer got testicular cancer. Dr Hamer would later understand that the day his son died he got a terrible shock[21], which caused his testicular cancer.

The tragic shooting of Dirk Hamer[22]

On the 18th of August 1978, the 19-year-old Dirk was on vacation with a group of friends on three boats cruising around Sardinia. They went on a short trip to the isle of Cavallo, which belongs to Corsica. They had intended to go back to Sardinia that evening, but, had deferred the trip till the following day because of a storm warning. They anchored their three boats together in the bay. A yacht belonging to an Italian aristocrat was anchored right beside these three boats.

His friends wanted to dine at an expensive restaurant on Cavallo. As Dirk had no money he couldn't go to the restaurant and went to sleep early that evening on the port (left) side of the boat Mapagia.

Dr Nikola Pende sat at a table with some of these young people who had travelled over from Sardinia. He was the son of the family doctor to this aristocrat. He did not know him personally. Also dining at the same restaurant with his own entourage was the aristocrat, who was seated at the table beside Dr Pende. Dr Pende and the young people were having a great time. There was a lot of laughter at the table. However, as events subsequently transpired, the aristocrat thought that Dr Pende was making fun of him, although this was not the case at all. They all left the restaurant at three o'clock in the morning.

The aristocrat was walking home with his friends and noticed Dr Pende get onto the boat *Coke* and then go below deck to his bunk. The aristocrat, apparently enraged by the alleged slight he had suffered from Dr Pende, rushed home to get a rifle.

His wife had the headlights of their jeep turned on to the bay so that her husband could see what he was doing. The aristocrat took a dinghy over to the starboard (right) side of the boat near the stern (back of the boat) where he guessed that Dr Pende was sleeping. His entourage were on the beach observing the whole scene and cheering him on, no doubt fuelled by too much alcohol.

The aristocrat shot twice through the starboard side of *Coke*. Dr Nikola Pende felt both bullets pass over his head and then hit the deck in order to protect himself.

Coke was the first of the three boats anchored in a row. It was the closest to the harbour. The two bullets went through the hull of *Coke*, through the hull of *Master*, entered the starboard side of *Mapagia*, and hit Dirk Hamer who was fast asleep mid-ship on the port side of the boat. Dirk was hit twice in the lower stomach. The bullets also ripped the right pelvic vein, which caused internal bleeding.

Dirk cried out for help in Italian, "Aiuto, aiuto". The aristocrat had a helicopter and a pilot at his disposal, which Dirk's friends were informed about. But after waiting for two hours for a helicopter that never appeared, Dirk's friends decided to bring him to Porto Vecchio, Corsica on *Coke*. An additional two hours later, they arrived at Porto Vecchio where Dirk was declared clinically dead. He had to be resuscitated and operated on for the internal bleeding. The next day he was flown to Marseilles, France where he had his right leg amputated. Two weeks later he was flown to Heidelberg, Germany where be battled for his life for a few months. After 19 operations, Dirk died three months later on December 7th 1978 in the arms of his father, Dr Ryke Geerd Hamer.

In 1991, 13 years after he inadvertently killed Dirk Hamer, the aristocrat was sentenced to a mere six month's probation for the illegal discharge of a weapon.

Dr Hamer's testicular cancer

The death of a child is the worst thing that could happen to any parent, particularly so young as in Dirk's case, and in such tragic and incredibly bizarre circumstances.

Dr Hamer was on his own at the hospital in Heidelberg with his dead son. The rest of the family were back at home in Rome. Dr Hamer suffered an enormous shock at the death of his son, which he would later describe as a "biological shock" or "psycho-biological shock" because it resulted in cancer. A biological shock concerning the loss or disappearance of a loved one results in testicular cancer in a man and ovarian cancer in a woman.

Within two months of Dirk's death, Dr Hamer's right testicle was enlarged. The significance of the fact that it was his right testicle would become apparent later.

Dr Hamer had a teratoma, which is a Greek word meaning monster tumour. This teratoma consisted of skin, bones, cartilage, glands, hair and teeth tissue. Ironically, his medical colleagues removed his right testicle with the Hamer-scalpel. This operation nearly killed him. They wanted him to undergo radiotherapy but Dr Hamer refused any further "treatment".

After two operations by March 1979, he was given a 20% chance of survival. Cancer was then discovered in his peritoneum, which was originally described as a metastasis from the original cancer in his right testicle. He was now given a 1% chance of survival. He somehow survived by the grace of God, and made a full recovery.[23]

He had been healthy all his life prior to his son's tragic death. Dr Hamer strongly suspected that there was a connection between him getting testicular cancer and the terrible shock he experienced. He resolved to investigate this connection as soon as he was able.

CHAPTER 4

Discovery of the Iron Rule of Cancer (IRC)

In 1981, Dr Hamer became the head of internal medicine at a Bavarian cancer clinic for women attached to the University of Munich. In this position he had the opportunity to study female patients with cancer and to compare his experience with theirs to see if the cause of their cancer was the same as his; if they had also experienced a terrible shock prior to getting cancer.[24]

By September 1981, Dr Hamer had discovered what he believed to be the origin or the cause of all cancers. He called it the Dirk-Hamer-Syndrome (DHS) in honour of his son Dirk. He had analysed about 170 patients. All of them, without exception, had experienced a terrible shock prior to getting cancer, which confirmed his personal experience and his hypothesis for the origin of all cancers. This seemed such an enormous discovery that he initially doubted it himself. Could it be true that all cancers are caused by a biological shock?[25]

At this stage of his life Dr Hamer dreamed almost nightly about his beloved dead son. Dirk seemed to speak to him in a dream and tell him that he was right, that he had indeed discovered the cause of cancer—a severe biological shock or a DHS. Dirk urged his father to keep going because he had to find out two more important things.[26]

One must understand what is meant by this biological shock. It is a sudden, unexpected event that has caught the patient off-guard, and all the patient can do is to think all the time about the events that caused such a terrible shock. Most of us have heard the tale of the person who one day had a full head of black hair and the next day their hair was completely grey. This loss of hair colour would have been caused by a biological shock. In this case the biological shock would be a brutal separation loss within the family: the sudden death of a parent, spouse or child. The complete loss of hair colour by the following day gives us an idea about the nature of the biological shock. Once the shock has occurred, as perceived by the person in their psyche, the effects are immediate and begin to occur simultaneously at the brain level and at the organ level.

Dr Hamer revised all these case studies and categorised the shocks that had led to these women getting a particular type of cancer. He made a breathtaking discovery: cervical cancer was always preceded by a biological shock of a sexual nature; breast cancer was caused mostly by a mother–child conflict or more generally a nest conflict. He had discovered that all cancers were caused by a particular type of biological shock. This must have been truly exhilarating for him. He had cracked it: firstly, he had found the origin of all cancers to be a biological shock or a DHS; secondly, he knew why people got a particular type of cancer.

Again, Dr Hamer doubted what he had discovered. Could this be true? Was there a definite link between the type of shock and the particular cancer that resulted from it? Dirk confirmed again in a dream that Dr Hamer was indeed correct, that a specific type of shock caused a specific cancer. Dirk told his father he was missing only one more thing.[27]

Dr Hamer now knew for certain that all cancers were caused by a biological shock (DHS) and that the nature or the theme of the biological shock determined the type of cancer that the patient got. His beloved son Dirk had confirmed all this to him in a dream and told him to keep researching for the third component of cancers.[28]

He worked feverishly through all his case studies and discovered that the patients who had been "cured" or who had in reality survived their cancer treatment, in each and every case, their conflict had been solved. Those who had died or whose condition had deteriorated, without exception, had not solved their conflict, the biological shock that had caused their cancer in the first place.[29]

His colleagues simply did not believe him and were uninterested in and dismissive of his findings. Dirk appeared again to Dr Hamer in a dream. Dirk was beaming with admiration. Dirk told him that he knew that what Dr Hamer had discovered was the absolute truth and that he had nothing to be afraid of.[30]

What Dr Hamer had discovered with the guidance in dreams from his dead son Dirk was that:

1. All cancers are caused by a most all-encompassing, most unbearable, acute, severe shock. This type of shock is called a biological shock or a psycho-biological shock.

2. The specific cancer caused depends on the nature of the shock.
3. The cancer can be reversed if the conflict that caused the shock is solved.

These three discoveries became the three criteria of the first Biological Law – the Iron Rule of Cancer (IRC).

We are predisposed to a particular DHS because of our past experiences, our vulnerabilities, our individual perceptions, our values and beliefs. We experience a DHS not because of the shock itself alone but because of who we are as a person, shaped by all our previous experiences, which makes this event or shock become a DHS for us. Animals experience a biological shock in concrete terms such as a deer challenged for control of his territory. Humans experience this type of "territorial-loss conflict" in a different way such as losing a job, a girlfriend, or wife.[31]

Dr Hamer investigated cases of ovarian cancer at the clinic and found that they too, like testicular cancer, occurred because of the death or disappearance of a loved one. Some examples of the events causing such a shock are:

1. An elderly woman walked into her living room one morning and found her canary dead.
2. A woman is told by her husband that they cannot have children because of his low sperm count: This was a loss-conflict for the children she desperately wanted, but could never have with her husband.
3. A young girl sees her beloved horse being put down because of a broken leg.[32]

Modern Medicine would never enquire into such events that have occurred in a person's life prior to getting ovarian cancer. The death of a canary and the subsequent occurrence of ovarian cancer would seem ridiculous to Modern Medicine. However, it takes a well-rounded soul-detective, a therapist with a real knowledge of humanity, to discover that the canary was very important in this elderly woman's life, and its death was a real loss for this woman: Hence her ovarian cancer.

The discovery that all cancers were caused by a biological shock or DHS is what Dr Hamer initially termed the IRC in 1981. At that time he thought that biological shocks only applied to cancers. He had no idea at this time that the IRC would become the central discovery for all of medicine. His point of view was very different from all the current medical theories, and when he presented these discoveries to his colleagues at the cancer clinic, they gave him an ultimatum: either to deny his findings or leave the clinic immediately. His findings went against conventional medical thinking. They were so outrageous that they had to be wrong.

Dr Hamer is a true scientist and a righteous person. He could not possibly deny his findings: He could not deny humanity the benefit of his momentous scientific discoveries. Dr Hamer had no choice but to leave the clinic.

By 1983, Dr Hamer determined that all diseases[33] were cancer or cancer-equivalent diseases: Hence possible alternative names would be the "Iron Rule of all Diseases" or the "Iron Rule of Medicine". By "cancer-equivalent", all Dr Hamer means is that the other diseases such as diabetes or MS are also caused by a biological shock, and can be explained by the New Medicine, just like all cancers. However, as Dr Hamer discovered the IRC originally in relation to cancer, his original designation the "Iron Rule of Cancer" stuck. He called it the Iron Rule because it works 100% of the time: It is the first of the five Biological Laws of Nature that work 100% of the time.

The Iron Rule of Cancer states that it is the theme of the conflict—the subjective experience of the conflict as it is felt by the individual—that is going to determine the precise area of the brain that is affected and consequently the afflicted organ. This theme boils down to fundamental emotions that are common to man and all animals. Conflict themes can be territorial, rejection, rivalry, or disgust.

Dr Hamer gives the example of the wife who catches her husband in bed with her best friend. The facts are obvious and undisputed; her husband has been caught in a compromising position by his wife and one can appreciate that this would cause a shock for any spouse. However the theme of the shock and resultant disease depends on the psyche or mind of the cheated wife.

The woman might feel that her family has been destroyed causing breast cancer. She might feel a sexual frustration conflict and get cervical cancer. She might feel herself plunged into an unbearable situation that she cannot get out of and get MS. She might feel herself to be worthless and get bone cancer/osteoporosis. The possibilities are as varied as the human psyche. She might have hated or disliked her husband and is now glad to be able to divorce him and sue him for every penny he has, with no health problems whatsoever.

The Iron Rule of Cancer has three criteria:[34]

The first criterion of the Iron Rule of Cancer states that every cancer or cancer-equivalent disease originates with a DHS. A DHS is a severe, highly acute, dramatic and isolating shock occurring simultaneously on the three levels of the human trinity:

1. Psyche.
2. Brain.
3. Organ.

This first criterion describes the conditions for the generation of a "biological conflict". The DHS causes a shock or biological conflict which results in a disease. The biological conflict is a severe, acute, dramatic and isolating shock for which we are not at all mentally prepared.

Obviously a DHS doesn't have to be as dramatic as the tragic death of a loved one. One could get a biological shock simply after hearing a bad remark.

We all have conflicts all the time; conflicts with our spouse, boss, children and work colleagues. The vast majority of these conflicts do not result in cancer. We manage these conflicts and are in fact mentally prepared for them. German New Medicine terms these normal everyday conflicts as "psychological conflicts". Psychological conflicts, as opposed to biological conflicts, are conflicts for which we have time to anticipate (even a few seconds) and consequently do not cause cancer. A psychological conflict is quite different from a biological conflict. We can usually master psychological conflicts over time; they may cause ongoing emotional distress but do not cause cancer.

The second criterion of the Iron Rule of Cancer (and all diseases) is that the conflict theme at the moment of the DHS or biological shock determines the location in the brain of the affected brain relay and the corresponding location of the cancer (or cancer-equivalent disease) in the body.

In the course of the evolution of the human, each brain relay was programmed with an emergency response program enabling the organism to combat an unexpected situation. At the moment the conflict shock strikes, the brain relay transmits a biochemical signal to the corresponding organ. The relation between the conflict shock, the brain relay and the organ is always unequivocal.

Depending on the theme of the shock, a specific brain relay is activated which controls a particular organ of the body. This activation is an emergency response programme. In the case of liver cancer, for example, the theme of the biological shock is a "starvation conflict"; the brain relay that controls the liver is activated and the liver expands or becomes cancerous.

An interesting observation is that one single DHS or biological shock can have several themes and impact several brain relays resulting in multiple diseases simultaneously. For example, if a businessman unexpectedly loses his business, he could simultaneously get angina pectoris (as a result of a "territory-loss conflict") and bone cancer (as a result of a "self-devaluation conflict").

The third criterion of the Iron Rule of Cancer states that the development of the conflict determines a definite development of the brain relay and a definite development of the cancer (or cancer-equivalent disease) in the organ. There is a direct correlation between the life-cycle of the conflict and the life-cycle of the cancer that develops in the body. The course of the cancer on all three levels of the human trinity, the psyche, the brain and the organ, always runs synchronously.

At the moment of the DHS (biological conflict) the brain relay is switched on at a specific location in the brain determined by the theme of the biological conflict.

Synchronously the afflicted organ (controlled by the brain relay) will either have a tumour (cell multiplication), necrosis/ulcer (cell decrease) or functional disturbances in the cancer-equivalent diseases in the conflict-active phase. The reverse will occur in the reparation phase. By functional disturbance, one means that diseases like MS or diabetes, which are clearly not cancers, but still respond in accordance with the Biological Laws, and are therefore called "cancer-equivalent" in the terminology of German New Medicine.

Mind-body connection

The mind–body connection can be represented by the following equation:

H(uman) = P(syche) + B(rain)+ O(organ)
H = P + B + O

In the case of a cancer, the biological shock in the psyche affects a particular brain relay and then the corresponding organ; or in equation format:

P = >B = >O

The following diagram illustrates the mind–body connection. Psychological conflicts, or normal everyday conflicts are manageable and do not cause disease. This is demonstrated by the arrows emanating from and terminating in the psyche. These conflicts may cause a great deal of mental distress but because there is no "shock", there is no biological conflict causing a cancer/disease.

However it is undoubtedly true that certain ongoing psychological problems can predispose a person to be more susceptible to a particular type of conflict shock.[35]

Biological conflicts are illustrated by the arrows going from the psyche to the brain. When a biological shock occurs, this will affect a specific brain relay, which in turn affects a specific organ of the body. Depending on which brain relay is affected, a specific organ (such as the heart, lungs or bowel) will be affected by the cancer or cancer-equivalent disease.

With this first Biological Law – The Iron Rule of Cancer, Dr Hamer has rediscovered, and has scientifically proven the mind–body connection. This is something which has always been suspected, has been discarded because of Modern Medicine, but nonetheless still exists.

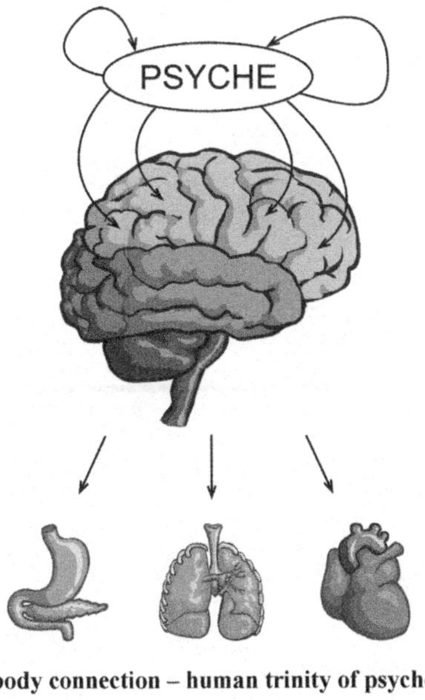

Figure 4.1 Mind–body connection – human trinity of psyche, brain and organ

CHAPTER 5

The Five Biological Laws of Nature

Having discovered the IRC, the first and most important Biological Law, Dr Hamer continued on with his research. In all, he would discover five Biological Laws of Nature. These natural Biological Laws individually and collectively turn everything we know from Modern Medicine upside down.

Dr Hamer attempted to copyright his body of work as "New Medicine" in 2003, but it was not possible. Dr Hamer eventually copyrighted his discoveries on 27th May 2004 as "German New Medicine". German New Medicine distinguishes his work from Modern Medicine and from all the other alternative therapies. Both of the terms, New Medicine and German New Medicine are used synonymously.

The five Biological Laws of Nature of the German New Medicine are essential to a scientific understanding of health. It will be necessary to re-read these several times in order to understand their true meaning.

Once you understand these five Biological Laws of Nature you will know more about medicine than any MD. This is a bold statement to make but as you will soon discover a true one.

A summary of these critically important five Biological Laws of Nature follows:

First Biological Law – the IRC

The first Biological Law is the Iron Rule of Cancer (IRC). It is the most important of the Biological Laws because it tells you why the person got a cancer or disease in the first place.

The important point to remember about the first Biological Law is to recall that a DHS is a severe, highly acute, dramatic and isolating shock occurring simultaneously on the three levels of the human trinity:

1. Psyche.
2. Brain.
3. Organ.

The shock occurs; the person thinks obsessively about it; a specific brain relay is switched on and a particular organ or part of the body is affected. For instance, a woman is walking on the pavement with her four-year-old child. Her child suddenly darts out onto the road and is knocked down by a car. The mother gets a DHS, a "mother–child worry conflict". The only focus of her attention is the safety and well-being of her child.

Second Biological Law – the two phases of every cancer/disease

The second Biological Law states that every cancer or disease has two phases provided the conflict is resolved. The first phase is called the "conflict-active phase", which occurs after a DHS or biological shock. The second phase is called the "reparation phase"[36] after the conflict has been resolved.

The conflict-active phase is also called the "cold phase". When the body is under stress the blood vessels are constricted, resulting in such symptoms as cold hands, cold feet, cold skin, chills, shivers and cold sweats.

In the conflict-active phase one thinks compulsively about the event that caused the biological shock. The conflict activity in the mind/psyche can be measured by the following vegetative parameters:

1. Constant compulsive thinking about the DHS. This is the most important clinical symptom of the conflict-active phase.
2. Loss of appetite.
3. Consequent loss of weight.
4. Cold hands and feet (cold extremities).
5. Cold skin.
6. Sleeplessness.
7. Waking up shortly after falling asleep.
8. Elevated blood pressure.
9. Fast heart beat.
10. Low blood sugar.
11. Intense urge to get out of bed early (4am or 5am) to do something.

Sleeplessness, biologically speaking, is vital because it allows the person extra hours during the day to focus on the conflict and find a resolution to it.

So if you know someone who is losing weight, who has cold hands and feet and has difficulty sleeping at night, you can immediately explain to them that they are in the conflict-active phase. They should be able to tell you the ongoing conflict that is causing these symptoms.

The reparation phase is also called the hot phase because the blood vessels are widened, resulting in warm hands, warm skin and a possible fever. There is a feeling in the mind/psyche of great relief that the conflict is finally over.

The reparation phase in the mind/psyche can be measured by the following vegetative parameters:

1. Feeling of intense relief in the psyche because the conflict is over. This is the most important clinical symptom of the reparation phase.
2. Good appetite.
3. Consequent increase in weight.
4. Warm hands and feet (warm extremities).
5. Warm skin.
6. Sleep disturbance until about 3–4am.
7. Fever.

Fever is a good thing. The body is returning to normal after a biological shock. A fever is designed by Mother Nature to cleanse the body and restore health. We don't have to fear fever anymore, particularly in young children.

A fever is not the symptom of a new disease, but the reparation phase of a particular conflict. The reparation phase of a conflict can often be the most dangerous part of the disease. This runs counter-intuitively: You would imagine that when you have solved the conflict that the person returns to normal. No. The person enters the reparation phase where the body recuperates, through rest and fever, and when this reparation phase is over the person has then returned to full health.

Third Biological Law – the ontogenetic[37] system of tumours and cancer- equivalents: the symptoms of disease

This third Biological Law states that the symptoms of a cancer or other disease in the conflict-active phase and the reparation phase are dependent upon the germ layer that the respective organ is made up from. This is what is meant by the term "ontogenetic".

There are three germ layers which are created in the first 15 days of the life of a newly created baby or embryo. These three germ layers are the endoderm or inner germ layer, the mesoderm or middle germ layer, and the ectoderm or outer germ layer.

Organs, whose tissue derives from the endoderm, experience tissue growth in the conflict-active phase and tissue destruction in the reparation phase. Organs whose tissue derives from the ectoderm experience tissue destruction or ulcers in the conflict-active phase and tissue reconstruction in the reparation phase. Organs deriving from the mesoderm experience a mixture of the symptoms from the ectodermal and endodermal layers, depending on which part of the brain controls the mesodermal tissue.

The classic case of tissue growth is the lump on a breast because of glandular breast cancer. It is mesodermal in origin and acts like the tissue of endodermal origin. It grows in the conflict-active phase and is destroyed by the microbes in the reparation phase.

Continuing with the example I gave earlier of the woman who got a DHS after witnessing her child being knocked down by a car. This DHS is a mother-child worry conflict which causes a tumour to grow on one of her breasts. There is an enormous significance as to which breast the tumour develops on, which will be explored later in detail.

A breast with a lump is seen as something awful. The tumour must be removed at all costs, possibly the entire breast may be lost, and further chemotherapy needed to prevent the "cancer cells" migrating to another part of the body through a process called metastasis by the MDs causing so-called secondary cancers. Now with the knowledge of the German New Medicine, we enquire into the preceding shock. If the woman is able to resolve the biological shock; the lump in the breast will degrade away gradually as it is destroyed by microbes in the reparation phase.

The woman's child makes a full recovery after a few weeks in hospital. The "mother-child worry conflict" has been naturally solved. A few days later the woman notices a lump on her breast. Shock! Horror! Panic! She visits her local MD, tests are done and her breast is removed; she endures a long course of chemotherapy and her life is destroyed. She is unlikely to survive five years later after having chemotherapy[38]. In reality her conflict was resolved; all she had to do was wait; the lump would have degraded naturally; there was no cause for alarm.

The brain can be divided into two key parts: the old brain and the new brain. The old brain is made up of the brain stem and the cerebellum. In the conflict-active phase, organs controlled by brain relays in the old brain exhibit a tumour growth. In the reparation phase they exhibit tumour degradation. The new brain comprises the cerebral medulla and cerebral cortex. In the conflict-active phase, organs controlled by brain relays in the new brain exhibit ulcers and necroses. In the reparation phase, the ulcers are replenished.

In this third Biological Law, all you need to remember is that all organs controlled by brain relays in the old brain exhibit tumour growth/cell multiplication in the conflict-active phase, and tumour degradation/cell destruction in the reparation phase. Whereas organs controlled by brain relays in the new brain exhibit ulcers/necroses in the conflict-active phase, and replenishment of these ulcers/necroses in the reparation phase.

Disease symptoms

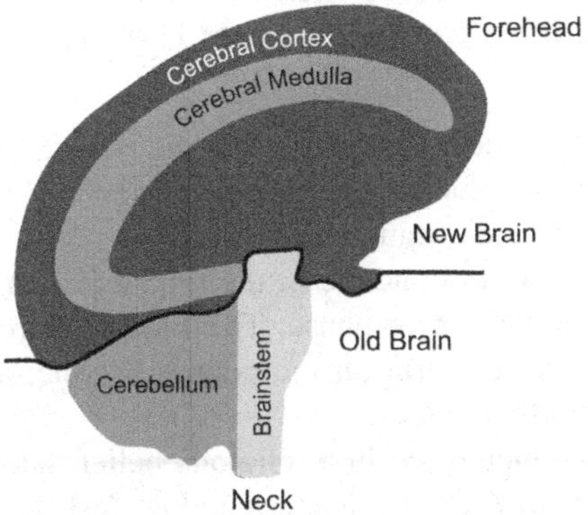

Brain Part	Conflict Active Phase Tumour Symptoms	Reparation Phase Tumour Symptoms
Old Brain	Cell Multiplication	Cell Destruction
New Brain	Cell Destruction	Cell Multiplication

Diagram 5.1 Major brain parts and tumour symptoms[39]

This information would be absolutely astonishing for any MD. They define cancer as a cell that has lost its normal control mechanism and thus has unregulated cell growth. What the MDs call "unregulated cell growth" can occur in the conflict-active phase and in the reparation phase depending on the affected organ. Thus endodermal organs such as liver parenchyma are diagnosed in the conflict-active phase and do indeed exhibit tumour growth or unregulated cell growth. In order to stop this uncontrolled cell growth the DHS causing it must be solved, otherwise the tumour keeps growing, the person remains in the conflict-active phase and the person eventually dies from cachexia. But the MDs define other diseases such as leukaemia as a cancer because of "unregulated cell growth" even though leukaemia is a disease that occurs in the reparation phase of bone cancer or osteoporosis. The solution to leukaemia is simply to do nothing, congratulate the patient on solving their DHS, reassure them but do absolutely nothing. The MDs cannot distinguish between cancers that occur in the conflict-active phase and cancers that occur in the reparation phase because they do not know this third Biological Law.

Fourth Biological Law – the ontogenetic system of microbes: the microbes that work in the reparation phase depend on the germ layer the organ is made from.

The fourth Biological Law states that the type of microbes operating in the reparation phase are dependent upon the germ layer that the diseased organ is made from.

The microbes are only active in the reparation phase and are not active in the conflict-active phase. The fungal microbes operate on endodermal tissue, bacteria on mesodermal tissue, and the smaller microbes on ectodermal tissue.

We have been inculcated in a religious belief that germs are bad, whereas in fact they are our helpers, either destroying the tumours that grew in the conflict-active phase or replenishing the ulcers that occurred in the conflict-active phase. We have no reason to fear these germs.

Because these microbes or germs are present in the reparation phase, when the patient had possibly a fever or other symptoms, it was assumed that the germs had caused the fever and the associated disease, whatever it was. Saying that germs are the cause of disease is like saying that snow is the cause of winter because it is present when it is very cold, or that firemen cause fires because they are always present at a fire, or that a traffic accident is caused by paramedics or ambulance men because they are always present when you drive past a car crash, or that flies cause manure because as soon as you see some manure you see flies around it...

Yes. Germs are present in the reparation phase of the disease or biological conflict. But the DHS or biological shock had occurred prior to the conflict. The germs had nothing to do with the DHS that caused the biological conflict. The germs did not cause the disease. The germs are used by the body to optimise the reparation phase.

Fifth Biological Law – the quintessence

The fifth Biological Law is the quintessence or the heart of German New Medicine. We do not get cancer or any other disease by chance or for no particular reason. There is no mistake by God or Mother Nature. Our cancer or other disease is merely in response to the biological shock that we got. Our cancer is a meaningful event. All so-called cancers and diseases are, in the German New Medicine, termed Meaningful Biological Programs of Nature (MBPs).[40] It tells us why we got a particular disease or cancer.

The biological shock causes a program alteration in a specific location in the brain, around the brain relay that had hitherto operated normally millions of times prior to the biological conflict. What is breathtaking and astonishing about this program switch is that (depending on the cancer) it can be a last resort by the organism or the person in the battle for survival. The disease or MBP occurs in order to allow the human body to override normal everyday operations and deal physically and biologically with the emergency situation. This programming switch is a meaningful event. It is a Meaningful Biological Program of Nature (MBP).

The MBP is an all-out effort by the organism to enable us to solve the DHS or the biological shock. In the case of some MBPs, if we cannot solve the DHS, then we may die of cachexia or simply waste away. In other cases we simply have to live with the symptoms of the disease in the conflict-active state such as diabetes or MS.

The first Biological Law states that a biological shock or DHS causes a cancer. The second Biological Law states that all MBPs have two phases: conflict-active phase and the healing or reparation phase[41]. The third Biological Law states the nature of the symptoms in the conflict-active and reparation phases depends on the germ layer the organism is made from. Organs made from the endodermal germ layer exhibit tumour growth in the conflict-active phase and tumour degradation in the reparation phase. The fourth Biological Law states the nature of the microbes in the reparation phase. The type of microbes operating in the reparation phase depends on the germ-layer origin of the affected organ. The fifth Biological Law encapsulates these four laws and answers the why or origin of disease: Why do we get cancer or a cancer-equivalent disease?

We get cancer or a specific disease to solve a particular problem of survival. With the exception of those organs controlled by brain relays in the cerebral medulla, the biological benefit of all other MBPs is in the conflict-active phase.

Organs comprised of mesodermal tissue, with their brain relays located in the cerebral medulla, have their biological benefit in the reparation phase. An example of such a disease is testicular cancer. The biological benefit of testicular cancer is that in the reparation phase you get testicular cysts or augmentation of the testicular tissue over-compensating for the necrosis in the conflict-active phase. This augmentation of testicular tissue results in a greater production of testosterone: The man becomes more masculine and is more capable of handling similar conflicts in future.

All other organs controlled by brain relays located in different areas of the brain have their biological benefit in the conflict-active phase. For example, in the worry conflict case of glandular breast cancer, the woman will get a tumour or growth on her breast because because of an archaic biological program to provide more milk for the injured child, even though the child could be well beyond the breast-feeding stage of its development.

We don't get cancer because the gods demanded it; we get cancer because of a shock, a biological shock, a psycho-biological shock, a DHS that we couldn't anticipate. Being ill is God's way or Mother Nature's way of saying we do have a second chance, a chance to discover why we got ill in the first place, and an opportunity to cure ourselves.

Germ Layer	Brain Part	Biological Benefit
Ectoderm (outer Germ Layer)	Cerebral Cortex	Conflict-active Phase
Mesoderm (middle Germ Layer)	1 Cerebellum 2 Cerebral Medulla	1 Conflict-active Phase 2 Reparation phase
Endoderm (inner Germ Layer)	Brain Stem	Conflict-active Phase

Figure 5.1 Biological benefits of diseases

Brain relays

When we get a biological shock a specific brain relay is switched on.

A CT scan is a more modern equivalent of the X-ray, offering a three-dimensional depiction of the body's internal organs. It is particularly useful for the examination of the brain. Dr Hamer has used it to great effect.

In the conflict-active phase these switched-on brain relays exist in target configuration. One can imagine the target configuration as having the same effect as that of a stone being dropped in a pond, with concentric rings surrounding the brain relay. When the conflict is resolved, when the patient is in the reparation phase, these concentric rings become oedematous: They fill up with fluid.

Thus if one is in perfect health, with no conflicts ongoing, the brain relays will not be observable on the CT scan. One can only observe the brain relays on a CT scan when they are in the conflict-active phase (target configuration) or in the reparation phase (oedematous).

One could argue that one cannot measure the effect of a biological shock on the psyche. This is not true. One can measure the effect with vegetative parameters such as an inability to sleep, lack of appetite, and all of these are indicators that the patient is in the conflict-active phase.

However in German New Medicine one can make a clear connection between a type of conflict such as a "loss conflict", (which is the loss or disappearance of a loved one) and the occurrence of testicular cancer in a man and an ovarian cyst in a woman. Dr Hamer has a Psyche-Brain-Organ disease chart which makes all these connections for every cancer and disease known to mankind.

I believe that the fact that one can observe the brain relays (when a disease is ongoing) on a CT scan provides sufficient scientific proof to convince people that there is something to these discoveries of Dr Hamer.

The three levels of the human trinity are mutually interrelated: the psyche, the brain and the organ. What happens on one level of the human trinity occurs synchronously on the other two levels. It is an over-determined system. By this, one means if one knows what is happening at the brain level through a CT scan, one can predict what is happening at the other two levels. If one knows which organ is affected, one can immediately tell which brain relay is switched on, and the nature of the biological shock.

Thus a biological shock resulting in a "loss conflict" because of the loss or disappearance of a loved one results in the conflict-active phase in compulsive thinking about the shock, causing either testicular cancer or ovarian cancer, and the affected brain relay controlling those organs is viewable on a CT scan of the brain.

One would imagine that if other MDs examined these CT scans they would be impressed and convinced that Dr Hamer had scientifically proven the mind–body connection?

CHAPTER 6

The Two-Phase Diagram of a Cancer/Disease

The second Biological Law can be pictorially represented using the two-phase diagram which illustrates the course of a Meaningful Biological Programme of Nature (MBP) from the DHS or biological shock resulting in the conflict-active phase, to the resolution of the conflict resulting in the reparation phase, and to a full return to normal health.

The four phases of a cancer/disease

A one-cycle disease is when you get a cancer or other disease and then fully recover from it. The two-phase diagram of a one-cycle disease, along with the five Biological Laws of Nature, is critical to the understanding of the origin of cancer/disease.

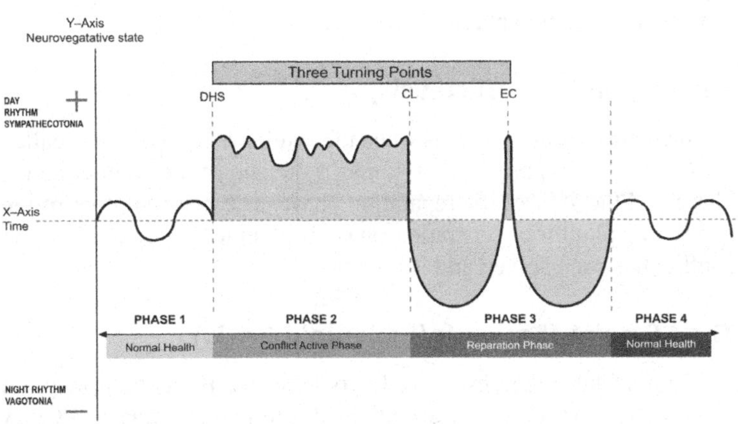

Figure 6.1 *Two-Phase Diagram of a Cancer/Disease*[42]

Using the above diagram of a one-cycle disease, one can see that there are four major phases in the state of health of an individual who has a one-cycle disease.

The first phase in the state of health of an individual with a one-cycle disease is the patient being perfectly healthy prior to the DHS or biological shock. This phase is important in that the patient (with an active conflict) has to try and recall when they felt well and thus place the DHS at a particular point in time.

Once the DHS occurs, the patient is in the second phase or the conflict-active phase. The third phase, the reparation phase, occurs when the conflict is resolved. When the conflict is completely resolved and the reparation phase is over, we enter the fourth phase, which is full health after the cancer/disease.

The DHS - Dirk Hamer Syndrome

The DHS is the pivotal point for all cancers and other diseases: They are all caused by an acute biological shock. The patient will always be able to recall the biological shock that caused the cancer. The nature of this biological shock is described in the first Biological Law, the Iron Rule of Cancer, which is the most important of all the Biological Laws.

Each one-cycle disease has three well-defined turning points. The first turning point is the DHS, the biological shock that is the instigator of the Meaningful Biological Program of Nature (MBP). Prior to the DHS, the patient was in full health. After the DHS, the patient is in the conflict-active phase.

The CL point (ConflictLysis)

The second turning point is when the conflict is resolved: It is called the ConflictoLysis point (CL). It marks the end of the conflict-active phase and the start of the reparation phase. The key symptom of the conflict resolution or reparation phase is complete mental relief: the conflict has been solved and is now over.

The EC point (Epileptic/Epileptoid Crisis)

The third turning point is the EC point or the Epileptic/Epileptoid Crisis. The reparation phase is divided into two sub-phases PCL-A and PCL-B. PCL meaning Post ConflictoLysis or after CL, so PCL is after the commencement of the reparation phase. The third turning point, the EC point occurs in the middle of the reparation phase.

The epileptic crisis is something Mother Nature devised a long time ago. It runs on all three levels of the human trinity (psyche, brain, and organ) at the same time. It happens at the height of the reparation phase, its purpose being to normalise the body again. What we usually call an epileptic cramp-spasm with muscle cramps is only one form of the epileptic crisis, namely, after resolving a motor conflict. The epileptoid crisis occurs for all other conflicts, which are not motor conflicts. It is called an epileptoid crisis because it is similar to the epileptic crisis for motor conflicts.

Epileptoid crises occur in every disease but with some variations in each. In the middle of the reparation phase, the patient experiences a recurrence of the physiological conflict, which means the patient experiences his conflict for a short time (sympathicotonia) all over again including cold hands, cold sweat, fast heart-beat and all the symptoms of the conflict-active phase. This happens so that the brain oedema gets suppressed and the fluid eliminated so that the patient can return to normal.

The best-known epileptic crisis is the heart attack. Strokes, brain haemorrhages and epileptic seizures are other example of events that can occur in the epileptic crisis.

Conflict Mass

Conflict mass = Conflict duration × conflict intensity

Dr Hamer lays great emphasis on the conflict mass. The conflict duration is determined from when the original DHS occurred. The conflict intensity is determined by talking with the patient and determining how all-encompassing the DHS was. The conflict mass is a product of the conflict duration and the conflict intensity as demonstrated in the equation above.

The person will die in the conflict-active phase if a conflict has lasted too long or has been too intense, or both. Even if the person solves the conflict and is in the reparation phase, the person will die if too much conflict mass has been built up. Examples of this are heart attacks and brain haemorrhages, both of which occur in the reparation phase.

The 21 criteria of a cancer/disease

Thus each cancer or one-cycle Meaningful Biological Program of Nature (MBP) has four clearly defined phases and three turning points or seven clearly defined states on the two-phase diagram of a disease. They are illustrated in Figure 6.1 but it is worthwhile to repeat them:

1. Phase1: Normal health prior to the onset of a disease.
2. First turning point: DHS or biological shock.
3. Phase 2: Conflict-active phase.
4. Second turning point: ConflictoLysis (CL) and conflict is now resolved.
5. Phase 3: Reparation phase.
6. Third turning point: Epileptic Crisis or Epileptoid Crisis (EC), which occurs in the middle of the reparation phase.
7. Phase 4: Normal health after a disease (one-cycle disease).

The three levels of the human trinity (psyche, brain and organ) run synchronously. Thus the four phases and the three turning points comprise seven specific criteria which can be observed on the three levels of the human trinity (psyche, brain and organ).

Each cancer, provided the patient recovers, has 21 fully testable and reproducible criteria, seven criteria for each of the three levels (psyche, brain and organ) of the human trinity. These can be reproduced for the same disease anywhere in the world. Thus one can say with absolute certainty that German New Medicine is a hard physical science just like chemistry.

Analysis of an MBP

The various conflict themes causing DHS and their associated symptoms in the conflict-active phase and the reparation phase are described in Dr Hamer's *Psyche-Brain-Organ Disease Chart* for all cancers and diseases known to mankind. This disease chart is the encyclopaedia for all Meaningful Biological Programs of Nature (MBPs). This disease chart allows the general public to understand all MBPs. It is absolutely wonderful.

With a good knowledge of the five Biological Laws of Nature, the diagram of the second Biological Law, along with the cause and theme of the DHS or biological shock, one has the necessary information to understand a particular MBP.

CHAPTER 7

Verification of German New Medicine

Dr Hamer submitted his discovery of the Iron Rule of Cancer (IRC) to the University of Tubingen, Germany in October 1981 as a post-doctoral thesis for qualification as a university lecturer. The objective of the thesis was to provide a university with Dr Hamer's results so that they could be publicly tested and verified and then be used to benefit every cancer patient worldwide. In May 1982 the university rejected the work without performing any tests of Dr Hamer's thesis. His findings were at direct variance with received medical wisdom. His empirical findings did not fit in with the current medical dogmas of the Biomedical Paradigm.[43]

In 1986, a German court barred him from practicing medicine on the basis that he "failed to deny the Iron-Rule-of-Cancer and failed to convert to the tenets of official medicine."[44]

Dr Hamer relied on other doctors to obtain brain scans and patients' records so that he could continue his ground-breaking research. By 1987, he was able to expand his discovery of the five Biological Laws of Nature of the German New Medicine to practically all diseases known in medicine.

To this day, the University of Tübingen refuses to test Dr Hamer's scientific work despite a court order in 1986 to do this work.

In 1997, Dr Hamer was arrested and sentenced to 19 months in prison for having given three people free medical information without a medical licence. When Dr Hamer was arrested, the police searched his patients' files. Subsequently, one public prosecutor was forced to admit during the trial that, after five years, 6,000 out of 6,500 patients with mostly 'terminal' cancer were still alive. And so, ironically, it was his opponents who provided the actual statistics attesting to the German New Medicine's remarkable success rate.

Most infamously in 1998, the Medical Faculty of the University of Trnava (Slovakia) tested seven patients with 20 specific medical conditions at the Sainte Elisabeth Institute of Oncology at Bratislava and the Oncology Unit of the Hospital of Trnva. Dr Hamer's GNM was found to be correct in all cases.

A number of university professors and lecturers observed the proceedings. Three university professors; an oncologist (Professor Krõméry), a psychiatrist (Professor Pogády) and a mathematician (Dr Mikloško) signed an affidavit to the effect that GNM was correct in all cases. The two MDs recanted when the full impact of what they were agreeing with became apparent to them. The third professor, the mathematician, and therefore unconnected with the Biomedical Paradigm did not recant. He was still convinced about the scientific truth of GNM. It was mathematically impossible to be incorrect. The five Biological Laws of Nature did work 100% of the time.[45]

Harald Baumann was present at the verification/non-verification/ infamous judgment, and told me that the oncologist recanted because he believed in the dogma of metastasis, and babbled on that cancer still had to be spread by malignant cancer cells. He couldn't accept the observed fact during the verification, that secondary and tertiary cancers are caused by subsequent biological shocks, and not by wandering cancer cells that nobody has ever seen, nor ever will see, because they do not exist. The oncologist was a white-coat,[46] a scientist in name only.[47]

The University of Trnava still teaches Modern Medicine despite having verified the five Biological Laws of Nature of the German New Medicine. This provides a terrible and conclusive confirmation of the power of the Biomedical Paradigm.

There have been many other verifications, but Modern Medicine refuses to recognise the validity of Dr Hamer's German New Medicine.

Dr Hamer was arrested in Spain on September 9th 2004 on a warrant issued in France. He was extradited there on October 18th 2004. The French judicial system had already sentenced Dr Hamer to three years in prison *in absentia* in July 2004. Dr Hamer's offence was "Agitation against Orthodox Medicine". Dr Hamer was freed from jail in February 2006. He was living at his home in Spain till March 2007 when he went into hiding. He is as of November 2007 on the run because an arrest warrant has been issued by a German magistrate. He is sure to be jailed again in a stupid attempt to quash his wonderful discovery of the five Biological Laws of Nature.

The crime of Agitation against Orthodox Medicine is revealing. It assumes that Modern Medicine with its Biomedical Paradigm and all its hypotheses and dogmas is absolutely correct. It is absolutely not. It is hopelessly flawed.

Anyone challenging these accepted dogmas must therefore be wrong and must be prosecuted. It would indeed be an "appalling vista"[48] to consider the possibility that Modern Medicine is wrong. Dr Hamer has to be wrong because he challenges the absolute truths that Modern Medicine promulgates.

This "appalling vista" judgment of the French judiciary directly affects the whole of humanity because we are all being denied the benefits of German New Medicine.

In essence the French judiciary are applying an absolute belief in the certain knowledge of science, and specifically Modern Medicine. The French judges are spectacularly wrong in their flawed belief in the absolute certainty of Modern Medicine.

Prior to being freed unconditionally in February 2006, Dr Hamer was offered conditional freedom if he recanted. This sounds suspiciously like what happened to Gallileo in the Middle Ages. Dr Hamer refused to recant. He had already suffered the trials of Job;[49] a few more years in a notorious French prison wouldn't kill him and certainly wouldn't kill off his work. The pen is indeed mightier than the sword.

The primary reason why Modern Medicine cannot accept German New Medicine is because of the belief system known as the Biomedical Paradigm which underpins Modern Medicine. Once this Biomedical Paradigm is proven to be wrong, it makes 95% of current MDs redundant.[50] More importantly, it cannot be accepted because once GNM is universally accepted, the full horror of the Ultimate Conspiracy will become apparent.

CHAPTER 8

Dr Lanka and the Non-Existent Viruses

By October 2005 (the third anniversary of my father's death), I had finally realised the true nature of the Ultimate Conspiracy. The reason why Modern Medicine could not verify the German New Medicine was because it would sign its own death warrant. The Ultimate Conspiracy would be over.

I had now reached my limit on what I could read on the internet in English about the GNM, and the non-existence of any so-called disease-inducing or pathogenic virus.

I had lived in Germany for six months in 1992. At that time I worked for Ericsson, and was an engineer charged with the operation and maintenance of a number of newly installed telephone exchanges in the former East Germany. They spoke no English there, so I had to learn basic German in order to get by. That was over 13 years ago.

In my resolution for the coming year, made in October 2005 just before my father's third anniversary, I resolved to relearn German in order to read the original works of Dr Hamer and Dr Lanka. By late 2005, with my rather limited German and an online dictionary[51], I was able to slowly read Dr Lanka's web-site[52] where he published details about his books and newsletter. I subscribed to the bi-monthly newsletter.

Dr Lanka and the missing evidence for the existence of viruses[53]

Dr Stefan Lanka was born in 1963. In his final year of high school, he studied biology because he wanted to learn more about the mystery of life. This inspired him to continue these studies at university. His ambition was to understand Nature and was emphatically not to change Nature.

During his undergraduate years at university, Dr Lanka came across a virus that had "infected" a sea algae. The virus didn't make the sea algae sick. In fact, the virus helped the sea algae to bloom and thrive, which was quite the opposite to what he had expected. He was really excited, because he had discovered what he thought was the first stable "virus host" relationship. The virus did not threaten the host, but was welcomed by the host/sea algae and both co-existed harmoniously or endo-symbiotically.

He had to isolate this virus, photograph it and biochemically characterise it in order to prove the existence of this virus. The photograph would be by an electron microscope originally invented in the 1930s, and the biochemical characterisation by techniques invented in the 1970s. By 1994 he had achieved this and had thereby obtained his doctorate.

In the mid 1980s, Luc Montagnier had claimed to have discovered a new virus: the HIV virus. As Dr Lanka had discovered a real virus infecting sea algae, he was deemed to be an expert on viruses and people naturally asked him about the HIV virus. Dr Lanka began researching the literature on the HIV virus.

Dr Lanka thoroughly checked the scientific publications and could not find any, where the HIV virus had been isolated, biochemically characterised and photographed. He publicised his discoveries at the university but the professors told him to keep quiet and finish his doctorate. They were not interested in the truth. They would not challenge the Biomedical Paradigm.

He couldn't believe that thousands of researchers were attending international AIDS conferences despite the fact that there was absolutely no evidence of the existence of the HIV virus that allegedly causes AIDS. It just didn't make any sense. He examined the literature further, and found there was absolutely no evidence of the existence of any virus deemed dangerous by the MDs, and against which our children are vaccinated.

Dr Lanka had discovered that there is no such thing as a disease-inducing or pathogenic virus. In fact the viruses that actually do exist are a good thing. He later discovered that in one litre of seawater there are about 100 million viruses.[54] He writes sardonically that it is just as well the MDs are not aware of this otherwise we'd have to wear a total body condom before we go for a swim in the sea! In fact, the viruses in seawater must be good for you otherwise these same MDs would not recommend sea-bathing as a general cure. Certainly, 100 years ago sea-bathing was a general cure for all sorts of ailments.

The Germ Theory of Disease states that microbes (bacteria or viruses) from an external source invade the body and are the cause of infectious disease. The concept of specific, unchanging types of bacteria (and subsequently viruses) causing specific diseases became officially accepted after the foundation of Modern Medicine and microbiology in late 19th century Europe.

Dr Lanka had scientifically proven, with 100% certainty, that these viruses did not exist because they have never been isolated, biochemically characterised and photographed. No scientist claims to have ever isolated these viruses. The isolation of a virus would be the first step in proving the existence of a virus. The reason why they cannot be isolated is because they do not exist.

Dr Lanka had discovered the fact that there was no such thing as a disease-inducing or pathogenic virus by the time he was 30 years old. He told everybody, but his colleagues and his professors were not interested. They were not true scientists willing to test every hypothesis or willing to query their own belief systems. The reason why they could not accept what Dr Lanka was saying was because they believed absolutely in the Biomedical Paradigm.

CHAPTER 9

The Ultimate Conspiracy – The Biomedical Paradigm

The Biomedical Paradigm

The word paradigm means a set of assumptions, concepts, values, and practices that constitutes a way of viewing reality.[55]

The Biomedical Paradigm of Modern Medicine is how doctors and other scientists view the medical world. It works fantastically well for any injuries or traumas caused by a car crash or fire. It also works brilliantly for plastic surgery. However Dr Hamer estimates that fully 95% of the procedures carried out by Modern Medicine will become redundant once GNM is universally accepted.

I read many articles in an attempt to understand why the medical profession, the scientific community, the governments, and more importantly, ordinary people, at least 99% of the population, currently believe in the Biomedical Paradigm. By this I mean if you are ill, you take a pill, have an operation, are basically "treated" by an outsider, an MD, and this is the way it should be.

Over the last few years I have discussed this with many people. Some friends have dropped out of contact because they don't want to hear about the GNM and I can't stop talking about it. They believed in the dominant opinion of the experts, the scientists and the MDs. Their common argument was that if the experts said it was true, it had to be true and I was wasting my time.

These are not stupid people. Most of them I would guess are intellectually smarter than me, with a higher IQ. But they don't "get it". I was particularly disappointed with a friend who said that he would still get his newborn baby vaccinated. He understood my arguments; we had discussed them many times, but he still didn't get it. How could this be?

We live in the age of experts. We are all specialists in our own particular field and most of us know very little about other areas of work. We defer to the experts and take their advice, particularly in the area of medicine. We are all very busy in our daily lives, work very hard, and unfortunately with all this work we have no time for reflection.

Most of us seem to have lost the ability to think for ourselves. That is my personal understanding as to why very few non-MDs question the Biomedical Paradigm. The MDs do not question the Biomedical Paradigm because they believe in it with a religious fervour. Modern Medicine is not a science for them; it is a religion.

Fritjof Capra, a physicist by profession, in his brilliant book, "The Turning Point", argues that physics changed its paradigm from the mechanistic paradigm of Newton to a more holistic paradigm in the early part of the 20th century in order to explain quantum theory and the theory of relativity. He argues that other disciplines such as medicine, biology and economics must also change their respective paradigms some 100 years after physics.

The Biomedical Paradigm is the world viewpoint of biologists and the medical profession. It has been the dominant paradigm for the last 400 years. In order to understand how the Biomedical Paradigm came about, one must understand the work of a few philosophers and thinkers, particularly René Descartes.

Philosophy and the mind–body connection

Hippocrates (460 BC–370 BC) is held to be the father of orthodox medicine. The Hippocratic Oath is the basis of the ethics of Modern Medicine and has as its famous dictum, "First do no harm". He rejected the views of his contemporaries that considered illness to be caused by supernatural or divine forces such as possession by evil spirits and disfavour by the gods. He held the belief that illness had a physical and a rational explanation. He argued that disease was not a punishment inflicted by the gods or God but rather the product of environmental factors, diet and living habits.[56]

Hippocrates also believed that the body has self-healing mechanisms and it was the physician's duty to aid these natural processes. His cures involved proper diet, rest and fresh air.[57]

In all of this Hippocrates was correct. Disease does have a rational explanation and is not a punishment from the gods. The body's natural state of being is to be in full health, so he was correct that the body had self-healing powers.

I do not know what Hippocrates views were on the mind–body connection, but Plato (427 BC–347 BC), a contemporary of Hippocrates, wrote in his chronicles in regard to the orthodox medicine of his day: "For this is the great error of our day in the treatment of the human body, that physicians separate the soul from the body". Presumably Plato doubted the received medical wisdom of the day, including that of Hippocrates.

Hippocrates is credited with the creation of clinical medicine or "symptomatic" medicine, which is what Modern Medicine is all about. Hippocrates made careful, regular note of many symptoms of a diseases, including complexion, pulse, fever, pains, movement and excretions. He extended his clinical observations into family history and environment. Symptomatic medicine means that the MD makes a note of all the symptoms and then diagnoses a medical condition to be treated by him.[58]

Since the time of Hippocrates, orthodox medicine has attempted to measure the symptoms of a disease and to allegedly cure them by various means. Modern Medicine has followed the orthodox route of classifying symptoms of diseases, claiming initially that diseases are caused by bacteria, then by putative viruses, and now by faulty genes. Modern Medicine is obsessed with symptoms and how to allegedly treat them. Modern Medicine has no explanation or interest in the cause of any cancer or any disease.

The fundamental problems with Modern Medicine: its complete focus on trying to treat symptoms (symptomatic medicine), and lack of interest in the cause of any cancer or disease can be traced all the way back to its founder: Hippocrates.

But the belief in the mind–body connection still dominated medicine in Europe despite the best efforts of the medical profession because of the rise of Christianity.

Cartesian philosophy[59]

The dichotomy between mind and body was firmly established by René Descartes during the Scientific Revolution or the Age of Enlightenment.[60] René Descartes (1596–1650) was a brilliant mathematician. He made important contributions to algebra and is the founder of analytic geometry. Descartes is also considered to be the father of modern philosophy. He maintained that one cannot accept anything as true unless one can clearly and distinctly perceive it. To achieve this, a compound problem is broken down into its constituent single-factor problems. Simple single-factor problems are solved first before the complex compound problems can be solved.

Descartes wanted to achieve certainty about the nature of life. He started by maintaining that one should doubt everything. Descartes doubted his senses, touch, hearing and smell because when we dream we feel we are experiencing reality. We can see what seem like real objects in our dreams; we can touch them and even smell them. So what separates our senses from reality, from being awake and from being asleep?

The fact that Descartes doubted his senses, the fact that Descartes doubted at all, led him to the conclusion that because he doubted, this meant that he was thinking and using his rational mind. He could not trust his feelings nor his senses, but he could trust his rational mind. Hence his famous statement "*Cogito, ergo sum";* "I think, therefore I am".

Descartes believed in two forms of reality:

1. Thought or mind.
2. Extension or matter.

He believed that mind, being purely consciousness, takes up no room in space, and cannot therefore be sub-divided.

Whereas extension or matter takes up room in space and can always be subdivided into smaller and smaller parts but has no consciousness.

He believed in God and that although thought and extension came from God, these two forms of reality have no contact with each other. Thought is independent of matter and matter is independent of thought. Descartes was therefore a dualist, believing in the sharp division between the reality of thought and extended reality or matter.

He believed that the mind is linked to the body through a special brain organ which he called the pineal gland. Thus the mind could be affected by the feelings and passions that are related to bodily needs. He believed that mind can rise above base impulses and operate independently of the body.

Our body ages and becomes bowed and weak and eventually we die. Reason doesn't age nor die: In this way mind is superior to matter or the human body, according to Descartes.

Descartes stated that extension or matter had certain quantitative properties that we can perceive with our reason or mind. Matter has certain quantitative properties such as mathematical properties that can be measured like length, breadth and depth. Matter, or outer reality, also has qualitative properties such as smell and taste, but because they are linked to our sensory perceptions they cannot be trusted to describe outer reality.

Descartes wrote that "all science is certain, evident knowledge". This belief in the certainty of scientific knowledge lies at the heart of Cartesian philosophy. The Cartesian method is analytical. A complex problem is broken into its constituent parts and arranged into a logical order. By solving the simpler problems one can then solve the more complex problems. The Cartesian method of breaking a complex problem down to its constituent parts, while a valid problem-solving method, has unfortunately led to the widespread use of reductionism in science.

Orthodox medicine and reductionism

The reductionist approach clearly has had great successes in the scientific and medical world; we now understand the different aspects of the human body, such as the digestive system and respiratory system. This is all well and good, but prior to the German New Medicine we did not understand how the organism worked as an entity. Why do apparently healthy people die from a heart attack or get cancer?

Clock-making had achieved an amazing degree of precision in Descartes' era.[61] Descartes compared a sick man with a badly made clock and a healthy man with a well-made clock. The Biomedical Paradigm is based on this notion of the body as a machine, of disease as the consequence of breakdown of the machine, and of the doctor's task as repair of the machine.[62]

In biology, the Cartesian view of living organisms as machines constructed from separate parts, still provides the dominant conceptual framework and is at the heart of contemporary biological thinking. In physics, this mechanistic paradigm was abandoned in the early 20th century in order to explain the very small atomic and sub-atomic physics, and at the level of the very large as in astrophysics and cosmology.[63]

This reductionism in medicine has led to the increasing specialisation of the medical profession, with a single doctor unable to view an illness as a disturbance of the whole organism, and unable to treat it as such. The analogy of comparing the work of an MD to a white-coat scientist with a microscope examining a few square millimetres of the body of an elephant vividly illustrates what the MDs do. The white-coat is great at telling you what is on this surface and can describe it in great detail but he doesn't know that what he is observing is in fact a very small part of an elephant. He simply doesn't get the big picture.

In the case of a cancer, the MD and his associated acolytes can tell you in tremendous detail about the tumour that is growing and all the different micro-organisms that are present and all the different tumour markers. The MD cannot tell you why that particular cancer happened in the first place, and sadly he doesn't even care because his entire focus is on attempting to treat the symptoms. All he can do is to attempt to treat the symptoms of the cancer and invariably he fails miserably to cure the cancer.

The pointless animal experiments that claim to prove that substance A, B or C is carcinogenic are in keeping with the Cartesian logic that these animals are nothing but machines with no psyche, and that testing these animals for carcinogens would prove that a particular substance was carcinogenic without taking the psyche (primitive though it may be) of the affected animal into account.

The medical therapy of Modern Medicine

Medical therapy is based on the principle of medical intervention, relying on outside forces for cure, or at least for the alleviation of suffering and pain, without taking into account the healing potential within the patient. The Cartesian division between mind and body has resulted in physicians treating the body and psychiatrists treating the mind, with little or no interaction between the two. Laboratory tests and the measurement of physical parameters, (purely because they are quantifiable), are deemed to be more important to the diagnosis than the assessment of the patient's emotional state. The emotional state of the patient, because it is a purely qualitative matter and hence cannot be measured, is not taken into account. When you visit an MD, they assess all the symptoms and attempt to measure and quantify them; they give the disease a name and then they attempt to cure it. This approach exemplifies the Cartesian method.

This celebrated dictum of René Descartes "I think, therefore I am" has encouraged the Western world to equate their identity with their rational mind rather than with their whole organism. The idea that one can remove a woman's breast, perform biopsies, chemotherapy and radiotherapy on her body, and these have no effect on the mind or psyche of the woman, is demonstrably false according to common sense and German New Medicine.

Twentieth-century physics has shown that there is no absolute truth in science. All concepts and scientific theories are limited and are approximations to the true nature of reality. Newtonian physics explains the tides and the movement of the planets around the sun: It does not explain quantum physics.

Modern Medicine, in adopting the reductionist approach of modern biology and adhering to the Cartesian division between mind and body, is therefore unable to treat the patient as a whole person. The fundamental problem of the reductionist model of Modern Medicine, the Biomedical Paradigm, is that it cannot explain the origin and the mechanism of disease. Transcending the Biomedical Paradigm of Modern Medicine will amount to a major revolution in medical thought, especially among the general public.

This Biomedical Paradigm is deceptive in its raw brutality. Every illness, cancer or disease must come from an outside force, like cigarettes, other so-called carcinogens, lifestyle, food, or infectious diseases.

The Biomedical Paradigm arrogantly and wrongly asserts that mind and body are separate: They do not interact. The fact that someone is worrying about something seemingly innocuous and irrelevant is not taken into account.

An old lady was correctly diagnosed by the MDs with ovarian cancer. Her beloved pet canary had died a few months earlier. The MDs will say that we have to get rid of this malignant ovarian cyst by chemotherapy and radiotherapy. There are no questions by the MDs concerning events in the patient's life prior to her getting this ovarian cyst. The death of her canary has absolutely no bearing on her ovarian cyst: How could there be any possible connection? Let's try to deal with the symptoms. Let's not investigate the why, the origin and the mechanism of cancer. The simple, harsh but beautiful truth is that all cancers and diseases are caused by biological shocks.[64] It's as simple as that. We need to understand the psyche of the patient in order to know them as a person so that we can treat them.

Modern Medicine cannot accept Dr Hamer's discoveries because of its absolute adherence to the Biomedical Paradigm. The Biomedical Paradigm is not only a pattern of thinking; it now has all the hallmarks of a world religion. The Biomedical Paradigm is indeed the Ultimate Conspiracy.

2

Medical Myths

When you tell a lie loud enough, often enough, and big enough, the people will eventually believe it.
Adolph Hitler (Fascist, 1889-1945)

A lie told often enough becomes the truth.
Vladimir Lenin (Communist, 1870-1924)

You may deceive all the people part of the time, and part of the people all the time, but not all the people all the time.
Abraham Lincoln (16th US President, 1809-1865)

If there is anything that human history demonstrates, it is the extreme slowness with which the academic and critical mind acknowledges facts to exist that present themselves as wild facts, with no staff or pigeon-hole, or as facts that threaten to break up the accepted system.
William James (American philosopher, 1842-1910)

In the sciences, people quickly come to regard as their own personal property that which they have learned and had passed on to them at the universities and academies. If someone else comes along with new ideas that contradict the Credo and in fact even threaten to overturn it, then all passions are raised against this threat and no method is left untried to suppress it. People resist it in every way possible: pretending not to have heard about it; speaking disparagingly of it, as if it were not even worth the effort of looking into the matter. And so a new truth can have a long wait before finally being accepted.
Johann Wolfgang von Goethe (German writer, 1749-1832)

Theories of science must be judged on the basis of fact and reason, not by the authority of dogma.

The great tragedy of Science—the slaying of a beautiful hypothesis by an ugly fact.
Thomas Huxley (English biologist, 1825-1895)

CHAPTER 10

The Myth that Modern Medicine is Scientific

The scientific basis of Modern Medicine

It is a truth universally acknowledged that Modern Medicine is scientific.[65] There are a number of possible terms that one could substitute for Modern Medicine: orthodox medicine, Western medicine or even scientific medicine. I personally prefer the term Modern Medicine.

A German professor, Dr Hans-Ulrich Niemitz from Leipzig, whose professional field is the "History and Ethics of Technology and Natural Sciences" wrote an excellent article[66] on the scientific basis of German New Medicine versus Modern Medicine in response to a query from Dr Hamer.

With regard to Modern Medicine, Dr Niemitz makes two central points:

1. Modern Medicine applies scientific methods such as observation and statistics but "the mere use of scientific method does not qualify an activity to be a science or a person to be a scientist".[67] Modern Medicine can only quote statistical survival chances to cancer patients.
2. Modern Medicine with its many hypotheses, or rather, unproven assumptions, is neither a science nor a natural science. It does not have one hypothesis-free theory concerning the biological events taking place in the individual patient. Modern Medicine is therefore not scientific and incapable of understanding the mechanism of any cancer or disease.

The scientific basis of German New Medicine

Dr Niemitz states that German New Medicine has a model of the disease that is "scientific, free of hypotheses and therefore demonstrable."[68] He further states that "An assertion or system of assertions can only be considered scientific if the assertion or assertions can be denied—technically speaking—or can be tested to determine whether or not they are false."

In simple language, this means that German New Medicine has made a series of assertions that can be tested to determine whether they are true or not. In opposition, Modern Medicine has a series of hypotheses such as the immune system and metastasis, which one cannot test because they are theories or mere guesses. These hypotheses have now acquired the status of dogmas within Modern Medicine and are accordingly revered as the absolute truth. Nobody has been able to observe the immune system directly. Nobody has been able to observe cancer cells in the blood stream or in the lymph nodes, yet these are the two suspected means of cancer transmission or metastasis, whereby cancer allegedly transfers from one affected organ to another according to Modern Medicine.

German New Medicine as a hard science

In hard physical sciences such as chemistry, the strength of a proof of a hypothesis is based exclusively on the public reproducibility of the experiment. Thus if one mixes hydrogen and oxygen in Ireland, the US or Germany, one always gets water, 100% of the time. Statistics are irrelevant: it either works or it doesn't work 100% of the time. One doesn't say that 50% of the time when you mix hydrogen and oxygen you get water. That would be absurd. It doesn't have to be the exact same hydrogen or oxygen molecules that are mixed, but an equivalent pair of hydrogen molecules and an equivalent oxygen molecule, anywhere in the world, mixed together in those exact proportions, will always produce water.

German New Medicine is an over-determined system consisting of the three levels of the human trinity: the psyche, the brain and the organ. "Over-determined" means that if one knows what is happening at one level, one can determine what is happening at the other two levels of the human trinity. Thus if one can ascertain the nature of the conflict from an anamnesis with the patient, one can determine from this psyche level what is happening at the other two levels, namely the brain level and the organ level. One can state where the concerned brain relay is and what is happening to the affected organ.

Conversely, if an experienced GNM therapist is given a CT scan of a patient's brain, the GNM therapist can determine from this brain part of the human trinity which organ is affected and the nature of the biological shock that caused the specific condition.

Modern Medicine: a new world religion

I always thought that science in general was open to new ideas, thoughts and discoveries. In a great article by Dr Rustum Roy entitled *Science and Whole Person Medicine: Enormous Potential in a New Relationship*, he debunks the idea of science being open to new ideas. Dr Roy is a materials scientist with over 50 years' experience. In his prescient article he argues that the next great breakthrough would be in the field of what he calls "Whole-Person Medicine".

He wrote:

From being the champion of discovery and innovation and newness, science as practiced today has become the main religious establishment of the West...From a deep curiosity about new facts, establishment science has become a "defender of the faith", a conserver of today's theories. No one denies that that is the purpose of one key element of the system: peer-review. This key procedure can only check new results by the single test of conformity to the true faith, that is, current theory. Indeed peer-review is most accurately characterised as the paradigm-police.[69]

Peer-review is the process by which a colleague's work is professionally examined. But as Dr Roy eloquently puts it, how do you test your colleague's work but by "conformity to the true faith", the accepted theories and dogmas of the day. By the "paradigm-police", he means that if the new discovery doesn't fit the current dogma or accepted theory, then by virtue of this paradigm it has to be wrong.

Dr Roy states that peer-review has in fact promoted bad science, because it was in accord with existing theories, and has rejected good science because it was counter to the existing theories.

Dozens of the greatest advances by Nobel laureates and others had been initially rejected by the peer-review system.[70]

Rightly have scientists held up Galileo's challenge to dogma with facts, as the quintessence of our trade. The cardinals who refused to look into the telescope because dogma had it that the moon's surface had to be perfect are, appropriately, scorned as unscientific.[71]

This behaviour is now commonplace in the conventional science-establishment.

Dr Roy quotes a philosopher (Alfred North Whitehead) who wrote that "Advance in detail is admitted: fundamental novelty is barred." Dr Roy adds that *"Peer review is the process which enforces this status."*[72]

This state of affairs that applies to science in general, most definitely applies to the medical world, and its absolute adherence to the sacred dogmas of the Biomedical Paradigm.

Modern Medicine is a new world religion founded by Louis Pasteur, and it has appropriated the rites of the Christian religion, specifically those of the Catholic Church.[73]

1. Louis Pasteur,[74] the father of Modern Medicine, has taken the place of Jesus Christ.
2. MDs have taken the place of priests and female and male nurses have taken the place of nuns and brothers, respectively.
3. The sacred scriptures of the Biomedical Paradigm that describe all the various dogmas the MDs must believe replaces the Bible.
4. The Germ Theory of Disease is the central dogma of Modern Medicine.
5. Vaccinations play the same initiatory role in Modern Medicine as baptism does in Christianity.
6. The search for health has replaced the quest for salvation.
7. The eradication of viruses and cancers has taken the place of exorcising demons.
8. The hope of physical immortality (cloning, genetic engineering) has been substituted for the hope of eternal life.
9. Pills/pharmaceuticals have replaced the sacrament of bread and wine.
10. Donations to cancer research or even better AIDS research have taken precedence over donations to the Church.
11. The never-ending search for a hypothetical universal vaccine that can save humanity from all its illnesses, just as Jesus Christ by his death has saved the world from all its sins.
12. Patients are alienated from their bodies, just as sinners used to be from their souls.
13. The regular medical check-up with our local friendly MD replaces confession with our parish priest.
14. There is an enforced conformity with medical dogma contained in the sacred scriptures of the Biomedical Paradigm, and anyone not conforming is branded a charlatan, just like the Church in the past branded people as heretics.

In fact, far from being scientific, Modern Medicine is a secular world religion, adopting Christian practices and rituals. There are a number of definitions of the word religion to be found in various dictionaries.[75] Two possible definitions are:

1. A set of beliefs, values and practices based on the teaching of a spiritual leader.
2. A cause, principle or activity pursued with zeal or conscientious devotion.

The basic belief of a Christian is that Jesus Christ is the Son of God, that he is our Saviour and that he suffered and died on the Cross to save us all from our sins. This basic belief is supported by the sacred scriptures contained in the Bible: the Old Testament proclaiming the Messiah to come and the New Testament proclaiming the Messiah as Jesus Christ. The Christian religion would correspond to the first definition of the word religion above: a set of beliefs, values and practices based on the teachings of Jesus.

In contrast, Modern Medicine as a religion is based on the belief system known as the Biomedical Paradigm which is followed with tremendous zeal and conscientious devotion by its principal advocates: the MDs. It would correspond to the second definition of the word religion as its cause, the Biomedical Paradigm, is pursued with tremendous zeal and conscientious devotion by the MDs.

The Biomedical Paradigm is based on a series of beliefs or dogmas such as:

1. There is no mind–body connection. The mind plays no role in a cancer or any other disease occurring in the body.
2. The body is like a clockwork mechanism. If part of it breaks down, we merely have to replace or fix that part and all will be well.
3. Animals do not have a psyche or a soul.
4. Intervention by MDs has prolonged life-spans and improved the quality of life.
5. Disease is caused by external factors such as germs, environment, or carcinogens and is not caused from within.
6. Cancer and other diseases are meaningless failures of Nature.
7. Vaccinations prevent infectious diseases.
8. And the list goes on and on.

The word dogma means: *An authoritative principle, belief, or statement of ideas or opinion, especially one considered to be absolutely true.*[76] This definition accurately describes what is meant by the dogmas that Modern Medicine follows. Any MD rejecting any of these dogmas will be deemed an apostate or charlatan and will be cast out of the medical profession and ridiculed.

It was only when I finally realised that Modern Medicine is a religion that I was able to understand that this belief system could never be overthrown from within by the MDs themselves.

This belief system, faith or religion known as the Biomedical Paradigm has created absolute dogmas like carcinogens, metastasis, vaccinations, Germ Theory of Disease, and immune system. The Biomedical Paradigm consists of about 5000 or so dogmas that have become the sacred scriptures of a new world religion, Modern Medicine, controlled by the MDs and the pharmaceutical industry, and provided with legal protection by our governments.[77] This is the Ultimate Conspiracy.

The reality that the Biomedical Paradigm is a false secular religion will not be revealed by the medical profession, the pharmaceutical industry, the cancer charities, your government and certainly not by the WHO (World Health Organization). It must be revealed by YOU as an ordinary member of the general public living in the free world.

CHAPTER 11

The Germ Theory of Disease Medical Myth

The most infamous of all medical myths

It is a truth universally acknowledged that germs cause disease. The Germ Theory of Disease medical myth is the key medical myth of the Biomedical Paradigm. Hundred of millions of people have been killed because of our collective belief in this insane and criminal medical dogma.

Modern Medicine has thousands of medical myths, just as in the Middle Ages there was a truth universally acknowledged that the Earth was the centre of the universe and consequently that the sun, moon and other planets revolved around planet Earth. This dogma existed that because God created man, Earth had to be the centre of the universe, the centre of all His creation.

Nicolaus Copernicus postulated that the Earth in fact revolved around the Sun. He waited until he was dying before he made his theories public because he was so afraid of offending the ruling dogma of the preceding 1000 years. Gallileo Gallilei was able to empirically prove with his telescope that in fact the Earth did rotate around the Sun as Nicolaus Copernicus had earlier postulated.

The central dogma of the Biomedical Paradigm is that there is a specific external agent that causes a disease or cancer and the job of the MD is to eliminate the symptoms of the disease and then the disease itself. The patient is not treated but the disease is. The disease is an entity in itself and the job of the MD is to eliminate it.

The Germ Theory of Disease is to Modern Medicine what the Resurrection is to Christianity. If Jesus did not rise from the dead three days after having been crucified, then He would not be the Son of God and Christianity would be meaningless. When the Germ Theory of Disease dogma is generally accepted to be false, the era of Modern Medicine will be finally over.

The Germ Theory of Disease is a theory that proposes that micro-organisms are the cause of many diseases. It claims that fixed species of microbes from an external source invade the body and are the first cause of infectious disease; for example, that the measles virus is responsible for measles. Although highly controversial when first proposed, this theory is now a cornerstone of Modern Medicine and microbiology. All mainstream MDs today subscribe to the Germ Theory of Disease.[78]

So how did the central dogma of Modern Medicine, the Germ Theory of Disease, come about?

The Miasma Theory of Disease

Prior to the Germ Theory, the predominant theory of disease was that of miasmas or that of bad-air. Therefore cholera or the black plague were caused by particularly noxious miasmas originating somewhere else (usually a foreign country or a remote place) and carried by the air.

However, by the late 18th century, the miasma/bad-air theory was being challenged by "contagionists" who claimed that disease was spread by human contact. Their viewpoint naturally underpinned the quarantine laws once a region was declared to be infected. Anti-contagionists generally subscribed to the miasma/bad-air idea.

A case in point of the contrasting viewpoints between contagionists and anti-contagionists is the yellow fever epidemic that occurred in Philadelphia in 1793.[79] It killed as many as 5000 people or about 10% of the population. Many of the city's famous residents, including George Washington, fled the city during the outbreak. Benjamin Rush, an MD and co-signatory of the US Declaration of Independence, stayed put and tried to help his fellow citizens. Rush angered his fellow MDs by arguing that yellow fever was not caused by contagion (passing from one person to another), but from poisoning by putrid matter.

In the case of yellow fever, Rush was correct. Yellow fever is not caused by infectious microbes, it is a water-borne disease caused by putrid matter or rotting substances such as dead animals in the water.

The Greek word miasma means pollution. The sanitation reformers in the mid-1800s in London, England, adapted the viewpoint of the miasma origin of disease from that of bad air to bad drinking water and non-existent sanitation/waste disposal systems. They were concerned to improve sanitation as a means of controlling disease and improving quality of life.

There were numerous cholera epidemics prior to this time. Cholera was endemic in places where the water smelt foul. Once these sanitary reforms were introduced, cholera and other infectious diseases were eliminated and death rates declined dramatically.

Origin of the Germ Theory of Disease[80]

The idea of the Germ Theory of Disease was around for at least 100 years prior to Louis Pasteur (1822–1895). In the late 1600s, a Dutch naturalist and lens maker, Anton van Leeuwenhoek, made the first recorded observations of micro-organisms.

In 1762, Marcus Antonius Plenciz, a Viennese physician, first published a germ theory of infectious diseases, which speculated that a special organism caused a particular disease, and that these micro-organisms might be conveyed from place to place by the air. This Germ Theory of Disease, which does seem to explain things like contagion and epidemics, would have been discussed widely in the medical and scientific circles of Pasteur's time.

The Germ Theory of Disease (the key dogma of Modern Medicine) developed from the Germ Theory of Fermentation as advanced by Louis Pasteur. A strongly held idea at the time was that the processes of fermentation or putrefaction and disease were similar. This meant that if one understood the causes of fermentation then one would understand the causes of disease. One must therefore understand how Pasteur got his ideas about the Germ Theory of Fermentation, and then applied them to so-called infectious diseases.

Béchamp and fermentation[81]

Pasteur's Germ Theory of Fermentation emanated from the original work done on the phenomenon of fermentation by Professor Antoine Béchamp (1816–1908). Fermentation typically refers to the conversion of sugar to alcohol using yeast.[82] A more accurate definition would be the chemical conversion of carbohydrates into alcohols or acids. Fermentation is the process used to produce wine, beer and vinegar, among other things.

In May 1854, Béchamp decided to investigate why cane sugar was transformed at room temperature into grape sugar when dissolved in water. The idea that prevailed at the time was that this transformation occurred spontaneously. Grape sugar is a solution of equal parts of glucose and fructose. The technical term for this change is inversion. Thus the grape sugar was also known as invert-sugar. This set of experiments was later referred to as his "Beacon Experiment".

Béchamp dissolved pure sugar cane in a glass bottle containing some air, but which was otherwise air-tight. As a control, he had several other glass bottles containing the same solution and some air but additionally with salts such as zinc chloride and calcium chloride and others with a small amount of creosote or mercuric acid added. All the capped bottles were left alongside each other in the laboratory.

In the bottle with no salts added, moulds appeared within 30 days and inversion of the sugar then developed rapidly. Creosote was particularly effective in the prevention of moulds and of alteration of sugar.

The appearance of the moulds increases the inversion of the cane sugar or the transformation of the cane sugar into grape sugar. Béchamp measured this process of inversion or fermentation by passing polarised light through the solution and observing the angle of rotation of this polarised light by a Polarimeter. The change in the plane of rotation with the other solutions was negligible but in the case of the solution with the moulds it was significant. Clearly the inversion did not occur spontaneously and the rate of inversion was directly related to the moulds. He published these observations in the Report of the French Academy of Science in February 1855.

But what caused the moulds? He started a second set of experiments in June 1856 in order to determine the origin of the moulds. In two bottles he had some air in contact with the solution. In nine other bottles there was no air. The results were conclusive. In the nine bottles without air, no moulds formed and no inversion of the sugar took place. In the other two bottles he observed again that the inversion changes were more rapid in the bottle in which the mould was also growing rapidly. These experiments proved beyond doubt that moulds and inversion of the sugar cane did not occur spontaneously in the water but must be because of something in the air. These moulds were living organisms and the cane sugar became inverted in proportion to the development of the moulds.

In 1856 it was generally accepted that fermentation could only occur with the presence of nitrogen. However Béchamp's solutions contained pure water and cane sugar. They did not contain nitrogen or any other minerals. Béchamp had proved that the mould grew because it had absorbed nitrogen from the air.

Proof that the solution contained nitrogen was obtained by heating the moulds with caustic potash. Ammonia was released which was proof that the moulds contained nitrogen. It would have been astonishing news at the time that these microbes absorbed nitrogen from the air, developed into moulds and fermented. This fermentation created moulds and a ferment that caused the inversion or transformation of the sugar.

Béchamp explained the phenomenon of fermentation as being due to the nutrition of living organisms; a process of absorption, assimilation and excretion. The airborne germs 'planted' themselves in the sugared solution, absorbed nitrogen from the air (because there was no nitrogen in the solution) and developed fungi or moulds. This is what Béchamp called the insoluble ferment because it did not dissolve in water. The soluble ferment, dissolved into the water and this caused the inversion or transformation of the solution. Fermentation is an effect accompanying the growth of the ferment or the mould.

The dates mentioned above for Béchamp's experiments are relevant because in 1860 Pasteur engaged upon a theatrical series of experiments to prove what Béchamp had already proved a few years earlier. He prepared 73 bottles of unfermented liquid to expose to the air in different places at various altitudes. He made his experiment public in advance.

He opened the bottles and then sealed them to capture the air at those locations inside the bottles. He opened the last 20 in a spectacular location, a glacier called Mer de Glace above Chamonix.

The results were as Béchamp had proved several years earlier. Pasteur had one interesting addition to this experiment. He borrowed the idea of a "swan-neck" bottle flask from a colleague. This specially made flask would only allow germ-free and dust-free air into the liquid solution; the air-borne germs settling in the horizontal part of the flask. No fermentation took place in the solution in the swan-neck flask proving that one needed air-borne germs for fermentation to occur.

In 1860, with his well publicised "high Alps" experiment, Pasteur had stolen credit for Béchamp's discovery that germs in the air caused fermentation. In 1861, at the Sorbonne in Paris, he had the audacity, in the presence of Béchamp himself, to take credit for what Béchamp had already proven.

Pasteur erroneously came to the conclusion that each kind of fermentation (milk, beer or wine) had one specific germ. At this time there was a widely accepted analogy between fermentation and disease. Even now this is not too hard to imagine. Fermentation and putrefaction are similar processes. Disease is a process of putrefaction, a process of breaking down the host organism, which results in possible contagion according to Modern Medicine. In this context it is not surprising that Pasteur made the unwarranted mental leap that if air-borne germs were the cause of fermentation that they had to be the cause of disease. The Germ Theory of Disease developed from this hypothesis.

In 1863 Pasteur was elected to the Academy of Science. Soon afterwards he had an audience with the French Emperor. Pasteur wrote in a letter the next day that "I assured the Emperor that all my ambition was to arrive at the knowledge of the causes of putrid and contagious diseases." And the rest, as they say, is history. Unfortunately![83]

Béchamp's microzymas[84]

However, Béchamp had discovered that fermentation did not always follow from air-borne germs. Béchamp discovered that the inversion of cane sugar did not occur when he mixed salts such as potassium carbonate in the solution. But when he used calcium carbonate (ordinary chalk), he found that the inversion of cane sugar did occur. This was an unexpected observation.

Béchamp had already proved that the creosote prevented external organisms from entering the medium. By adding creosote in with ordinary chalk the inversion still occurred. So the addition of creosote had not prevented this inversion occurring in this case?[85]

When chemically pure calcium carbonate ($CaCO_3$) was added to his sugared solutions, no inversion occurred. When ordinary chalk chipped off from a rock was used, inversion always occurred. The chalk found in Nature contained what he called "little bodies" or "microzymas". They were smaller than anything he had seen in moulds before. Because they moved and caused fermentation, he regarded them as living organisms. The block of limestone that he got the chalk from was very old. These ferments had remained dormant in the limestone for millions of years, and were the survivors of living beings from long ago.

If these ferments found in ordinary chalk were living beings, it must be possible to kill them. Béchamp heated chalk to 300 degrees centigrade and found that the microzymas were killed and no fermentation took place.[86]

In early 1868, Professor Béchamp and his colleague Professor Estor tested their theories on the origin of these microzymas or little bodies that they had discovered in the chalk found in Nature. They obtained the body of a dead kitten and buried it in pure carbonate of lime, which was specially treated so as to exclude airborne external germs. They placed this entombed dead kitten in a glass jar. They covered the top of the jar with several sheets of paper, placed so as to allow air but to prevent dust or other airborne germs to enter. This jar was left on a shelf in the laboratory for seven years until the end of 1874.

When they opened it they found that the kitten's body had been almost entirely consumed with the exception of some small fragments of bones. There was no smell and the carbonate of lime was not discoloured. There were no microzymas to be observed above the kitten's body but there were thousands in the part of the carbonate of lime below the kitten's body.

Béchamp thought there might have been air-borne germs in the kitten's fur, lungs, or intestines. He repeated the same experiment using the carcass of a kitten in one case, the liver only in another, and the heart, lungs and kidneys in a third. These experiments started in 1875 and ended seven years later in 1882.

Again, with the possibility of air-borne germs that could potentially have caused these changes excluded, Béchamp and Estor discovered seven years later that microzymas were also present.

These series of experiments proved that these microzymas are the living remains of plant and animal life in which these microzymas had been the constructive cellular elements. They are the primary anatomical elements of all living beings. The organism might die but the microzymas remain indestructible.

Béchamp was the first scientist to explain the fermentative power of air-borne germs. He also demonstrated how this fermentation could occur without the presence of air-borne germs. These air-borne germs were the microzymas released from animal and plant forms.[87]

Béchamp and bacteria[88]

Professor Béchamp and Professor Estor found bacteria present in both sets of experiments. Because they had taken care to exclude air-borne germs, they deduced that bacteria develop from microzymas. Bacteria are in fact a scavenging form of these microzymas; developed when tissue needs to be repaired or broken up. These bacteria were not created externally, but developed from the microzymas, which in turn developed from the decomposing body of the dead kitten.

In 1869 Béchamp wrote that in cases of typhoid fever, gangrene and anthrax one had discovered bacteria in the tissue and blood. People like Louis Pasteur and Robert Koch interpreted the presence of these bacteria as having caused these diseases, and that these bacteria or germs invaded the organism from outside. However the interpretation of Béchamp and Estor was that the cells in the body itself had changed and produced bacteria in response to the conditions of the host organism.

Béchamp's microzyma, including specific bacteria, could take on a number of forms during the host's life-cycle and these forms depended primarily on the chemistry of their environment, on the biological terrain, or on the condition of the host.[89] This idea of the cells changing and producing bacteria and virus-like particles is called pleomorphism (from the Greek meaning many shapes). The idea of the cells having one shape only is called monomorphism (from the Greek meaning one shape). If one believes in the medical dogma called monomorphism, it is easy to explain changes in the shapes of the cells that occur during measles, mumps, or rubella by external viruses.

Béchamp argued strenuously against vaccines, asserting that "The most serious disorders may be provoked by the injection of living organisms into the blood."[90] Bacteria in man or animal do not cause disease. They have the same function as those found in the soil, in sewage or elsewhere in Nature. They exist in order to rebuild dead or diseased tissues or eliminate body waste. Bacteria do not attack healthy tissue.

Bacteria, fungi and virus-like particles (but definitely not viruses because they do not exist) are available for repair work/rebuilding of tissue or for caseating or breaking down tumours in the reparation phase of a particular disease or MBP. Béchamp's work confirms in advance the scientific truth of the fourth Biological Law of GNM.

Claude Bernard and Pasteur

In 1878, Claude Bernard, a friend and scientific colleague of Pasteur, died. One of Bernard's colleagues instigated the production of his laboratory notes which disputed Pasteur's purely "air-borne" germ theory of fermentation. Claude Bernard had never challenged Pasteur's theory while alive.[91]

Pasteur was then 55-years-old; a French hero with a reputation to protect. Pasteur repeated Bernard's experiments and produced a devastating critique of Bernard in both tone and substance. Part of his critique was about the dangers of preconceived ideas, or of believing what you want to believe to be true. By contrast, Pasteur presented himself as a true scientist, working empirically and having no preconceived theories.[92]

In fact, any analysis of Pasteur's own work, shows that he conducted his own experiments according to his own preconceived ideas and rejected experiments that did not fit in with the result he had expected—the exact opposite of what a true scientist should do. As a result of the posthumous publication of Bernard's notes and the furore caused, and probably influenced by worries over being called a fraud and a plagiarist, Pasteur instructed his family to keep his laboratory notebooks private.

Pasteur died 18 years later in 1895. This incident over his diatribe against Claude Bernard must have been on his mind on his deathbed. He is alleged to have said "Bernard is right: the microbe is nothing: the terrain is everything."[93] In other words, microbes don't cause disease; they are merely present during disease. However it was too late. The Germ Theory of Disease that he had promulgated was now in the ascendancy.

Koch's postulates

Robert Koch MD (1843–1910) is celebrated as the founder of modern bacteriology. He discovered tubercular bacteria and cholera bacilli, which are present during these diseases and which allegedly caused these diseases. He is also famous for his postulates:

1. The pathogenic microbe can be observed in the body fluids of a host suffering from the disease. This pathogenic organism is not present in a healthy host.
2. The pathogenic microbe can be isolated from the diseased host and cultured in the laboratory.
3. The cultured pathogenic microbe causes the same disease when introduced into another host.
4. The microbe can be re-isolated from that experimentally infected host.

The theory behind these postulates is that you can observe these microbes in a sample of blood from an infected host; you can isolate them and grow them in the laboratory; you inject them into another host and cause the same disease; and you can then isolate the same microbe from the newly infected host. These postulates would all make perfectly good common sense if pathogenic microbes existed. Unfortunately for Modern Medicine they don't exist.

You cannot even isolate viruses because they do not exist. There is no scientific paper available where any scientist has isolated any virus. In relation to bacteria you can isolate bacteria and culture them, the first two of Koch's postulates. However, you cannot inject say tubercular bacteria or cholera bacilli into somebody and cause tuberculosis or cholera. This means that the Germ Theory of Disease does not work for viruses because they do not exist; it also does not work for bacteria because you cannot cause the same disease by injecting the bacteria that allegedly cause that disease into another person. Koch's third and fourth postulates do not work for bacterial diseases. Bacterial diseases like tuberculosis are not contagious.

The Germ Theory of Disease was hotly debated at the time, but because of the dominance of the Biomedical Paradigm it became generally accepted. It was indeed a lost chapter in the history of biology and medicine that the original scientific work of Professors Béchamp and Estor was discarded in favour of the plagiarist and scientific fraud Louis Pasteur.[94]

CHAPTER 12

The Myth that Vaccinations are Necessary

Modern Medicine's theory of vaccines

It is a truth universally acknowledged that vaccinations have a scientific basis, and are necessary to prevent infectious diseases.

The "immune system" is, according to Modern Medicine, a complex network of cells and organs that work together to defend the body against attack by "foreign invaders" or nasty and potentially deadly viruses like measles, mumps and rubella.

Vaccination is the process of administering weakened or dead pathogens to a healthy person or animal, with the intent of conferring immunity against a targeted form of a related disease agent.[95]

Taking measles as an example, the measles vaccine is called an antigen and allegedly stimulates the immune system to produce antibodies against the weakened or dead measles "virus" contained in the vaccine. The supposed advantage of being vaccinated is that your immune system remembers the measles virus and can quickly create antibodies in the future to destroy a real live dangerous measles virus. In this way you are protected from the measles virus.

Proof that the measles virus works according to Modern Medicine is:

1. Most children in the free world don't get measles because they have been vaccinated;
2. Antibodies can be measured, which prove that the measles vaccine has been effective.

The immunity dogma

The whole theory of vaccinations is rooted in the belief or medical dogma that immunity is conferred by a non-fatal attack of a disease.[96] This theory arose for two reasons. Firstly, Modern Medicine considered disease to be an entity, a definite thing in itself, instead of being due to events that have occurred within the individual person's life. Secondly, Modern Medicine obtained the idea of immunity from the observed facts over many thousands of years that most children only get real diseases such as measles, mumps, rubella or chicken pox once and that some kind of protection has been given to them to prevent any further occurrences. This belief in immunity from a real naturally occurring disease (such as measles) occurring more than once was then transferred over to a belief in vaccinations, that the perceived immunity that occurs from ordinary diseases could be manufactured and replicated in the form of vaccinations.

Thus the theory of Modern Medicine is that by injecting a child with a mild form of the "virus", the immune system is stimulated. It produces antibodies against this weakened or, in technical terms, attenuated form of the virus. These antibodies are present so that in future when the child's immune system comes across the real measles, mumps and rubella viruses, for example, it can immediately fight them off providing immunity to these so-called deadly viruses.

Over thousands of years, human experience would indicate that the child (or host organism) has learned from having real diseases such as measles, mumps and rubella and is most unlikely to get these diseases again. However it does not preclude their reoccurrence.

Harald Baumann (an experienced GNM therapist) has come across a person who has had mumps three times. MDs, if they are honest, will also have come across similar situations such as kids who have had measles twice or three times whether vaccinated or not vaccinated.[97]

Measles, mumps, rubella and tuberculosis are not diseases or entities that we pick up from the measles, mumps or rubella viruses and tubercular bacteria, but are caused by events that have occurred in our lives.

A brief history of vaccinations

The evil practice of vaccinations long predated the Germ Theory of Disease. The driving impetus behind the perceived need for vaccinations arose because of the disease called smallpox.

Smallpox is, according to Modern Medicine, a highly contagious disease unique to humans. It apparently has two variants: Variola major with a typical mortality from 20% – 40% of those infected; and Variola minor, which kills 1% of its victims. Many survivors are left blind in one or both eyes. The main symptoms are persistent skin scarring in very visible pockmarks all over the body. Smallpox was responsible for millions of deaths in the 20th century alone.[98]

Lady Montagu had lost a brother to smallpox and had her own face scared by the disease. In 1716–1717 her husband was the British Ambassador to the Ottoman Empire based in the city of Constantinople (modern-day Istanbul). She witnessed the widespread practice of inoculation there and was greatly impressed. In 1718 Lady Mary Wortley-Montagu had her son "vaccinated" in Istanbul. The word vaccination had not yet been invented. The term used to describe this procedure was variolation or inoculation.

Variolation involved purposely infecting a person with smallpox (variola). This procedure involved transferring the smallpox postule or pus from a person suffering from a mild form of smallpox onto a scratch between the thumb and forefinger of a healthy person. The idea was to cause a mild form of the disease because of a mistaken belief in the Immunity Dogma: if you get the disease once, even a weakened form of it, you are now immune for life. This Immunity Dogma had been prevalent in Asia for over 3000 years and is now deeply ingrained worldwide.[99]

There clearly is some truth in the old wives' tale that normal childhood diseases like measles, mumps and rubella only occur once. This may be, say, 95% true. However it is still possible that they may occur more than once. But it was this belief in a form of natural immunity being obtained from an occurrence of these childhood diseases that led the orthodox medical profession of the day to believe they could manufacture or artificially create this immunity by the practice of inoculation in relation to smallpox.

On her return to England, Lady Montagu campaigned for the introduction of this so-called prophylactic or preventative procedure. Six prisoners due to be hanged were given the option of this procedure which was witnessed by a number of prominent MDs. The experiment succeeded and the daughters of the Prince of Wales were inoculated in 1722. This practice spread among the royal houses of Europe and was naturally adopted by their respective peoples.[100]

Thousands more people died in London from this procedure than from the occurrence of smallpox itself. By 1727 there were descriptions of smallpox outbreaks as a result of inocculation. But despite all the evidence to the contrary, there was this mistaken belief in the Immunity Dogma fortified by the MDs and others carrying out this procedure, but also as a generally accepted belief by the people being vaccinated. The practice of inoculation (from person to person) continued until the discovery of "vaccination" by Edward Jenner in the late 1700s. This led to the decline and eventual banning of smallpox inoculation.[101]

Edward Jenner (1749–1823) can be regarded as the father of vaccination. He got the idea of protection from smallpox by using cow pox from a farmer, Benjamin Jesty. Jenner called his discovery *vaccination,* coming from "Vacca", the Latin word for cow. The pus from cowpox was injected directly into the person's vein. In 1790, Jenner vaccinated his 10-month-old son in this fashion. His son was thereafter mentally handicapped and died at the age of 21. Jenner's belief in his discovery blinded him against the terrible consequences and he continued with his vaccinations. At the end of his life he expressed doubts about what he had done, but the practice of vaccination was a much too profitable a business for his fellow MDs.[102]

Dr Archie Kalokerinos, an Australian MD and ardent vaccine critic, states that the death rate and the severe damage from Jenner's vaccinations would be enormous if carried out today.[103] There is a huge body of evidence to support the reality that the practice of inoculation and vaccination enormously increased the death rate from smallpox.[104]

The New Medicine and germs

The underlying dogma supporting the practice of vaccinations is the Germ Theory of Disease. This dogma explicitly states that the measles virus causes measles and that the polio virus causes polio. All these viruses come from air-borne germs or from direct human contact. Once you believe this central dogma of Modern Medicine, then the idea of vaccinations to prevent these viruses becomes necessary.

The fourth Biological Law of Nature states that the relevant microbes only become active in the reparation phase of a disease. The microbes did not cause the disease; they become active in the reparation phase of the disease. They are the optimisers of the organism; they work to rebuild the cells broken down in the conflict-active phase or to caseate or break down the tumours or excess growth that occurred in the same conflict-active phase.

In other words, the microbes or germs are only active in the reparation phase, the second phase of the disease process. Every disease is caused by a biological shock. Every disease has two phases: the conflict-active phase and the reparation phase. Using the example of measles; in the conflict-active phase (invisible to the eye) the cells in the top layer of the skin are broken down. In the reparation phase of measles, the cells that were broken down are now rebuilt. The so-called viruses that cause measles are in fact internally generated microbes that maximise healing and are not malignant. Contrary to popular opinion they are not contagious. It is in this reparation phase that the measles spots appear.

Viruses

Modern Medicine believes as an absolute dogma that the measles virus causes measles. The reason why vaccinations are wholly unnecessary for so-called viral diseases is because the so-called viruses that causes allegedly infectious diseases like mumps, measles, rubella, hepatitis and AIDS do not exist! There is no scientific publication available in which a scientist states that he has proven a pathogenic virus to exist!

When I first came across the idea that pathogenic viruses simply do not exist, I was absolutely stunned. We hear the word virus every day. Viruses even affect our computers. But computer viruses at least exist. There is no proof whatsoever for the existence of any virus said to affect humans.

According to current scientific standards, to prove that a virus exists, it must be isolated, photographed and biochemically characterised. If, for example, the measles virus really did exist, it should be possible to extract the measles virus from a child (by taking a blood sample), and then to isolate the measles virus from the ordinary cells and to photograph and biochemically characterise it.

Dr Stefan Lanka assures us that any amateur can learn within a few days how to isolate, photograph and biochemically characterise those viruses that do exist and which are completely harmless. The photographs produced in medical text books and scientific publications that allegedly represent the viruses are fraudulent. When you ask the relevant authors and scientific authorities, they will eventually admit that they are not pictures of isolated viruses. They are usually pictures of what they consider a virus to look like.

The MDs and scientists believe in the medical dogma called "monomorphism". All cells only have one particular shape. They do not consider the possibility that the cells can change shape, for example, when the patient has measles. Instead of the measles virus coming from the air or human contact, the cells of the patient change shape when the patient has measles. This concept of cells changing shapes has been around for over 100 years (thanks to Professor Antoine Béchamp) and is called pleomorphism (pleo meaning many and morph meaning shape).

The MDs state that the measles virus comes from outside the human organism and infects it, which causes measles. This idea of the existence of a virus affecting humans, animals or plants has been refuted by Dr Lanka. Viruses do not exist in humans, animals or plants. They only exist in more simple life forms such as sea algae.

What German New Medicine says very clearly is that measles is caused by a particular type of shock; in the conflict-active phase, the cells in the outer skin layer are broken down and are rebuilt in the reparation phase, which causes measles. When the person has measles, the cells change shape to deal with this situation (pleomorphism) and the MDs and other white-coats believe that this changed shape is because of the measles virus.

Bacteria

It is very easy to refute the myth that vaccines are necessary in relation to viruses because viruses do not exist. There is no need to vaccinate against something that does not exist. However bacteria do exist. So what about infections allegedly caused by bacterial diseases?

The 74-year-old German hygienist Max von Pettenkofer wanted to prove his theories on the true causes of cholera. He got a cholera culture from the Koch Institute without revealing his true intention. On the 7th October 1892 he drank a millilitre of these cholera bacilli. He didn't get sick nor did he get cholera. His assistant repeated the same experiment on the 17th October 1892. He got slightly sick but recovered rapidly. He did not get cholera.[105]

The Bio-Chemical Society of Toronto, Canada carried out similar experiments in which pure cultures of typhoid, diphtheria, pneumonia, tuberculosis and meningitis were consumed in large quantities by a group of volunteers. No ill-effects were observed.[106]

The cholera bacilli did not cause cholera; they are present when the host is suffering from cholera after drinking bad water over a period of time. Tubercular bacteria do not cause tuberculosis. Just as the presence of firemen at a fire does not necessarily mean that they caused the fire. Just as snow is present during Winter does not mean that snow causes Winter. Just as flies are present on a dung-heap does not mean that they caused the dung-heap.

Microbes are present during disease but are not the cause of the disease. There are no diseases as entities in themselves, only disease conditions.[107] Disease is born of us and in us.[108]

The real necessity for vaccinations

Vaccinations are only necessary if one wants to turn the human being into an easily controllable person that believes that all factors concerning their health come from external sources: germs, the MDs and pharmaceuticals. Such people do not believe that health comes from within and they believe that they have very little personal control over their own health.[109]

If you allow your children to be vaccinated (and I did) you will tend to allow anything in the name of Modern Medicine. If you get cancer, you will probably allow the MDs to treat you with chemotherapy and radiotherapy. You will agree with the white-coats (the scientists and MDs) who want to do stem cell research using human embryos and start experimenting with genes. You will agree with euthanasia in the interests of pain relief and so-called humanity for the patient. You will agree to almost anything in the name of science, progress and Modern Medicine.

Vaccinations do indeed play the same initiation role in Modern Medicine as baptism does in Christianity.

CHAPTER 13

The Myth that Vaccinations are Safe and Effective

It is a truth universally acknowledged that vaccinations caused the elimination of infectious diseases, are harmless in themselves, and are responsible for preventing any further epidemics.

Modern Medicine believes as dogma that vaccinations are effective because of the reduction in the incidence of infectious diseases since the introduction of vaccinations, because the vaccines are meant to be prophylactic or preventative. If, for example, you get the measles vaccine, the MDs believe that the measles vaccine is prophylactic or preventative, and you cannot get the real disease measles.

Secondly, they believe as an absolute dogma, that vaccinations are safe despite overwhelming evidence to the contrary. Any MD deviating from these dogmas will be ostracised by the medical profession and will probably eventually lose their right to practise medicine.

The reduction in the incidence of infectious diseases

The myth that vaccines are effective arose primarily because of the real reduction in both mortality and incidence of so-called infectious diseases. We are repeatedly told this by the MDs and the media, so much so that we nearly all believe it as an absolute truth, which proves Lenin's point that a lie repeatedly told becomes the truth.

The MDs themselves believe this and write in their text books and brochures that vaccines have been the most effective action of Modern Medicine in reducing death rates among children.

Ian Sinclair, author of V*accination – The "Hidden" Facts*, discovered in the course of his research that in most medical text books and journals the graphical evidence on the decline of infectious diseases starts from 1940 when antibiotics and certain vaccinations commenced.

Ian shows in his excellent book one graph of the measles death rate in the US starting from 1960 and running through to 1970. The measles vaccine was introduced in the US in the early 1960s. The graph shows a continuous decline in the death rate from the introduction of the measles vaccination. This graph would mislead MDs, student doctors and others examining it to conclude that the steep decline in the death rate from measles is because of the measles vaccine.[110]

Ian shows side-by-side with the graph dating from the 1960s a graph dating from 1900 to 1980 illustrating the death rate from measles. The death rate from measles had been falling dramatically long before vaccinations were introduced, and has simply continued its long-term decline after the introduction of vaccinations. The death rate from measles had fallen by 98% before the introduction of the vaccine.[111]

The only conclusion one can draw from these two graphs is that the measles vaccine had clearly nothing to do with the dramatic decline in the death rate from measles before its introduction, and probably had nothing to do with the continued decline in the death rate from measles after its introduction.

This graphical evidence is true for all of the other so-called infectious diseases that we vaccinate our children against. The decline in the death rate from all of these diseases long preceded the introduction of vaccinations against them.

Despite overwhelming evidence to the contrary the HPSC (Health Protection Surveillance Centre, Irish vaccine experts) in one of their brochures, aptly named *Vaccination – your child's best shot* state that: "In Ireland the benefits of vaccination are clear: fewer children develop serious infectious diseases and fewer die from these diseases."

The proposition in that statement is clear. Vaccines are responsible for the reduction in the incidence of infectious diseases and are also responsible for the fact that fewer children die from these infectious diseases when they get them. The myth that vaccines are responsible for the reduction in infectious diseases is easily revealed by reading any anti-vaccine book and there are hundreds if not thousands of these books. Let's examine this myth by examining a few "infectious" diseases.

The authorities only keep record of mortality from infectious diseases and do not even now keep accurate records of the incidence of these diseases. In almost all cases of infectious diseases, a decline in mortality rates has been accompanied by a commensurate reduction in the incidence of these diseases. Unless otherwise stated, the reduction in mortality will also be taken as a proxy for the reduction in the incidence of these diseases.

Tuberculosis

Tuberculosis (TB) was one of the biggest killers of people in England up till the mid 1800s. It killed around 3000 people per million of the population. The decline in mortality from tuberculosis started around 1850 and continued on. By 1954 the death rate from tuberculosis had declined by 95%, when the Bacille Calmette Guerin (BCG) vaccine was introduced. Death rates from TB merely continued their decline after the introduction of the vaccine.[112]

The BCG vaccine had absolutely nothing to do with this continued decline. There has never been a vaccination against TB in the US. The decline in the incidence of the disease there is analogous to those European countries that have the vaccine.[113]

In the 1970s, WHO ran a large field trial with the BCG vaccine in Southern India. One sub-group was vaccinated; the other was not. The group that were vaccinated against TB using the BCG vaccine had higher rates of TB than the group that were not vaccinated. Despite this study, Ireland, Britain and many other countries continue to use the BCG vaccine.[114]

Measles

In 1900 in the US, the death rate from measles was of the order of 133 per million population. This death rate had declined by almost 98% to less than 1 per million population by the time of the introduction of the measles vaccine. These figures are mirrored in England and Wales with a death rate of 318 per million population around 1900 to less than 1 per million population by the time the vaccine was introduced.[115]

Smallpox

It is estimated that smallpox deaths had reduced from 5000 to 2000 per million population between the years 1600 and 1800. It had declined to 400 per million by the time compulsory vaccination was introduced in England in 1852. There is an enormous body of evidence that proves that the smallpox vaccine increased the incidence of smallpox after the vaccine was introduced. Nonetheless, despite the smallpox vaccinations, smallpox deaths continued their long-term decline even after the introduction of the smallpox vaccine.[116]

Whooping cough (pertussis)

The death rate in the 1860s in England from whooping cough was about 1372 per million children. It had fallen to 815 per million children by 1910 and to 140 per million children by 1940. By the time the vaccination program had started in the late 1950s, the death rate was 5 per million children. The vaccination was introduced when the death rate had already declined by well over 99%.[117]

Diphtheria

The death rate in 1860 in England from diptheria was 1300 deaths per million children, and fell to fewer than 300 deaths per million in 1940 when the diphtheria vaccination was introduced. The death rate from this disease had already declined by 75% when the vaccine was introduced.[118]

Scarlet fever

There were 4000 to 5000 deaths per annum from scarlet fever in 1900. By 1923, the number of deaths had declined to fewer than 33 per annum. There never has been a vaccine for scarlet fever.[119]

Et cetera

Measles, mumps and rubella

It is very clear that the mortality rate from measles, mumps and rubella has declined dramatically over the last 100 years. It has been well established that vaccines had nothing to do with this reduction in mortality. What has not been determined is why the incidence of these three diseases has declined so dramatically in the last 40 years.

It would appear that my generation all got measles as children. I have noticed that in Ireland the incidence of measles, mumps and rubella has declined dramatically. None of my kids or their peer group have had measles. Why? It cannot be because the vaccines are effective because the measles virus doesn't exist. One would expect the incidence of diseases like measles, mumps, rubella and chickenpox to be constant from one generation to the next. I do not definitively know why the incidence of measles, mumps and rubella have declined so dramatically in the last 40 years.

The antibody dogma?

Antibodies are proteins in the blood. They can be made to coalesce or bind with other proteins in laboratory tests and in this way can be manipulated arbitrarily. The efficacy of a vaccine is determined by an appropriate level of antibodies. Vaccines are said to be effective for two reasons: the reduction in the incidence of infectious disease and the level of antibodies after the vaccination.

The antibody dogma was exposed over 50 years ago in a study published by the British Medical Council. Nine MDs determined antibody levels in people who developed diptheria and those who didn't but were in close contact with those same diptheria patients.[120]

If the antibody dogma is correct then those with diphtheria would have low levels of antibodies and those without diptheria would have high levels of antibodies.[121] The reverse was found. The antibody dogma was proven to be scientifically wrong.

This study, and I'm sure countless others, were ignored because they did not fit in with the antibody dogma, which is a key dogma in the vaccination fraud.

The true cause of the decline of these "infectious" diseases

In the early 1800s, in London England, almost 50% of children died before the age of five. The reasons for these deaths were attributed to poor housing conditions, polluted drinking water, inadequate sewage disposal and malnutrition.

Edwin Chadwick, a London lawyer, suggested that if improvements were made in the quality of drinking water and sanitary reform, effective waste disposal and if a clean-up of the environment were carried out, that most epidemic diseases would disappear. As a result of Chadwick's work, the Public Health Act was introduced in 1848 in Britain.

Dr Snow MD is hailed as the first epidemiologist. He discovered that the source of cholera in London during an epidemic in 1854 was a particular water pump. The areas of London supplied by the relatively clean upper Thames had much less incidences of cholera than those sections of the city supplied with water from the lower Thames which was fouled by human sewage. Sanitary reform eliminated cholera, typhoid and other diseases in London. Chadwick was absolutely correct.[122]

Max von Pettenkofer iniated a similar clean-up in Munich providing clean drinking water to all houses and setting up an effective waste disposal. As a consequence of this work, the death rate from typhoid declined from 72 per million population in 1880 to 14 per million in 1898.[123]

Since 1893 in Hamburg there has been a general decrease in infant mortality (with noticeable increases during both world wars) from a peak of almost 30% of live births to almost zero today. The sand-filtration of the water from the river Elbe started in 1893 and is responsible for the general decline and elimination of diseases like cholera, typhus, smallpox and even polio in the city of Hamburg. The reduction in these diseases is caused by an improvement in the hygiene of the drinking water and also of the waste water.[124]

Clean water and good sanitation prevents water-borne diseases like typhoid, cholera and yellow fever. But how do we explain the reduction in mortality from other so-called infectious diseases?

From the beginning of time hunger would have been an everyday occurrence for most people. It was only banished by the introduction of intensive farming, which ensured adequate production of food in the mid 1800s throughout Europe.[125]

Interestingly the Irish famine of 1845–1848 was caused by the failure of only one single crop, the potato, which was a staple food for the Irish peasants of the time: other crops did not fail and there was still enough food produced in Ireland in the mid 1800s to feed the population.

If a malnourished child in the 1840s in Ireland died from measles, is it the measles that killed the child or the fact that the child was malnourished over a prolonged period of time? The reality is that the child died from the effects of starvation and not from measles. These so-called infectious diseases like measles, mumps and rubella against which we vaccinate our children are not to be feared in a well-nourished and well-loved child living in the First World.

The vaccination industry and MDs take credit for the decline in infectious diseases. In reality we should honour the campaigners for sanitary reform and clean drinking water and the civil engineers who designed and built these facilities.

The myth that vaccines are safe

There is overwhelming evidence which proves that vaccines are not safe. They never have been safe and they never will be safe. All vaccines contain toxins. Vaccines were introduced initially to combat smallpox. The elimination of smallpox is always given as proof of the efficacy of vaccination. The safety concerns and the millions of deaths that arose as a result of the multiple smallpox vaccination campaigns should have been enough to kill off the concept of vaccinations forever. The reality that vaccinations have continued since the smallpox debacle provides eloquent proof about the power of the Biomedical Paradigm and our collective unimaginable stupidity.

The Chief Medical Officer of England stated in May 1871 that 97.5% of the population had been vaccinated against smallpox. In 1872, England experienced its worst ever smallpox epidemic which killed nearly 45,000 people. The death rate from smallpox rose during the period of compulsory vaccination from 280 to 460 per million population between 1871 and 1880.[126]

The Philippines had a death rate from smallpox of about 10% in 1905 prior to the US takeover. Systematic vaccination by the US government caused the mortality rate to range from 25–50% in different parts of the islands. In 1918-1919 a smallpox epidemic occurred in Manila, (the capital of the Philippines) which was by then almost totally vaccinated, which had a mortality rate of 65%.[127]

Et cetera.

Vaccines are dangerous and unnecessary

Vaccines are unnecessary because germs such as bacteria do not cause disease. Vaccines are unnecessary against viruses because viruses do not exist. Vaccines are dangerous. They always have been and they always will be.

CHAPTER 14

The HIV-AIDS Myth

It is a truth universally acknowledged that we have an immune system and that the HIV virus causes AIDS (Acquired Immune Deficiency Syndrome), or a breakdown in our immune system.

The immune system dogma

The medical myth of the *immune system* came about in the early 1970s to explain why some people are susceptible to disease/cancer, whereas others survive.

The immune system has been presented to us as a type of army in our body whose job is to eventually destroy the malignant cancer cells and malignant germs.[128]

There is no such thing as malignant cancer cells. They exist when one is suffering from cancer; they do not cause cancer. Cancer is caused by a biological shock, a DHS (Dirk Hamer Syndrome). There is also no such thing as malignant germs; they are active in the reparation phase of all diseases (according to the fourth Biological Law).

The medical myth of an immune system is another dogma invented by Modern Medicine to explain why the Germ Theory of Disease dogma does not work. If I were to drink or breathe in a huge quantity of tubercular bacteria isolated from somebody with tuberculosis I would not get this disease. I would bet that if 1000 people fully understood what is being advanced in this book and drank or inhaled huge quantities of isolated tubercular bacteria, not one of them would get tuberculosis.

Modern Medicine would explain this by stating that the observation that the Germ Theory of Disease dogma as advanced by Pasteur does not work, is because of a new dogma called the immune system. The immune system dogma is a necessary refinement of the Germ Theory of Disease dogma: One dogma to explain another dogma to explain the unexplainable within the pattern of thinking known as the Biomedical Paradigm.

We know from GNM that there is no such thing as the immune system. If we get a biological shock we get a cancer or disease. There is no other reason. Our immune system has not weakened, nor broken down. We have simply had a biological shock.

If there is no such thing as the immune system then there is certainly no such thing as AIDS or Acquired Immune Deficiency Syndrome. Our body does not suddenly become susceptible to new diseases caused by a new virus called HIV.

The HIV medical myth

The HIV virus supposedly occurs in many body fluids, and its transmission, especially in semen and blood to a new person, triggers a slow but inexorable progression to AIDS and finally death.[129]

AIDS is allegedly caused by the HIV retrovirus. What exactly is a virus? Dr Lanka provides an excellent definition of viruses with the following:

> *Viruses are essentially just packages of genetic information enclosed in a coat which consists of proteins. They can reproduce themselves only by infecting a suitable host cell and appropriating the chemical machinery they find there. The proteins making up the viruses are characteristic for each species of virus. Apart from enveloping and transporting the genetic information intact, the composition of proteins for a given virus results in a specific shape for the virus particle.*[130]

This definition of a virus by Dr Lanka would not be controversial. The definition of a retrovirus used by MDs is any virus belonging to the viral family *Retroviridae*.[131] A retrovirus is simply a particular type of virus.

The HIV virus, in common with other viruses such as mumps, measles or rubella, does not exist. However, there is a fundamental difference between the so-called HIV virus and other alleged viruses like measles, mumps or rubella. The disease called measles does exist, even though this disease is not caused by any virus, let alone the measles virus.

However the disease AIDS does not exist. AIDS is simply the name given to a collection of different diseases and clinical symptoms that are said to occur because the immune system has weakened because of the action of the alleged HIV retrovirus.

AIDS was discovered in June 1981 when the CDC (Centre for Disease Control and Prevention) in the US reported a cluster of Pneumocystis carinii pneumonia in five homosexual men in Los Angeles. It was originally thought to be exclusively related to homosexual men, hence its original name GRID (Gay Related Immune Deficiency). In 1982, the CDC introduced the term AIDS to describe this newly recognised syndrome because AIDS did not affect just homosexuals. It's now an equal-opportunity disease![132]

Because of this belief in the Germ Theory of Disease, the race was on to find the virus that caused AIDS. In 1983, Luc Montagnier led a team of scientists at the Pasteur Institute in France that allegedly discovered the HIV virus.

If Luc Montagnier had isolated the HIV virus, it should be possible to photograph the isolated HIV virus in an electron microscope. It should then be possible to compare the virus observed in this photograph with the virus as it exists in cells, body fluids or cell cultures in order to distinguish them from other cellular particles which look like viruses but are not viruses.[133]

If the HIV virus exists, it should be possible to biochemically characterise it. The biochemical characterisation would involve separating and photographing the proteins that make up the viral coat surrounding the virus. This produces a pattern which is characteristic of a particular virus. A similar biochemical characterisation procedure must be carried out for the core of the virus which contains DNA or RNA. A good analogy of a biochemical characterisation would be that of a viral signature/finger-print.

No such definitive evidence has been produced for the existence of the HIV virus nor for any other virus. There are no photographs in existence of an isolated HIV virus. None! The reason why is because the HIV virus does not exist.

Dr Lanka discovered a real virus in sea algae in the late 1980s. As the AIDS hysteria was at its peak he decided to read the scientific journals and specifically scientific papers produced by Luc Montagnier, the real inventor of the HIV virus and Bob Gallo, a would-be inventor of the HIV virus. Nowhere in these publications did these two gentlemen claim that they had isolated, photographed and biochemically characterised the HIV virus.

The photographs that have been produced of the AIDS virus are photographs of virus-like particles in cell cultures, but not of the isolated HIV virus.

The only basis by which the HIV virus is said to exist is because of an international scientific consensus, which is formed because of a secular-religious belief in the Germ Theory of Disease medical dogma.

Definition of AIDS

So if the virus causing AIDS, HIV, does not exist, what then is AIDS? AIDS itself is defined as a collection of separate diseases[134] such as:

- Pneumocystis carinii pneumonia.
- Kaposi's Sarcoma.
- Toxoplasmosis.
- Tuberculosis.
- Clinical symptoms such as extreme weight loss and wasting, exacerbated by diarrhoea, which can be experienced in up to 90% of HIV patients worldwide.
- Meningitis and other brain infections.
- Fungal infections.
- Syphilis.
- Malignancies such as lymphoma and cervical cancer.

The HIV theory of AIDS is that HIV causes Acquired Immune Deficiency (AID) by destruction of the T4 lymphocytes. AID then leads to the development of the clinical syndrome AIDS, with the various separate diseases outlined above.[135]

To solve the AIDS conundrum all we have to do is solve these individual diseases. A simple control experiment applying GNM therapy, would enable one to treat a group of Western homosexual males or/and intravenous drug users, who are the two largest AIDS infected population groups in the Western world, for their respective diseases.

In sub-Saharan Africa, the MDs rarely test for HIV antibodies because it is too costly. They diagnose AIDS by a combination of clinical symptoms such as chronic fevers, diarrhoeas, coughs and weight loss.[136] In reality, these symptoms are diseases of poverty. One would treat a group of sub-Saharan Africans who have been diagnosed with AIDS for the respective diseases that make up AIDS. The "treatment" in nearly all of these cases would be to provide clean water, good food and hygienic conditions. Mostly these Africans, as with the HIV-positive people in the West, would be assured that they do not have AIDS because the HIV virus does not exist. The result of this experiment would be to prove conclusively that AIDS is a name given to a collection of separate diseases and that in the case of sub-Saharan Africa they are mostly diseases of poverty.

Unlike Africa, the cause of AIDS diseases in the Western world, like Kaposi's sarcoma, is more complex in the case of Western homosexuals. However we solve all these diseases by solving the respective shocks that caused them.

AIDS inconsistencies

There are many AIDS inconsistencies that would make any intelligent person wonder if they spent a few minutes thinking about it. My favourites are:

1. The prediction when the alleged HIV virus was first discovered was that AIDS would infect a large percentage of the heterosexual population of the Western world as it has subsequently done in sub-Saharan Africa. This has never happened, and as we now know, never will happen.
2. In the Western world, the AIDS virus has predominantly affected two groups in society: homosexuals and drug-users. How come heterosexuals in sub-Saharan Africa are predominantly affected by AIDS? Various explanations are given by the MDs such as the HIV retrovirus changing form, but they defy common sense. This point has been made by people like President Mbeki of South Africa. How can the same virus affect one population group in the Western world and a different population group in Africa?
3. How come people have been diagnosed as HIV-positive and have lived for a long time but have not developed AIDS? The explanation offered will be that they have a strong immune system. This is a circular argument and is impossible to falsify.
4. How come people that were previously diagnosed as HIV-positive have had their diagnosis reversed and are now deemed to no longer have the HIV virus? I heard one American gay man talk about this on an Irish radio station. His life had been destroyed by this original diagnosis. He was very angry and was in the middle of a lawsuit.

The reason for AIDS in sub-Saharan Africa

The reason for AIDS in sub-Saharan Africa is because most of the population do not have clean drinking water, effective sanitation and adequate food. All we need to do to remedy the situation in Africa is ensure that the population get clean water, effective sanitation and are not malnourished. The last things these poor Africans need are the former US President Bill Clinton or the software billionaire Bill Gates or the Irish pop singer Bono pushing them HIV drugs, however well-intentioned they are. The road to Hell is paved with good intentions.

Kampala is the capital of Uganda and is a city of about 1.3 million people. Many of the poorer people live in a flood zone. There are "heaps of unclaimed garbage" strewn around these houses. During the floods this rubbish is presumably swept away into the river. There are basic toilets in these areas built above water streams. This raw sewage is released into the streams, the same streams that people use for drinking water. Those that do not have access to these basic toilet facilities use "flying toilets"; they defecate into a plastic bag and throw it into the stream. There are stagnant water holes around these shanty towns in the flood zones, which provide a good breeding ground for mosquitoes. According to the Ugandan National Water and Sewage Corporation in 2003 only 55% of Kampala is provided with treated water and only 8% with effective sewage disposal.[137]

The situation is not much better in rural areas. Most have no clean water. They wash clothes, bathe and dump their sewage upstream and downstream from where they get their drinking water. Water wells are shared with animals, which being animals, defecate and urinate at these water holes.[138]

This description of life in Uganda describes a perfect breeding ground for disease. Instead of tagging clinical symptoms in Kampala like chronic diarrhoea, weight loss, dysentery, or cholera as being symptomatic of AIDS and then causing further misery to these people by pushing them anti-retroviral drugs, one should initiate a plan for clean drinking water, proper sanitation and adequate food for these people. Let's help Africa today to do what Europe started to do in the 1850s.

The reason for AIDS in the Western world

Homosexuals[139]

Any homosexual presenting to an MD with Kaposi's sarcoma and pneumonia will be told that they have Acquired Immune Deficiency Syndrome (AIDS) caused by the phantom HIV virus. The fact that they have these two diseases will be regarded as proof that their immune system has broken down. However they do not have AIDS, because the HIV virus does not exist. They have suffered a number of biological shocks, and have acquired these individual diseases.

Pneumonia occurs in the reparation phase of a fear-of-loss-of-territory conflict. Examples of a loss of territory could include the potential loss of a sexual partner. This partner had belonged to the patient and now that he might go, it is a real shock, a potential loss of his territory. Or the fear-of-loss of territory could be for a job, house, wife or children. In the reparation phase of this Meaningful Biological Program of Nature (MBP) one gets pneumonia.

Kaposi's sarcoma occurs in the conflict-active phase of a defilement conflict. A possible example of a defilement conflict would be for example, if a homosexual had sex with a man he didn't like, and felt defiled or dirtied by the experience.

In the original cases of the handful of homosexuals who presented with both Kaposi's sarcoma and pneumonia, the MDs (because of their belief in both the Germ Theory of Disease and immune system dogmas) diagnosed that a new virus must be the common factor behind these two separate diseases. The search was on for this new virus, which is how the HIV virus was invented.

Instead of a phantom HIV virus being the cause of these two separate diseases, the true cause was the life-style of the men concerned. Apparently the original cohort of homosexual men who presented with both pneumonia and Kaposi's sarcoma had a common lifestyle. They took drugs at the weekend to keep them awake, and capable of partying non-stop, and having sex with multiple partners. They then took other drugs to enable them to function during the working week. It is not too difficult to imagine how such a lifestyle would predispose one to the biological shocks that cause both pneumonia and Kaposi's Sarcoma.

Disease is not a separate external entity. It is born within us.

Drug users

Intravenous drug users do not eat enough food and generally have extremely bad living conditions. All their energies are devoted to getting money to support their drug-habit. It is not too difficult to imagine that they living in these squalid conditions they can get a number of shocks causing various diseases. Because they are also drug users and have various diseases that indicate a breakdown of the so-called immune system, they are now deemed to be HIV-positive by the MDs.

The AIDS tests

HIV-positive is an abbreviation for HIV-antibody positive. The HIV test is performed upon a specimen of the patient's blood where the test kit registers the presence of antibodies. The HIV test is used to verify if these antibodies are caused by the presence of the HIV virus. If so they are called HIV antibodies and the patient is said to be HIV-positive. Antibodies are proteins made by cells called lymphocytes. They are switched on when something foreign such as a bacterium or alleged virus or protein is introduced into the body.[140]

The AIDS test allegedly detects antibodies produced by the immune system in response to infection by the HIV virus. But how can one have a reliable test for existence of the HIV virus if the HIV virus itself has never been proved to exist?

The leaflet on an AIDS test kit eloquently proves this point:

> *The test for the existence of antibodies against AIDS-associated virus is not diagnostic for AIDS and AIDS-like diseases. Negative test results do not exclude the possibility of contact or infection with the AIDS-associated virus. Positive test results do not prove that someone has AIDS or pre-AIDS disease status nor that he will acquire it.*[141]

In other words the AIDS tests are absolutely worthless.

Resolving the issue of the existence of the HIV virus

The Perth Group of HIV/AIDS dissidents was formed in 1981 at the Royal Perth Hospital, which is a teaching hospital for the University of Western Australia. The original members are the leader, biophysicist Eleni Papadopulos-Eleopulos, emergency physician Val Turner and Professor of Pathology John Papadimitriou.[142]

The Perth Group suggest that there are three ways to resolve the debate of whether the HIV virus exists or not:

1. One approach would be to isolate the HIV retrovirus from an AIDS patient.
2. A second approach would be to have a public debate between a small number of mainstream MDs and scientists and medical dissidents.
3. A third approach would be for alleged HIV patients to have the evidence for their diagnoses examined in courts of law.

It is impossible to isolate either the HIV retrovirus or the measles, mumps and rubella viruses, or any other virus from any patient, because these viruses do not exist. I believe the argument put forward by Stefan Lanka, Karl Krafeld and the Klein-Klein-Aktion[143] team to prove the existence of the viruses in the first place is much more compelling.[144] This will be the natural outcome of the first approach favoured by the Perth group and would be an essential prerequisite for their second and third approaches.

There is a long-established scientific tradition that those who propose theories provide the proof. According to this scientific tradition it is up to the HIV protagonists to come up with proof that the HIV retrovirus exists. A scientist cannot employ the "Martian argument" which states that Martians exist because there is no proof that they do not exist. You cannot prove a negative, you cannot prove that Martians and HIV do not exist. However you can at the very least expect that anyone who states with certainty that they do exist to provide proof for their existence.[145]

The problem with their second approach of having a public debate between the proponents of HIV and the medical dissidents is that the ground rules would have to be made very clear. The basic question for the debate would be: What proof is there for the existence of the HIV virus?

The third approach favoured by the Perth group could be promising. If a person diagnosed HIV-positive, with all the trauma that such a diagnosis, treatment and prognosis entails, were to have their diagnosis proved in a court of law, it could begin to unravel the comprehensive fraud that is HIV-AIDS. Again, the first question would be: What proof is there for the existence of the HIV virus?

With all the three approaches advocated by the Perth Group I believe we come back to the key question asked by Dr Lanka, Karl Krafeld and Klein-Klein-Aktion: In which scientific journal is published proof of the existence of the HIV virus; where the HIV virus is isolated, photographed and biochemically characterised? There is no such publication. But we must get the relevant authorities to admit there is no evidence for the existence of these viruses. The approach by Klein-Klein-Aktion to ask the authorities for evidence of the existence of the HIV virus will in time engender sufficient public awareness to demand a public debate and a scientific debate between the MDs and other white-coats about the non-existence of the HIV virus and all other viruses said to affect humans and animals.

CHAPTER 15

The Bird Flu Myth

It is a truth universally acknowledged that viruses exist, and that a variant of the flu virus, the bird flu virus H5N1, could potentially cause a mass pandemic killing many tens of millions of people.

The flu myth

Before we get into the bird flu myth it is important to understand exactly what the flu is. The "flu" is a common name for influenza. Influenza is an alleged virus that causes fever, sore throat, muscle pains, severe headache, coughing, and general weakness and fatigue.[146] The common cold is caused by a different putative virus, but it is a much less severe disease. In reality, the only difference between flu and a cold is in the severity of the symptoms. However, there is a vaccine against the flu virus but there is no vaccine against the common cold virus.

The Irish vaccine authority recommends annual vaccinations for high-risk groups because the influenza virus allegedly changes variant every year.[147]

Regardless of when you get a bad cold/flu in winter or summer, it takes about a week to fully recover from it, whether you go to an MD or not.

The outcome of all of this is that if you happen to have a bad cold in the middle of winter, the local MD is likely to diagnose that you have the flu. The same bad cold occurring during the summer is simply a bad cold and not a flu. It might feel like a flu, because it feels as bad as a flu, but the MD will diagnose a bad cold, and you will probably believe him.

The bird flu myth

The bird flu myth is a horror story that most of us believe. The white-coats have persuaded the politicians and the media to make us believe that migratory birds in Asia have been infected with a deadly virus. These mortally diseased birds then fly thousands of kilometres for several weeks. They then apparently infect, in Romania, Greece, the UK and elsewhere hens, geese and other poultry, with which they have had no proven contact, and which, within a very short period, get diseased and die. But the migratory birds do not get diseased and do not die, but keep on flying and apparently infecting poultry at will. Anyone who believes this will believe almost anything. Do you still believe it?[148]

Bird flu used to be called bird plague. Since the end of the 1800s, diseased poultry have been observed in mass poultry farming with the following symptoms: blue-colouring of the crest, decrease in egg-laying performance and lacklustre plumage. Some died, after displaying these symptoms allegedly of bird plague and now in our so-called scientific age, bird flu or H5N1.[149]

Intensive poultry farming, for example, when hens are being raised in small cages, with a tiny amount of space allocated to them, living in massive sheds with only artificial light will inevitably cause some birds to die each day as a result of this alien manner of living for them. It doesn't take a genius to work out that hens might not be very happy living in a small cage even though they are well fed. Incarcerated in these cages, it is not surprising that they are not healthy; they would like to be outside in the fresh air, in their normal habitat with the freedom to move around and be normal hens, like they have been for millions of years.

The problem is that when an abnormally large number of them die, the vets are called in. Because veterinarians operate under the Biomedical Paradigm, with the major dogma being the Germ Theory of Disease, they state that these poultry diseases are caused by a contagious virus, maybe even the dreaded H5N1, which is confirmed of course by arbitrary laboratory tests.

Instead of killing off thousands of these birds because of the fear that the virus has spread to all the other birds in the shed, one should investigate the blatantly obvious, which is their living conditions. The farmer probably can only economically survive by this intensive poultry farming because of the low prices paid by the supermarkets. The solution is simple: we need to raise our poultry and all our farm animals in appropriate conditions. It will mean paying more for our food, but it will be worth it.

Poultry need significantly more free space; they need to spend most of their time out-doors. They do not want to be incarcerated in huge sheds with a constant, strong and nauseous smell of bleach and other disinfectants. The poultry have souls and their living conditions need to be improved considerably. Once this occurs, there will be far fewer mysterious deaths of poultry and the quality of meat produced will be better, but it will certainly be more expensive.

Bird flu and backyard farming[150]

Most of the Southeast Asian bird flu outbreaks have occurred in three countries: Thailand, Indonesia and Vietnam. Chicken production in these countries has jumped eight-fold in only 30 years with most of this production taking place on factory farms.

The bird flu outbreaks occur on these factory farms and do not occur in what is called backyard farming. The white-coats (because they are pseudo-scientists) in the United Nation's Food and Agriculture Organization (FAO) and of course the World Health Organization, do not even consider the possibility that there is something wrong with industrial-scale intensive poultry farming even though there are no mysterious deaths of poultry in backyard farming.

Instead the white-coats blame backyard chicken producers. The TV pictures show the white-coats in their space suits running around chasing frightened chickens on these backyard farms. The TV pictures never show the white-coats in the factory farms; do they?

In backyard poultry production, the chickens wander outdoors and are in contact with migratory-birds that are allegedly infected with the bird flu virus. These farms are thus said to be a magnet for the alleged HVN1 virus according to the white-coats.

The absolutely crazy thing about all of this is that even though the bird flu symptoms only occur on factory farms, these small-scale producers are blamed and are forced to close down. The big poultry corporations use these bird flu outbreaks as an opportunity to finish off small-scale poultry production.

English white-coats use bird flu as a pretext for creating genetically modified bird flu-resistant chickens. If this continues to its logical conclusion we will only be allowed to eat poultry from factory-farmed chickens that have been genetically modified against a non-existent bird flu virus. This is a horrific vision.

This plan to have all poultry produced in factory farms is a catastrophe for hundreds of millions of rural poor in Southeast Asia and throughout the world. Backyard farming is essential for their daily food intake as well as their income. Rural households in Southeast Asia for example normally keep a few chickens for meat, eggs, and fertiliser. The UN's FAO are well aware of this but they still talk about the alleged risks from backyard poultry farms.

The real human tragedy about the death of migratory birds by the phantom bird flu virus in Qinghai lake, Northern China in 2005 was that the entire local stock of 20,000 poultry located within a 30-mile radius was culled without compensation. One poor farmer named Zhang Gi-hua whose income was less than €210 per year, and who depended on his small flock of poultry is quoted as saying: "Our family had five chickens and we were told we had to kill them all or we would be fined. It was a real blow. I used to buy my children's pens and schoolbooks with the money from the eggs."[151]

Louise Fresco, Assistant Director-General of the FAO states the problem from the white-coats' viewpoint: *The backyard chicken is the big problem and the fight against bird flu must be waged in the backyard of the world's poor.* The FAO issued a statement in November 2005 confirming this horrible propaganda: *The movement of migratory birds has caused outbreaks to emerge in several countries and regions simultaneously.*

This medical myth that the bird flu virus H5N1 exists is being used as a pretext to destroy backyard farming which is the only means of survival both from hunger and from absolute poverty for hundreds of millions of people worldwide.

Migratory birds and the bird flu myth

The white-coats repeatedly tell us that bird flu is spread by migratory birds. Despite assurances from those august pseudo-scientific bodies, the WHO and the FAO, there can be no scientific evidence at all that migratory birds spread bird flu because the bird flu virus does not exist.

The actual geographical spread of bird flu does not match the migratory routes and the seasons that these migratory birds travel. Dr Richard Thomas from Birdlife International[152] states authoritatively that: "When plotted, the pattern of outbreaks follows major road and rail routes, not flyways. And the absence of outbreaks in Africa, South and Southeast Asia and Australasia this autumn is hard to explain, if wild birds are the primary carriers."[153]

There was an outbreak of H5N1 confirmed on a factory farm in Nigeria in February 2006. The FAO and international white-coats pointed to migratory birds, even though the infected factory farm was nowhere near migratory wetlands and there was no evidence of infection or deaths among wild birds in the area. Even a white-coat in the FAO admitted, "If it's not wild birds, it will be difficult to understand." Right![154]

Migratory birds and a potential pandemic

Thousands of migratory birds died from an apparent mass outbreak of H5N1 on Bird Island in Qinghai lake, Northern China in May–June 2005. They were mostly geese (bar-headed geese), but also other migratory birds including gulls, shelducks and cormorants.[155]

The white-coats came up with the theory of the phantom bird flu virus, but could not conceive of the obvious explanation that the geese were poisoned. The white-coats were worried that the migratory birds would spread the H5N1 virus. Julie Hall, the WHO official in charge of communicable diseases in China said that that "This is an international issue. We need to give an early warning to countries on the birds' routes."[156]

But bird conservationists, and notably the organisation, BirdLife International, pointed out that Qinghai lake has many surrounding poultry operations. They also noted that there is a fish farm in the area that the FAO helped construct. They also noted that chicken faeces are commonly used as food and fertiliser in fish farms in China.[157]

Is it not possible, in fact is it not probable, that these migratory birds were poisoned by either the intensive fish-farming or poultry-farming? Chicken faeces would be high on my list as a possible source for the mass-poisoning of these migratory birds.

H5N1

A well known trick employed by the white-coats and the media is to give us a bit of science so that we know the disease isn't just bird plague or bird flu but is in fact H5N1. This seems to be very specific and scientific. It must be right. Once we read that the bird flu is in fact H5N1 our eyes glaze over. It's enough information; it must be real; the scientists have identified it.

What do these pseudo-scientists mean by "H5N1"? The 'H' in H5N1 stands for haemagglutinin and the 'N' stands for neuraminidase. The pseudo-virologists allege that the protein haemagglutinin and the enzyme/protein neuraminidase are found in the coat of the bird flu virus.[158]

The pseudo-virologists have agreed among themselves that there are supposed to be 15 different variants of haemagglutinin in the coat of the bird flu virus. The 'H5' is for type 5 of an alleged protein which somehow has only been indirectly proven.

It is exactly the same story with the enzyme neuraminidase, which is alleged to be a component part of the coat of bird flu viruses. There are nine different types of this enzyme alleged to exist by the pseudo-virologists. The 'N1' is for the first type of this enzyme said to exist in the coat of the bird flu virus.

The laboratory tests for H5N1

There is a laboratory in Weybridge, Surrey, England that is the reference laboratory for all of Europe with regard to the bird flu virus. They determine whether humans or birds have died from the dreaded bird flu: H5N1.

Before we examine the detail of what they do we must be clear on one critical point. Viruses do not exist in humans, plants or animals. If the bird flu virus did exist in these birds, Dr Lanka assures us that it could be determined in a matter of hours by a scientist in an ordinary laboratory. They could also tell whether the virus came from a live or dead bird.

But the testing that does actually take place in Weybridge seems to take a week to determine whether the bird died from H5N1 or not.

Indirect test methods, which tell absolutely nothing are being used to determine the alleged existence of this virus. These pseudo-virologists at Weybridge allege that there are specific antibodies which would combine with the body of the alleged H5N1 virus and only with this H5N1 virus. The evidence of a successful combination between the body of the H5N1 virus and the specific antibody determines the existence of the alleged H5N1 virus.

In reality, those alleged antibodies are soluble blood proteins, which play a central role in the sealing of cells which are growing and dividing and in the healing of wounds. These soluble blood proteins, also called globulins, will combine arbitrarily with other proteins in test tubes containing appropriate concentrations of acids and bases, minerals and solvents.[159]

These scientists are using indirect means to prove the existence of the bird flu virus, which only exists because of their adherence to the Germ Theory of Disease medical dogma. The only way to uncover this fraud is to ask these pseudo-scientists for the scientific publication in which the bird flu virus H5N1 was isolated, photographed and biochemically characterised.

In this way, according to Dr Lanka, you can take a sample from any bird or person, decide what result you want, and then get the desired result from the test. This is not just a matter of scientific error: It is much more than that. If a lot of people this winter get a bad cold, and because it is winter the MDs diagnose the bad cold to be a flu, or if somebody living near a poultry farm, or better still working on a poultry farm, is diagnosed initially with flu and then further diagnosed to be suffering from bird flu, the results could be absolutely catastrophic.

Photographs of the bird flu virus

There are no direct photographs of a bird flu virus. They do not exist because the bird flu virus itself does not exist.

The pictures that are shown in the media of the bird flu virus are recognisable by any biologist as normal component parts of cells, or even of complete cells. To verify this, all one has to do is to ask the scientists for the scientific publication which describes how this would-be virus was isolated, and from which the photograph was taken. No such scientific publication exists.

The bird flu virus has never been isolated, photographed in an electron microscope and its component parts biochemically characterised in processes which are called electrophoresis.

The Spanish flu, bird flu and Tamiflu

The great fear propagated by the white-coats (the MDs and pseudo-scientists) is that the bird flu virus H5N1 will spread from human to human causing a mass pandemic similar to the Spanish flu of 1918–1920 when up to 50 million people died. More people will die because of the increased mobility of humanity through air travel. We should be all afraid of this horrible new virus that could kill up to a 100 million people.

Dr Jeffrey Taubenberger claims that he has reconstructed the Spanish flu virus from the frozen corpse of a woman who died of the Spanish flu in 1918 in Alaska. Dr Taubenberger claims that the bird flu virus H5N1 caused the Spanish flu.[160]

The problem with all of this is that there is no scientific paper produced whereby the Spanish flu virus was proven to exist in any corpse.

If no virus was isolated, photographed and biochemically characterised then how can he claim to have produced a genetic model of the virus?

Rather than debate the intricacies of how he produced a genetic model of a non-existent virus it would be simpler to ask him for the proof that the bird flu virus he allegedly isolated actually exists in the first place.

The BBC (British Broadcasting Corporation) aired a 90 minute TV program on November 7th 2006 called "Pandemic", based on the premise that the bird flu virus spreads from human to human. It was a masterpiece of propaganda for the proponents of the Biomedical Paradigm. This show had the product Tamiflu (an anti-viral drug) prominently displayed. During a flu pandemic people would be assaulting each other in order to get anti-viral drugs such as Tamiflu.

Tamiflu is supposed to act as neuraminidase-restraining agent. By restraining neuraminidase it is supposed to prevent new viruses emerging from infected cells.[161]

The side-effects of taking Tamiflu are almost identical to the symptoms of a serious flu. These side-effects are clearly described on the instruction leaflets for Tamiflu.

Tamiflu is marketed by Hoffman-La Roche using this same trade name. The drug's scientific name is Olsetamivir and it was developed by Gilead Sciences. Tamiflu/Olsetamivir is used for the treatment and prevention of flu.[162]

Donald Rumsfeld, the former US Defense Secretary, is a former chairman and significant shareholder in Gilead Sciences. President George W Bush, in November 2005, announced a set of domestic measures to fight the phantom pandemic which included an envelope of up to US$1.4 billion for Tamiflu.[163]

These facts have spawned a number of interesting conspiracy theories about Tamiflu. But they all divert from the real conspiracy, the Ultimate Conspiracy which is the Biomedical Paradigm.

CHAPTER 16

The Lung Cancer – Smoking Myth

It is a truth universally acknowledged that smoking causes lung cancer and that even passive smoking[164] also causes lung cancer.

I had the greatest personal difficulty in rejecting this medical myth. In my late teens, I smoked one cigarette and I inhaled.[165] I was violently ill and retched repeatedly. I have witnessed the smoker's cough and thought that it was a sure indicator of cancer or other diseases. While I could accept Dr Hamer's New Medicine, and even his explanation that lung cancer is caused by a particular type of biological shock,[166] surely smoking had something to do with lung cancer?

In Defense of Smokers[167]

There are thousands of articles on the internet challenging the HIV–AIDS medical myth. There are very few articles challenging the dogma that lung cancer is caused by smoking. One of the very few is a challenging internet book called *In Defense of Smokers* by Lauren A Colby, a US trial lawyer and smoker. Lauren Colby, who is definitely not an MD, was applying his common sense, life-experience and real science to all the falsehoods behind the myth that lung cancer is caused by cigarette smoking.

He makes a number of salient points in his short and excellent book on the smoking myth:

1. Anecdotally we all know of heavy smokers who live long lives and do not die from lung cancer, and conversely non-smokers who die from lung cancer.[168]

Modern Medicine naturally has a convenient explanation that the 95-year-old smoking 20 cigarettes a day for over 80 years must have a strong immune system. The non-smoking, non-drinking, vegetarian and good-living Christian, who dies from lung cancer at the age of 39, must have had a weak immune system. This is simply one hypothesis to support another, to support another, to support all the dogmas of the religion known as the Biomedical Paradigm.

2. If there was a clear link between smoking and lung cancer one would suspect that the countries with the highest per-capita consumption of cigarettes would have the highest lung cancer death rate (LCDR) and a lower life-expectancy because smoking is allegedly a causal factor in a number of diseases. A Dutchman, Kees van der Griendt, compiled data for 87 countries in 1994, using data from the WHO and the CIA (Central Intelligence Agency) World Fact Book. He found that countries like Iceland, Japan and Israel have a higher percentage of smokers than the US but also a higher life expectancy. In 1994 the percentage of male Japanese smokers was 2.7 times higher than Swedish males (59% versus 22%) although the average Japanese male had an increased life expectancy of one year over the average Swedish male.

So how can the anti-smoking lobby claim that smoking reduces your life expectancy by between 20 and 25 years? This is propaganda and absolute fiction.

3. Cigarette smoking peaked in the US in 1961 with a per capita rate of 3986 cigarettes per annum. In 1961, 68% of all males in the US were smokers. There is no correlation between the decline in the per capita cigarette consumption and the increase in the LCDRs. These LCDR figures are not given in percentages, but in death rates per 100,000 age-adjusted. Instead between 1970 and 1990 the LCDR increased despite a falling rate of cigarette consumption.

This apparent increase in LCDR rates is probably because of better detection rates and a predilection by the MDs to diagnose lung cancer for a smoker.

4. A British medical researcher, Professor Philip Burch, plotted cigarette consumption in England and Wales against LCDRs. He also stated that many cases diagnosed as being primary lung cancers were in fact secondary or tertiary cancers. Burch concluded that the rise in LCDR was due to improved diagnosis and not due to smoking. Burch also refuted the "incubation theory" argument.[169]

According to GNM, lung cancer is a "Fear of Death" biological shock. So if you have already been diagnosed with one form of cancer and get a subsequent shock because of the diagnosis, and believe that you are going to die, you will get alveolar lung cancer or more simply, lung cancer.

5. Other studies indicate that poorer people are more likely to be heavy smokers than richer people. However no correlation is made between lung cancer and poverty but rather between lung cancer and smoking.

We know from the GNM that alveolar lung cancer is caused by a Fear of Death biological shock and this is naturally going to be much more prevalent in poorer people. Poorer people do not have the financial means to survive the trials and tribulations of life such as losing a job or getting divorced and these events can possibly cause a biological shock or DHS. Richer people can survive these tragic events more comfortably without them necessarily causing a shock at all.

If poorer or lower-income people are more likely to be smokers, then the fact that the person is a smoker should be in the jargon of statistics an "associative factor" and not a "causative factor". The causative factor of lung cancer, being a Fear of Death biological shock, is likely to be more prevalent among poorer people.

I would bet everything I have that all things being equal, a rich smoker will, on average, live longer than a poor non-smoker. Smoking is not a causative factor in lung cancer as was clearly demonstrated by Lauren Colby. Lung cancer is usually caused by the diagnosis from an MD that you have another type of cancer, and being in fear of death you get a secondary cancer, the lung cancer caused by the MD's news.

6. The basic science in proving that lung cancer is caused by smoking was set out in the Surgeon General's report in the US in 1964. A committee was established which examined seven prospective studies. A prospective study is when a population is sampled and their smoking habits are observed and this is repeated for a number of subsequent years to determine the respective death rates from lung cancer. All the participants knew that the purpose of the various studies was to prove that lung cancer was caused by smoking. This introduces detection bias into the equation, whereby lung cancer will be more readily detected in a smoker than a non-smoker. The responses from the studies were flawed in that the group being monitored apparently was much healthier than the general population as a whole. How could one rely on the results of this study when the participants were significantly healthier than the population as a whole?

There were no statisticians on the panel of experts although statistical expertise was essential to a proper analysis of the epidemiological studies. In 1965, a prominent statistician, KA Brownlee of the University of Chicago, wrote a scathing review of the report, which pointed to the many discrepancies in the data.[170]

7. The experiments that allegedly proved that passive smoking/environmental tobacco smoke (ETS) were carcinogenic were flawed. They were carried out on the partners of people who smoked. The idea was to prove that the partners of people who smoked were more likely to get lung cancer than the partners of people who did not smoke. At the time of the Environmental Protection Agency (EPA) study, there were about 30 studies from around the world involving human populations exposed to second-hand smoke. Twenty-four studies showed no significant correlation between ETS and lung cancer. Six studies reported weak statistical associations between exposure to second-hand smoke and lung cancer.

The primary data was manipulated (by merging the studies and reducing confidence levels) in order to prove that ETS does indeed cause lung cancer. This report was published in 1993 by the US EPA.

Writing in *Toxological Pathology*, Alvan Feinstein, a Yale University epidemiologist, quoted another epidemiologist about the EPA report: "Yes, it's rotten science, but it's a worthwhile cause. It will help us to get rid of cigarettes and become a smoke-free society."[171]

In an article entitled *Second-hand Smokescreen* published in 2001, Steven Milloy elaborates the point on second-hand smoke made by Lauren Colby and explains that the tobacco industry challenged the EPA determination in court. The federal judge disputed the EPA's main conclusions. This ruling should have destroyed the myth that second-hand smoke causes lung cancer except that it came more than five years after the EPA issued its report. The anti-smoking lobby exploited that time to convert the EPA's flawed report into conventional wisdom.

Steven Milloy further reported that the WHO's International Agency for Research on Cancer published in 1998 the largest-ever study on second-hand smoke and lung cancer and reported no statistically significant increase in lung cancer risk associated with exposure to second-hand smoke.[172]

8. In an autopsy there is no way of distinguishing the lungs of a smoker from the lungs of a non-smoker, assuming that neither of

them had lung cancer. This is hardly surprising because almost all of the cigarette smoke is filtered out before it reaches the lungs. Those pictures of the ravaged lung of a smoker would be the same as those of a non-smoker with alveolar lung cancer.

Lauren Colby asked Dr Ed Uthman, MD, a pathologist practicing in Dallas, Texas, whether a surgeon, at autopsy, could determine from an examination of the deceased's lungs, if the deceased was or was not a smoker? Dr Uthman's response is revealing:

> "I don't think one can tell if the deceased were a tobacco smoker or not by the appearance of the lungs. The absence of any black pigment suggests that the person was either a nonsmoker or a very light smoker. Heavy black pigmentation suggests that the person was either a heavy smoker, or lived in a city with heavy particulate air pollution, or was a coal miner, or some combination of the three. The black pigment in question is elemental carbon, which most investigators believe to be inert in its effects on the lungs."[173]

German New Medicine and the lung cancer medical myth

If 30% of the population of a country smoke, then according to GNM one would expect that 30% of the people with lung cancer are smokers and that 70% are non-smokers. This would assume that both smokers and non-smokers are equally wealthy. If smokers are poorer than non-smokers, then one would expect a higher death rate from lung cancer among the smokers. The statistics that allegedly show that smokers are eight times more likely to get lung cancer than non-smokers are flawed. Flawed is a polite way to describe these statistics; they are pure propaganda allegedly for a noble cause.

1. The first issue is what is the definition of a smoker? If you are an ex-smoker of 1, 2, 10, 12 years' standing are you classified as a non-smoker or a smoker? In some of the studies, anyone who had ever smoked was classified as a smoker.
2. The second issue is how do we define lung cancer? Do we include throat cancer and bronchial cancer? Or is lung cancer to be defined as simply alveolar lung cancer? In the case of a smoker these separate diseases are invariably lumped together as lung cancer.
3. The third issue is that MDs are more likely to diagnose lung cancer in the case of a smoker than in the case of a non-smoker

because they are pre-disposed to do so. This is the so-called detection bias.

4. A fourth issue is whether the lung cancer is the primary cancer or is it a secondary or tertiary cancer probably as a result of the diagnosis of a primary or secondary cancer. This is the most significant issue from a GNM viewpoint.

Once these issues are scientifically resolved it will become apparent that smokers are no more likely to get alveolar lung cancer than non-smokers.

Dr Hamer emphatically makes the point about correlation. Apparently shepherds in the Caucasus, Russia live long lives. They eat, naturally enough, a lot of goat's milk cheese. A pseudo-scientific study was done that claimed on this basis, that goat's milk cheese is anti-carcinogenic. But is the fact that shepherds eat a lot of goat's milk cheese the primary causal factor behind them living a long life? Or is it possible that shepherds are less likely (because of their lifestyle) to have a biological shock resulting in a cancer and therefore more likely to live a long life?[174]

British case-law and lung cancer

A British judge, Lord Nimmo Smith, examined the arguments about lung cancer being caused by smoking in a case brought by Alfred McTear.

Alfred McTear, who smoked 60 cigarettes a day, died of lung cancer in 1993 at the age of 48. Just before his death he had launched a case against Imperial Tobacco. His widow Margaret carried on the battle, asking for £500,000 damages in the first case of its kind in Britain.

Lord Nimmo Smith issued his ruling in June 2005. He determined, after hearing from all the expert witnesses, that the general causal connection between cigarette smoking and lung cancer has not been established by any branch of scientific inquiry other than epidemiology.

Specifically, laboratory experiments on animals had not established that exposure to cigarette smoke caused alveolar lung cancer.

Epidemiology is the study of patterns of disease occurring in human populations and the factors that influence these patterns. An epidemiologist may collect primary data, by conducting a survey, or secondary data, derived from other researchers' primary data.

The following paragraph of Lord Nimmo Smith's judgment is revealing:

[6.162] I can say with confidence that no evidence was led about the primary literature which was sufficient to impart to me special knowledge of the relevant subject-matter and to enable me to form my own judgment about it and the conclusions to be drawn from it. This could have been done: it is clear that the survey of British doctors, on which Sir Richard Doll and colleagues have worked for many years, is regarded as a classic of its kind, both because of the pioneering Nature of the research, a preliminary report of which was published as Doll and Hill 1950, and because this has been followed up with subsequent papers over several decades. I could at least have been shown these papers, which I assume disclosed the data, the statistical techniques and all the other considerations which led to the authors' conclusions, so that I could see for myself whether these conclusions were soundly based. The opportunity was there, with Sir Richard Doll in the witness box, and indeed Professor Friend for one thought that evidence would be given about this survey. Warning had been given on behalf of ITL, as early as the specification of documents referred to at para.[1.24], that Sir Richard Doll's data were of potential interest to the court. But in the event, no attempt was made to show me the data.[175]

In paragraph 6.166 Lord Nimmo Smith states baldly "*But however often a conclusion may be repeated, it is only as sound as the research on which it is based, and of this I have seen none.*"[176]

In this landmark case, the prominent MDs who did the primary research that allegedly established the epidemiological evidence that smoking causes lung cancer did not show the judge the primary evidence, and therefore the judge could not determine for himself whether the conclusions that the MDs drew from this evidence were in fact correct.

The key question here is why did these eminent MDs refuse to present the primary evidence on which they concluded that lung cancer was caused by smoking? I would boldly suggest that they know if their primary evidence is re-evaluated by proper mathematicians and statisticians and even by a judge with only a legal training, they will be found to be just more junk-science obtained from falsified-statistics.

As Lauren Colby has clearly demonstrated, the primary evidence is flawed and no such conclusion that smoking is caused by lung cancer could be adduced from it.

Smoking – what it really causes[177]

Smoking gives you bad breath and makes your clothes smoky with an unpleasant odour. Smoking increases your metabolism and your heartbeat because the body must do more work to eliminate the toxins in the cigarette. Therefore smoking does reduce your vitality but it does not cause alveolar lung cancer, nor indeed any other kind of cancer, nor any other disease.

It is legitimate to ban smoking if you want to prevent people from having to smell people with bad breath or getting their clothes all smoky and dirty after a night out. It is not legitimate to ban smoking because it is alleged by the MDs and other white-coats to cause lung cancer as well as other cancers and diseases.

CHAPTER 17

Other Cancerous Myths

It is a truth universally acknowledged that cancer spreads from one part of the body to another by a process called metastasis, and that when a cancer is detected by the MDs, it must be immediately aggressively treated by chemotherapy, radiation treatment, or radical surgery to prevent it from spreading any further.

It is a truth universally acknowledged that certain substances cause cancer, especially so-called carcinogens such as cigarettes.

It is a truth acknowledged (even if not universally acknowledged), that certain foods such as apricots and goat's milk cheese are anti-carcinogenic, whereas other foods such as chips[178] or French fries and fast food in general are carcinogenic.

The metastasis medical myth

The word metastasis is defined by the MDs as a secondary cancerous growth formed by transmission of cancerous cells from a primary growth located elsewhere in the body.[179]

This definition of metastasis is based on a hypothesis or guess of Modern Medicine that cancer spreads from a primary site to a secondary site. This hypothesis is considered to be absolutely true despite the fact that no-one has ever observed cancerous cells being transmitted from a primary site to a secondary site. The suspected mechanism of this alleged transfer is via the blood-stream or the lymph nodes. However despite the fact that this transfer mechanism has never been observed, this hypothesis of metastasis has acquired all the characteristics of a dogma and is a required belief for all the MDs and oncologists.

German New Medicine states emphatically that the second cancer is not the result of metastasis but is the result of a second biological shock. If Modern Medicine took its hypothesis of metastasis seriously it would prohibit blood transfusions because they could contain potentially cancerous cells.[180] Of course, they don't.

Metastasis is a medical myth invented by Modern Medicine to explain that people who have a cancer and are treated by an MD invariably get a second or third cancer because of the medical treatment by the MDs themselves. Dr Hamer estimates that 90% of secondary and tertiary cancers are caused by the misguided and deadly actions of the so-called experts, the oncologists or cancer-MDs.[181]

Animals are fortunate and rarely get secondary cancers. Dr Hamer emphasises this point repeatedly. Luckily animals don't understand the vets and do not get an iatrogenic cancer caused by the announcement that they have a primary cancer.

Metastasis example

An example of metastasis would be if one is diagnosed with osteoporosis or bone cancer by the MDs. Bones are mesodermal in origin, controlled by the new brain and in the conflict-active phase suffer decalcification, which is called osteoporosis. The bone becomes decalcified or develops holes and becomes brittle: They are much easier to fracture. Osteoporosis or bone cancer is caused by a major self-devaluation biological shock.

Faced with a diagnosis of osteoporosis by the MD, and then having to undergo cancerous treatment such as chemotherapy and radiotherapy, it would not be surprising that one would get a second biological shock that one is about to die, a "Fear of Death" biological shock. The alveoli of the lungs are endodermal in origin causing them to multiply in the conflict-active phase.

Osteoporosis and lung cancer have nothing to do with each other. They are both caused by different biological shocks with completely different themes. They are not caused by migrating cancer cells in a process called metastasis by the MDs.

Lung cancer is a common secondary cancer caused by the MDs; the diagnosis of a primary cancer and then the subsequent medically induced secondary cancer.

One has to ask oneself how can the same migrating cancer cells cause osteoporosis or cellular breakdown or necrosis in the bones, and then travel up to the lungs and cause the alveoli of the lungs to multiply? It doesn't make any kind of sense.

These migrating cancer cells that nobody has ever seen allegedly cause bone cancer or necrosis/decalcification/cellular breakdown of the bones and then transform and migrate across germ layers (from the mesoderm to the endoderm) and allegedly cause the alveoli of the lungs to multiply. The same migrating cancer cells cause cellular breakdown in the bones and cellular multiplication in the lungs, which is what the MDs call metastasis. This irrational belief in wandering cancer cells is a major dogma of the Biomedical Paradigm and all cancerous MDs (oncologists) are obliged to believe in it.

The carcinogenic medical myth

Certain substances, such as cigarettes, are said to be carcinogenic or cause cancer. Other substances, such as particular foods, are said to prevent cancer or to be anti-carcinogenic.

Carcinogens are usually determined by performing cruel and insane experiments on animals. Dr Hamer cites an experiment using rats to prove that formaldehyde is carcinogenic in order to illustrate the insanity of these experiments.[182] Rats have an extremely keen sense of smell, and in their normal environment would avoid anything that smells like formaldehyde. In this experiment the rats were sprayed with formaldehyde on their nose several times a day. Naturally enough, they absolutely hate the smell of pure formaldehyde. Not surprisingly, they all got a biological shock of not wanting to have to smell the pungent odours of formaldehyde. Their nasal mucous membrane ulcerated because they simply did not want to smell this awful odour any more. After a few months of this insanity, the white-coats stopped the torture, and some of these rats were immediately killed and examined by the white-coats. They found no cancer. Four weeks later another group of these rats were killed and examined. They found cancer in the nasal mucous membrane. Why? Because the biological shock causing this DHS had now been over for four weeks, and the nasal mucous membrane was healing, causing the ulcers to be replenished. But the white-coats stated that this was proof that formaldehyde was carcinogenic! I bet that this is the first time you felt sorry for a rat!

Formaldehyde is poisonous but it is not carcinogenic. With an understanding of GNM we know there is no such thing as a carcinogenic substance. Cancer, like every disease, is born in us and from us,[183] and is directed by our psyche via our brain.

A few years ago I was extremely sceptical of the animal rights lobby. Surely these experiments on animals were being performed for the benefit of humans and were therefore good? However the animal rights people are correct: Animal experiments are cruel and insane. Moreover, because they are conducted under the auspices of the Biomedical Paradigm, with the belief that all carcinogens work locally (like formaldehyde and cigarette smoke) and that animals have no soul or psyche, they are also unnecessary and pointless.

Dr Hamer jokingly suggests that one could perform a similar type of experiment on humans (preferably white-coats and, even better, oncologists, who are cancerous MDs) and spray their nose several times a day with human excrement for a few months. A few weeks after this insane torture ended, just like with the rats, one would also observe cancer in their nasal mucous membrane, proving that shit is carcinogenic![184]

There are no such things as carcinogens. All animal experiments are therefore pointless and should immediately end.

The cancer and food medical myth

There are thousands of scientific papers and books on the myth that certain foods cause cancer or are carcinogenic or prevent cancer and are anti-carcinogenic.

There are two disparate groups of allegedly primitive people who before the onset of "civilisation" lived their allotted time-span. They are the Hunza in northern Pakistan and the Inuit in the Arctic regions.

The Hunza eat almost exclusively fruit and in particular apricots. The Inuit eat all kinds of fish, seal and whale. These two geographically separate groups of people, who have completely different diets, lived long, healthy lives.

There have been scientific papers on the fact that goat's milk must be anti-carcinogenic because shepherds in the Caucasus live to an old-age; that eating chips or French fries increases the incidence of breast cancer later in life; that because the Hunza eat a lot of apricots, that apricots must be anti-carcinogenic… The list is endless and unfortunately increasing all the time.

The reason why the Hunza currently live longer is because they manage their conflicts (biological shocks) better than so-called civilised people, but not because of the apricots or other fruits that they eat.

The real danger with food is with processed food. It is dangerous (but not carcinogenic) because of the toxic additives contained within it. A good rule of thumb is that if something is advertised on TV you shouldn't eat it.

The reality is that with a good natural diet, that gives us all the necessary nutrients, we should all live to our allotted time-span.

Placebo effect – medical reality

The Latin word "placebo" means "I shall please".[185] The placebo effect is the measurable, observable, or felt improvement in health not attributable to the treatment itself that is administered by the MD. The classic case is that of the patient receiving a sugar pill to solve a problem such as depression or blocked arteries. The patient believes that the drug will work and then it does work even though it was a placebo. The placebo effect is proof of the control exerted by the mind over the body. It is the greatest clue that Modern Medicine is following the wrong paradigm.

Spontaneous healing – medical reality

Spontaneous healing is not a modern medical myth but is in fact an awkward reality. In fact, this has to be the second greatest clue that Modern Medicine is following the wrong paradigm. The tumour has faded away, the ulcer is gone, the germs have disappeared. It seems to be a miracle. MDs don't call it a miracle of course, but instead call it a spontaneous healing.

GNM has a simple explanation for spontaneous healing. The person has solved the conflict that caused their cancer/disease and consequently has been spontaneously healed.

Modern Medicine – cancerous reality

Modern Medicine is the greatest worldwide threat to our health and our lives. Modern Medicine is an awful cancerous reality that must be overcome. If we do not overcome Modern Medicine, it will eventually destroy all of us.

3

The Iatrogenic Effect

Hell is paved with good intentions.
Saint Bernard of Clairvaux (Cistercian Abbott, 1091 – 1153)

Doctors are men who prescribe medicines of which they know little, to cure diseases of which they know less, in human beings of whom they know nothing.
Voltaire (French writer, philosopher, 1694–1778)

God heals and the doctor takes the fee.
Benjamin Franklin (Founding father of the US, 1706-1790)

The medical establishment has become a major threat to health.
Ivan Illich (Catholic priest, writer, philosopher and polymath, 1926–2002)

In summoning even the wisest of physicians to our aid, it is probable that he is relying upon a scientific 'truth', the error of which will become obvious in just a few years' time.
Marcel Proust (French writer, 1871–1922)

Nearly all men die of their medicines, and not of their illnesses.
Molière (French writer, actor 1622–1673)

The greatest threat of childhood diseases lies in the dangerous and ineffectual efforts made to prevent them through mass immunization.
Dr Robert Mendelsohn MD (American paediatrician, 1926–1988)

The only real mistake is the one from which we learn nothing.
Sir John Powell (British jurist, 1633–1696)

Only two things are infinite, the universe and human stupidity, and I'm not sure about the former.
Albert Einstein (American physicist, 1879–1955)

CHAPTER 18

The Financial Cost of the Biomedical Paradigm

The financial cost of Modern Medicine

As a means of illustrating the nature of the Biomedical Paradigm, I examined the media stories in Ireland concerning Modern Medicine on the 19th October 2005. Most medical stories that day were false. Two medical stories that day were true; the unnecessary death of Patrick J Murphy at a small local hospital in Monaghan, Ireland and a brief story about the escalating costs of health care in the US damaging US manufacturing industry.[186]

Patrick J Murphy died because of a bleeding ulcer because the MDs wouldn't operate on him at a small hospital in Monaghan. Why? Because of the financial costs associated with the Biomedical Paradigm, we must have a small number of hospitals in large urban centres where we can have all the specialists in the various divisions and sub-divisions of Modern Medicine. The case of the bleeding ulcers of Patrick J Murphy, is one where external intervention is absolutely necessary to prevent death. Afterwards one can discover what caused the ulcers in the first place and solve the underlying problem.

In Ireland and I'm sure worldwide, people naturally campaign strongly against the closure of their local hospital. We will continue to need local hospitals for emergency cases such as trauma (car accidents, etc) and life-threatening conditions like bleeding ulcers. But the financial logic of the Biomedical Paradigm is that we need to close down or curtail the services provided by these local hospitals because it is only economic to provide these services at much larger hospitals.

It is interesting to examine the escalating financial costs of the Biomedical Paradigm and whether there is any noticeable improvement in health by this continuous increase in health costs.

The biomedical model of Modern Medicine is extremely costly. In 1962, the US spent 4.5% of its income (Gross National Product) on health care; in 1975, the US spent 8.4% of its income on health care; in 2005, the US spent 15% of its income on health care; and this percentage is expected to reach 17% of US income by 2011.

There are new and expensive drugs and therapies that hold out the elixir of a longer and healthier life. Following the Biomedical Paradigm, one simply has to get these latest and incredibly expensive treatments. Governments and health insurers are morally obliged to provide these in the interests of public health care and medical costs continue to escalate faster than income earned. We simply cannot financially afford the continued escalation in health care costs for little or no improvement in life expectancy nor in the quality of life.

Health story of the day in Britain – 21st August 2006

An example of the latest pharmaceutical elixir was the medical news story of the day in Britain on the 21st August 2006. There are apparently two drugs called Avastin and Erbitux that allegedly prolong life by up to five months in patients suffering from bowel cancer. These drugs are widely available in the US and much of Europe. Patients suffering from bowel cancer naturally enough want the latest medical treatment and demand it as a right.

A married couple, two retired teachers, appeared on a British TV nightly news show that night. The woman had bowel cancer and her husband felt that the Government was morally obliged to provide this treatment to his wife and others free of charge. The problem was that this treatment cost from £15,000–20,000.

Avastin, known generically as bevacizumab, works by starving tumours of blood supply, while Erbitux, or cetuximab, stops the proliferation of cancer cells.[187]

In an effort to contain health costs in Britain (within the constraints of the Biomedical Paradigm) the British Government set up a cost-effectiveness watchdog with the interesting acronym, NICE: the National Institute for Health and Clinical Excellence. The folks at NICE are responsible for deciding which medicines are cost effective for use by the National Health Service (NHS) in Britain.

The experts at NICE decided that the high cost of these two medicines was incompatible with the best use of resources. Neither drug provides a cure for bowel cancer, but the treatments have shown in clinical trials to extend life expectancy by around four to five months in some patients! This is what I find funny in a tragic way about all this. Clinical trials have shown extended life expectancy in some patients for up to five months? But in other patients has it reduced their life expectancy?

Hilary Whittaker, chief executive of the charity Beating Bowel Cancer, condemned the NICE decision:

> "The decision by NICE not to make these drugs routinely available on the NHS to appropriate patients is a scandal and we strongly urge NICE to reconsider its decision," she said in a statement.
>
> "Why should patients in the UK be worse off than patients in the rest of Europe?"
>
> "Beating Bowel Cancer campaigns hard to ensure that patients have access to the best treatments available, regardless of their ability to pay for them, and we feel extremely disappointed that bowel cancer—the second biggest cancer killer—is not being given the attention or funding it deserves."[188]

The arguments on both sides are compelling.

The married couple, both teachers, hard-working decent citizens and in their hour of need cannot get a drug costing "only £20,000" which could give the wife possibly an extra five months of life. They have paid a lot more than £20,000 in taxes over their lives, surely they deserve it?

The other argument is the financial argument: The taxpayer will be forking out £20,000 to treat this woman for only a possible extra five months of life. Resources are limited and should not be wasted on these drugs. The financial argument concerns the broader picture. There is not an infinite amount of tax-payers money; hard choices have to be made.

The most compelling argument in favour of the Biomedical Paradigm is from the pharmaceutical companies. They are making a fortune out of these drugs. The stock market expects them to continue making steady profits from these drugs. In previous decades pharmaceutical companies traded with a significantly higher valuation than the stock market average. They are currently trading at the stock market average, meaning that the market still values them in line with all the other companies quoted on the stock market.

If the Biomedical Paradigm continues to dominate, the pharmaceutical companies can again in the future outperform the general stock market. There have been many articles written in the business section of newspapers in late 2006, early 2007 outlining this thesis. When enough of us see through the Biomedical Paradigm, pharmaceutical companies will start to under-perform the general stock market average and become eventually as financially bankrupt as they are now morally and scientifically bankrupt.

The pharmaceutical industry is in a healthy state because our governments help buy these drugs or subsidise these drugs on our behalf. Both the cost of these drugs are increasing and the numbers of drugs we are consuming are escalating to provide a positive outlook for the pharmaceutical industry,

Capping the cost of the Biomedical Paradigm[189]

As the costs of the Biomedical Paradigm continue to escalate, the government authorities in the US, Ireland, Britain and the rest of the world are doing their best to cap the escalating costs of providing health care within the confines of the Biomedical Paradigm.

The cover story article on Business Week (a US Business magazine) on May 29, 2006 was called Medical Guesswork. The sub-heading is: *From heart surgery to prostate care, the health industry knows little about which common treatments really work.*

People who work within the confines of the Biomedical Paradigm, freely admit that they do not know what they are doing. They admit that there is no scientific or evidence-based or empirical basis for most of the procedures carried out by Modern Medicine.

The person who is the focus of this article is Dr David Eddy. Dr Eddy coined the phrase "evidence-based" medicine. He believes passionately that MDs must have evidence that their proposed procedures and treatments are actually effective.

Dr Eddy was a fourth generation MD who took up heart surgery because it was at the cutting edge of medicine at the time. But he clearly had doubts about what he and the other MDs were doing. Was there evidence to support the procedures that were being carried out by the MDs? Medical decisions were being made concerning procedures which were not rational and did not suit the needs of the patient but suited the needs of the MD making this decision.

He returned to school and did a PhD thesis at Stanford. His thesis made front-page news in 1980 by overturning the medical guidelines of the time. It proved that the annual chest X-rays and yearly PAP smears for women at low risk of cervical cancer were a waste of resources, and it won the most prestigious award in the field of operations research, the Frederick W Lanchester prize. Based on his results, the American Cancer Society changed its guidelines.

Now clearly the MDs performing these annual chest X-rays and pap smears did not want to give up this lucrative source of income. But as Dr Eddy proved it was a complete waste of resources.

We know from GNM that all cancers including cervical cancer are caused by a particular type of shock. There is simply no point in screening for any kind of shock. It makes no sense.

Dr Eddy traced the common practice of preventing women from giving birth naturally if they previously had had a caesarean birth to the recommendation of one particular MD. Naturally the MDs are in favour of caesarean operations; it keeps them busy and pays well.

Dr Eddy testified for a health insurance company (Blue Cross) in high-profile court cases concerning the provision of expensive medical treatment such as bone marrow transplants for breast cancer. The women were told by their MDs that this procedure worked. They naturally wanted it. The MD performing the surgery wanted it. He was making a lot of money from it. But there was no evidence that it actually worked. The health insurance company did not want to provide the procedure because it cost them a lot of money for no proven benefit. When clinical trials concerning this procedure were finally done, they showed that the treatment, costing from $50,000 to $150,000, didn't work. It cost a huge amount of money for no proven benefit. The only people who benefited from these procedures were the MDs.

Modern Medicine recognizes this problem but cannot solve it. It cannot solve this problem because it is operating within the confines of the Biomedical Paradigm. Modern Medicine has no understanding of the origin or the mechanism of disease. When new procedures are technically possible like bone marrow transplants and they allegedly help to cure breast cancer then why not give them a go? Nothing else works!

MDs routinely test for prostate-specific antigen (PSA), which is a tumour marker for prostate cancer. Even within the Biomedical Paradigm, there is no evidence that this test improves survival. This is also true for all other prophylactic or preventative screenings carried out by Modern Medicine.

Clearly when one accepts that all cancers are caused by severe shocks or biological shocks/DHSs, the whole concept of screening will be seen to be pointless. In fact it will be seen to be positively harmful as the screening itself can cause a biological shock leading to a cancer, further proof of medically induced cancers.

People in their hour of need are desperate for anything that can help prolong life. The new treatment mentioned by the MD seems to offer great promise. The MD believes that this new treatment will work, but this is a belief as there is no evidence that it will work.

Because Modern Medicine does not understand the origin of disease; it cannot tell us why somebody got the cancer in the first place; it cannot have any definitive answers to any particular disease. The answers you get depend on the MD and his speciality. If he is a surgeon, he will recommend surgery. If he is a radiologist, he will recommend radiotherapy. The MDs will recommend what they know best, their own particular speciality. This is not only because this is their area of expertise, it is also because they have a huge financial incentive if the patient opts for their particular type of treatment.

When an MD or a hospital purchases an expensive machine, they have to pay back the cost of this new machine and thus have a huge economic incentive to refer people for this new procedure on this new machine. Instead of demand from the consumer causing supply to become available, which is the normal rule of economics, the normal laws of economics are turned on their head. The supply of these new machines and the corresponding availability of new procedures means that the supply is now available so the MDs have to stimulate demand for these new procedures.

The US spends 2.5 times more money per person than any other country in the world on health care. Are Americans 2.5 times healthier than any other country on the planet? The article quotes a study which indicates that "middle-aged Americans are in far worse health than their British counterparts, who spend less than half as much and practice less intensive medicine."

There is a tacit admission in the US health care industry that there is an enormous amount of money spent on procedures that do not help patients. There is also an understanding that these unnecessary procedures put the patient's life at much greater risk. However, the health care professionals are not willing to publicly discuss these matters.

Dr Eddy likes to cite that only about 15% of what MDs currently do is backed up by hard evidence. Presumably vaccinations and other procedures currently deemed to be effective fall into the 15% category cited by Dr Eddy?

Dr Hamer reckons that once GNM is implemented worldwide, only about 5% of what Modern Medicine currently does will be deemed to be effective.

Heart surgery[190]

The heart surgery industry is worth an estimated $100 billion dollars per annum in the US alone. The typical scenario is that the patient has trouble climbing stairs and walking any kind of distance. The MD does a scan which reveals that the arteries feeding the heart have severely narrowed. The MD refers you to another MD who does the coronary bypass surgery. You can now climb the stairs and walk again without running out of breath. Heart surgery is portrayed as another great success story of Modern Medicine. Or is it?

The two main procedures involved in heart surgery are bypass surgery and angioplasty. Bypass surgery uses blood vessels to go around or "bypass" clogged coronary/heart arteries so blood can flow through these new blood vessels to the heart. An angioplasty is when narrowed blood vessels are expanded and kept open with metal tubes called stents.

Most people would be under the impression that these kinds of procedures like widening/bypassing the arteries are the medical equivalent of the plumber inserting a new pipe to replace the blocked pipe and everything working as new again.

But it fundamentally doesn't fix the problem.

Again, the data from clinical trials (conducted under the current Biomedical Paradigm) are clear. Dr Nortin M Hadler MD, professor of medicine and author states that the results of clinical trials on bypass-surgery in the late 1970s proved that bypass operations have not been proven to prolong life or prevent future heart attacks except in a small minority of patients. There is a 1% to 2 % chance of dying during a bypass operation. There is a high risk of complications and a 40% chance of cognitive defects. The healthy, active post-bypass surgery patient is an "urban legend" or medical myth. Many of these patients never return to work or feel themselves to be healthy.

More recent trials with angioplasty show bypass surgery reduces deaths mainly in emergencies.

These clinical trials have proved that the reasons for heart attacks are not because of "bad plumbing" as they originally thought. The raison d'être of these procedures was that the slow accumulation over time of plaque inside arteries gradually narrows the vessels. This reduced blood flow causes chest pain, or angina. As the arteries narrow further, they eventually become blocked, which triggers a heart attack.

Newer evidence (within the Biomedical Paradigm), however, pins the blame not on this gradual narrowing but on unstable plaque that breaks off and causes clots. The clots are what obstruct the arteries, which is called a thrombosis by the MDs. There is no evidence that opening up these chronically narrowed arteries reduces the risk of heart attacks.

This newer evidence ties in with German New Medicine. Heart attacks are not caused by bad plumbing or chronically narrowed arteries. Heart attacks are directed from the brain. Even with "bad plumbing", one can live for a long time; one may not be able to run or walk fast, but nonetheless one can live for a long time without getting a heart attack. Narrowed arteries do not cause heart attacks.

Dr Elliott S Fisher, professor of medicine at Dartmouth Medical School, examined regional differences in health care spending in the U.S. He assumed that people in areas with lower expenditures would have worse health than people in regions where spending was between 1 1/2 to 2 times higher because they were failing to receive the required care. The opposite was true. His assumption was wrong. Patients treated in high cost intensive-care systems have a substantially increased risk of death. Additional visits by MDs in these intensive-care units often lead to unnecessary procedures and operations, all of which carry risks.

There is also evidence that the procedure itself can have a placebo effect. In June 2005 Dr Roger J Laham reported on the results of a randomized trial concerning laser surgery to improve blood flow. Patients who had the procedure reported significantly less pain and improved heart function. But patients who had a sham operation, a placebo, also reported the same results 30 months later. Dr Laham's conclusion was that the placebo effect might explain most of the benefits associated with angioplasty and bypass surgery.

Financial interest in overcoming the Biomedical Paradigm

Even MDs practicing medicine according to the Biomedical Paradigm admit that about 15% of what they currently do is evidence-based and effective. Many procedures are carried out because they are in the MD's specialist field. There is no evidence to justify most of these procedures. One thing for sure is that the cost of the Biomedical Paradigm is increasing every year with no additional benefit for the patient. In fact the reverse is the case. The MDs also have a strong financial interest in maintaining the Biomedical Paradigm.

However industry in general (apart from the pharmaceutical and biomedical companies) has a strong financial interest in significantly reducing its health care costs in order to aid its ability to survive and compete internationally. This situation is most acute in the US, which has the highest health care costs in the world. Many companies and industrial sectors in the US will not be able to compete internationally because of these unnecessary health care costs.

Governments also have an incentive to reduce health care costs but they have a much stronger incentive to support the status quo and not to question the Biomedical Paradigm.

Governments in the free world will continue to support the status quo—the Biomedical Paradigm—until they are eventually forced by public opinion to verify German New Medicine. Once GNM is verified and accepted, health care costs will decline dramatically.

CHAPTER 19

The Full Extent of the Iatrogenic Effect

Death by Modern Medicine

The Iatrogenic Effect could also be called the human cost of the Biomedical Paradigm: It describes the death and injury toll inflicted by the MDs on us, their patients. The word "iatrogenic" comes from the Greek words "iatros" for physician and "genesis" for origin. Thus "iatrogenic" means "originating by the physician". Iatrogenic diseases are induced in a patient by the activity, manner or therapy of an MD.

The Iatrogenic Effect is the number one killer of people in the First World.

"*Death by Medicine*"[191] is an illuminating study compiled by Gary Null and associates where they quantified the iatrogenic effect of the US health care system into various categories:

1. In-hospital, adverse drug reaction (ADR).
2. Medical error.
3. Unnecessary procedures.
4. Surgical error.
5. Bedsores.
6. Malnutrition.
7. Nosocomical Infection (Hospital acquired iatrogenic infection).
8. Outpatient ADR.

Their conclusion using conservative means of measuring the Iatrogenic Effect is stark: "It is evident that the American medical system is the leading cause of death and injury in the US". The second leading cause was heart disease and the third leading cause was cancer (all cancers combined).

In the US in 2001 the death rate from heart disease was 699,697. The death rate from cancer (all possible cancers) was 553,251. The death rate from the Iatrogenic Effect using the above categories was estimated to be 783,936.

They have used a conservative estimate of the Iatrogenic Effect because it is well known that it is grossly under-reported in hospitals because of peer-pressure. Don't admit a colleague made a mistake because it could be your turn some other time and you will want your colleagues' backing.

This extremely interesting study attempts to quantify the extent of the Iatrogenic Effect while operating within the confines of the Biomedical Paradigm. When we take into account the knowledge given us by Dr Hamer and Dr Lanka we will have to consider specifically the Iatrogenic Effect caused by vaccinations and the treatment of cancer. More generally, most therapies currently employed by the MDs will turn out to have been worthless and to have greatly shortened the individual patient's life-span.

Doctors' strikes

With a knowledge of GNM, one knows that Modern Medicine kills (even if inadvertently) a lot more people than the figures produced by Gary Null and associates. The proof of this statement is that there have been a number of strikes by MDs in Israel and while the strikes were ongoing the subsequent death rate had fallen.

The Israel Medical Association began strike action on the 9th of March 2000 to protest against the proposed imposition of a new four-year wage contract. The strike action kept the emergency rooms and other vital medical services working but cancelled or postponed tens of thousands of elective procedures. Meir Adler, manager of the Shamgar Funeral Parlour in Jerusalem, when questioned about the death rate falling because of this strike by MDs, emphatically stated:

> *"There definitely is a connection between the doctors' sanctions and fewer deaths. We saw the same thing in 1983."*

In 1983, the Israel Medical Association also had a strike or sanction lasting for four and a half months.[192]

Whenever MDs strike, death rates go down! In 1976 in Bogota, Columbia, MDs went on strike for 52 days, with only emergency care available. The death rate dropped by 35%. In 1976 in Los Angeles County, a similar strike by MDs resulted in an 18% drop in the death rate. In another strike by MDs in Israel, a 50% decrease in mortality occurred in 1973 during a one month stoppage.[193]

The examples from Israel are positive proof of the Iatrogenic Effect. However, Modern Medicine can explain it all away. Avi Yisraeli, director general of the Hadassah Medical Organization explains this real reduction in the death rate: “Mortality is not the only measure of harm to health. Lack of medical intervention can lead to disability, pain, and reduced functioning. Elective surgery can bring about a great improvement in a patient’s condition, but it can also mean disability and death in the weakest patients. And patients who do not undergo diagnosis or surgery now could decline or die in a few months due to the postponement.”[194]

This is simply further convoluted reasoning to explain the unexplainable within the straitjacket of thinking known as the Biomedical Paradigm.

Official recognition of the Iatrogenic Effect

Clinical misjudgments or mistakes mean that the odds of dying as a result of being treated in hospital are 33,000 times higher than those of dying in an air crash, according to the British Chief Medical Officer, Sir Liam Donaldson. “In an airline industry, the evidence from scheduled airlines is the risk of death is one in 10 million. If you go into a hospital in the First World, the risk of death from a medical error is one in 300.”[195]

This quote from Sir Liam Donaldson did not cause any controversy. It is clearly generally accepted that even within the confines of the Biomedical Paradigm, there is an extremely deadly Iatrogenic Effect. It clearly is not unacceptable to the medical profession and, more importantly, the general public.

Why is flying an aeroplane 33,000 times safer than going into hospital? Would you fly an aeroplane if there was a 1 in 300 chance of dying? Most people wouldn’t fly in similar circumstance but yet most of us continue on with the Biomedical Paradigm despite the awful iatrogenic death rate.

The good done by Modern Medicine in areas such as plastic surgery and emergency medicine is more than outweighed by the harm done by Modern Medicine. The MDs have become the greatest threat to our collective health and well-being.

CHAPTER 20

Vaccinations

Vaccinations are how we are initiated into the Biomedical Paradigm. Vaccinations are the equivalent of the sacrament of baptism in Christianity. Once a child is vaccinated, it has a possibility of getting diseases such as autism, encephalitis, SIDS and SBS. Some of these diseases require consequental, regular visits to the MDs, creating an iatrogenic condition known as Patients For Life Syndrome (PFLS).[196]

Vaccination schedule in Ireland

I thought the best way to examine the current Iatrogenic Effect of vaccinations would be by considering the various vaccinations that we willingly allow to be given to our children. The Health Protection Surveillance Centre (HPSC) have approved the following vaccination schedule for the Republic of Ireland. I am sure that, with the exception of the BCG vaccine, it is similar to that of most countries in the free world.

Vaccination Timetable for the Republic of Ireland[197]

Age	Vaccine
Birth to 1 month	BCG
2 months	DTaP/IPV/Hib ("5 in 1") and Meningitis C
4 months	DTaP/IPV/Hib ("5 in 1") and Meningitis C
6 months	DTaP/IPV/Hib ("5 in 1") and Meningitis C
12 to 15 months	MMR, Hib[1]
4 to 5 years	DTaP/IPV ("4 in 1") and MMR
11 to 12 years	MMR (in cases where 2 previous doses have not been given)
10 to 14 years	BCG[2]
11 to 14 years	Td (Tetanus and low dose diphtheria)

[1]A single dose of Hib vaccine is also recommended if the child presents after age 13 months and has had no previous Hib vaccine.

[2]Only for those who are known to be tuberculin negative and have had no previous BCG.

The BCG vaccine is given between birth and one month in Ireland. The BCG vaccine is against tuberculosis. Its efficacy is disputed even within the limited thinking of the Biomedical Paradigm with the US and Holland never having used the BCG vaccine.

At the ages of 2-months, 4-months and 6-months of age, babies in Ireland are given two separate shots, the 5-in-1 vaccine and the Meningitis C vaccine. The 5-in-1 vaccine is also called the DTP/IPV/Hib vaccine. It vaccinates against diphtheria, tetanus and pertussis (DTP) and polio (IPV) and haemophilus influenza B (Hib).

The 'DTP' grouping in the vaccine name is because these three separate diseases used to be vaccinated together in a 3-in-1 shot called the DTP vaccine.

The 'IPV' abbreviation in the 5-in-1 vaccine stands for Inactivated Polio Vaccine. This vaccine replaced the oral polio vaccine which is now admitted to cause paralytic polio in a few cases.[198] Another advantage of the IPV vaccine is that it does not contain thimerosal (a mercury-based toxin). They did not admit these problems at the time, did they?

The 'Hib' abbreviation in the 5-in-1 vaccine stands for haemophiluhs influenza B.

At 12–15 months, children are recommended to get the MMR vaccine and a booster Hib vaccine. Prior to 2006, a single dose of Hib vaccine was also recommended if the child did not previously get the Hib vaccine (which is currently included in the 5-in-1 vaccine). In 2004, a small number of cases of Hib disease occurred in children in Ireland who were fully vaccinated. The HPSC in 2006 now recommend that all children reaching 12 months of age are offered the Hib booster vaccine.

It is interesting to note that 3 doses of the Hib vaccine at the ages of 2-months, 4-months and 6-months does not provide immunity against this disease but now another vaccine, a fourth dose of the same vaccine, is required at the age of 12–15 months. When will they realize that vaccines are ineffective, always have been and always will be and do not provide any kind of immunity?

At 4–5 years old, the children receive 2 booster vaccines, the MMR again and a 4-in-1 booster which covers the same diseases of the 5-in-1 vaccine with the exception of Hib.

At 11–12 years of age, the MMR vaccine is recommended if the child has not received two previous doses of this vaccine. At 10–14 years of age the BCG vaccine is recommended if the child had never had this vaccine or if the child has no proven "antibodies" to tuberculosis. At 11–14 years of age the Td vaccine is recommended; a combination of tetanus and diphtheria vaccines.

The Iatrogenic Effect of vaccinations

If you examine the anti-vaccine web-sites, they nearly all focus in on the dangers of vaccinations and in particular, the "combo-vaccines" (the 5-in-1 and 3-in-1 vaccines). They also focus on the toxic content of the vaccines and the ensuing toxic overload because of the quantity of shots given. They rarely question the need for vaccines. This point must be repeatedly made; vaccines are unnecessary. Vaccines are particularly unnecessary against viral diseases because viruses do not exist in humans, animals or plants.

Vaccines are only necessary if you want to poison children, permanently damage them, or even kill them: They are only necessary because of their proven Iatrogenic Effect.

In most countries these vaccines are provided free of charge by the government. We are being poisoned by our governments who are supporting the lifestyle of the MDs and guaranteeing a captive lucrative market for the pharmaceutical industry.

Thimerosal – Vaccine preservative[199]

One particular component of vaccines that has received a lot of attention in the US is thimerosal. Thimerosal is a mercury-based preservative developed by Eli Lilly back in the 1930s and has been used in as many as fifty different vaccines. From the very beginning, the scientific case against the mercury additive has been overwhelming. The preservative, which is used to stem fungi and bacterial growth in vaccines, contains ethyl-mercury, a potent neurotoxin.

Thimerosal enables the pharmaceutical industry to package vaccines in vials that contain multiple doses, which require additional protection because they are more easily contaminated by multiple needle entries. The larger vials cost half as much to produce as smaller, single-dose vials.

In 1982, an expert panel at FDA reviewed thimerosal and found it toxic, caused cell death, and called for its removal in over-the-counter products. In 1991, the FDA considered banning it from animal vaccines. But tragically, also in 1991, the CDC recommended that infants be injected with a series of vaccines containing thimerosal.

By the late 1990s in the US, children received a total of 22 separate immunizations.

Despite the known toxicity of thimerosal, nobody worked out the cumulative effect of thimerosol in all the vaccines that these children had received.

Dr Boyd Haley heads the chemistry department at the University of Kentucky. He states that: "You couldn't even construct a study that shows thimerosal is safe. It's just too darn toxic. If you inject thimerosal into an animal, its brain will sicken. If you apply it to living tissue, the cells die. If you put it in a petri-dish, the culture dies. Knowing these things, it would be shocking if one could inject it into an infant without causing damage."

One of the CDC scientists claimed that *"science is best left to the scientists"*. Georges Clemenceau, a former French Prime Minister, is quoted as saying that "War is too important to be left to the generals." Our health is much too important to be delegated to the scientists and the MDs.

The estimated number of cases of autism had increased fifteen-fold in the US, from one in every 2,500 children in 1991 to one in 166 children in 2005. The suspicion for this increase is down to the increasing number of vaccines given since 1991 that contained thimerosal.[200]

The vaccine manufacturers had obviously realised there was a particular problem with thimerosal and began to phase it out of vaccines. However they continued to sell off old thimerosal vaccines as late as 2004 in the US. These tainted vaccines not suitable for US babies were now being exported to the third world.

However bad the effect of these vaccines are on well nourished children in the US, the effects are more devastating in the third world.

Congressman Dan Burton from Indiana oversaw a three-year investigation of thimerosal after his grandson was diagnosed with autism. His committee concluded that "thimerosal used as a preservative in vaccines is directly related to the autism epidemic and that "This epidemic in all probability may have been prevented or curtailed had the FDA not been asleep at the switch regarding a lack of safety data regarding injected thimerosal, a known neurotoxin."

The committee added that the FDA and other public-health agencies failed to act, the committee added, out of "institutional malfeasance for self protection" and "misplaced protectionism of the pharmaceutical industry."

The problem with the argument concerning the thimerosal preservative/neurotoxin contained in vaccines is that the pharmaceutical companies can wriggle out by stating they no longer use this deadly toxin; shell out a few dollars to the thousands of permanently damaged victims; say sorry, and continue on poisoning people with other toxins, perhaps less toxic than thimerosal but nonetheless toxic. The problem with vaccines is not just with one mercury-based component, thimerosal. The problem is with all the components of vaccines.

Vaccine components

Vaccines contain a number of substances which can be divided into the following three groups:[201]

1. Antigens.
2. Adjuvants.
3. Preservatives.

Antigens are whole-cell proteins or just the broken-cell protein envelopes of the micro-organisms, either bacteria or what they consider to be viruses, that are believed to cause specific infectious diseases and which the vaccine is supposed to prevent.

Adjuvants are chemical substances which are supposed to enhance the so-called "immune response" to the vaccine.

Preservatives and tissue fixatives are chemical substances that are supposed to halt any further chemical reactions and putrefaction of the live or attenuated or killed biological constituents of the vaccine.

Thimerosal is a particularly toxic preservative, but all the constituents of vaccines (antigens, adjuvants and preservatives) are toxic. Replacing thimerosal with a less toxic preservative does not solve the problem.

Injecting foreign matter into the blood stream results in a wide range of diseases creating more work for the MDs – the aptly named Patients For Life Syndrome (PFLS).

Iatrogenic Effect of the combination 5-in-1 vaccine DTP/IPV/Hib vaccine[202]

Pediacel is the name of the 5-in-1 vaccine licensed in Ireland and the UK. It is called Pentacel in the US.

Results of medical trials by the manufacturer of the 5-in-1 vaccine Sanofi-Pasteur have revealed that this "super-dose" vaccination can have serious side-effects. The manufacturer prepared a report on this vaccine for the regulatory authority in the UK for vaccines, the Medicines Healthcare Regulatory Authority (MHRA).[203]

Evidence from the vaccine's manufacturers shows that, in clinical trials, 64 per cent of 451, (almost 2 out of every 3 babies) given the Pediacel vaccine experienced what the manufacturer terms "bad reactions". Ten per cent of these reactions were "moderate to severe". The reactions included convulsions, loss of consciousness and high-pitched, persistent and inconsolable screaming.

Other studies showed that components of the vaccine can cause breathing difficulties, blue discolouration of the skin due to lack of oxygen, swelling of the brain, low blood pressure and extreme allergic shock.

Nicholas Kitchin, medical director of Sanofi Pasteur, tellingly stated that "there are fewer side-effects with the five-in-one than were reported with the older four-in-one vaccine". This means that there were possibly unacceptable side-effects with the previous vaccine? But my strong hunch is that these side-effects of the previous vaccine combination were fobbed off in the same way as the side-effects of the new vaccine. The trick here is that it is ok to issue official concerns about a vaccine once it is no longer used; but it is not ok to issue official concerns about vaccines in use. It has always been so.[204]

Nicholas further added that all vaccines have side-effects of which parents should be made aware. Naturally, the manufacturers have covered themselves by stating these side-effects on the information leaflet included with every vaccine. He stated that "severe reactions are rare and the benefits of vaccination far outweigh the risks."

Parents are never made aware of the information leaflets. I certainly wasn't and I'm sure the vast majority of parents are not told about the possible side-effects of vaccines. I'm certain the reason why the MDs/nurses do not show the information leaflets to the parents is because they do not want to scare them.

Iatrogenic Effect of the 3-in-1 MMR vaccine

In 1998 the gastroenterologist, Dr Andrew Wakefield, was the lead author of a report stating that there was a causal link between the MMR vaccine and autism and painful gut disorders suffered by twelve autistic children.[205] Irish Professor John O'Leary confirmed this in 2002. American researchers have revealed that 85 per cent of samples taken from autistic children with bowel disorders contain a "virus" similar to the one used in the measles, mumps and rubella 3-in-1 vaccine.

The American parents say their children were developing normally until they had the MMR vaccine at the age of 12 months to 18 months old. The children now suffer from regressive autism. More than two thousand British families believe their children suffered damage as a result of the MMR vaccine. Who knows a child best, the MD or the mother and father? If the parents noticed the child was damaged in some way after a vaccination I would be strongly inclined to believe them.

MMR and me

The MMR booster vaccine is recommended in Ireland for 4–5 year olds as is a 4-in-1 booster vaccine for diptheria, tetanus, pertusis and polio (but not Hib).

In Autumn 2005 (just after he started primary school), my then 4-year old son was due to be given these booster vaccines in Northern Ireland. At that time I only knew about the dangers of these vaccines and nothing much else. A little bit of research confirmed what I had been told about vaccine safety concerns. I declined permission for my son to be vaccinated/poisoned. I informed the nurse/health visitor of my decision by telephone. She never asked me why. Even now when I think about it, I cannot believe that I had previously allowed my children to be vaccinated because I trusted the medical profession and the relevant government agencies. I had believed them. Surely they knew what they were doing?

Dr Gerhard Buchwald MD and the Iatrogenic Effect of all vaccines

Dr Gerhard Buchwald used to be a regular MD who believed in the efficacy of vaccines. Until he was nearly 40-years-old he believed the medical myths he had been indoctrinated into at medical school concerning vaccinations. He believed these medical myths until his eldest son, born in 1957, received a smallpox vaccination at the age of 18 months. Until then, his son had developed normally. Eight days after the small-pox vaccination his son could no longer stand up in his cot.[206] His son had post-vaccination encephalitis and Dr Buchwald has since then had a "completely destroyed human being at home."[207]

Dr Buchwald has spent over 40 years researching the iatrogenic effect of all vaccines. He has documented these in his book: *Vaccination a Business based on Fear*. As an example, in relation to the BCG vaccine: Possible complications from the BCG vaccine include abscesses at the injection site which appear about 6-weeks after vaccination. Lymph nodes can swell and form abscesses. This occurs 1–3 months after vaccination. Inflammation of the bones (osteitis) and bone marrow (ostemyelitis) can occur from 6 months to 4 years, and in most cases after 12 months following the vaccination.[208]

Dr Buchwald has examined all the other vaccines in detail. They all damage, some more so than others. The combination-vaccines are certainly more dangerous than the single-dose vaccines, but they are all dangerous.

The damage caused by vaccinations is either hidden from the public or is denied. The Iatrogenic Effect of vaccinations (vaccine damage and death) are written off as being coincidental, something that would have happened anyway even without vaccinations. The possibility of vaccine damage is trivialised by stating that vaccine damage occurs extremely rarely or naming the ensuing vaccine damage as a new obscure disease or syndrome. For these reasons the vaccines damage claims that are officially registered are the tip of the iceberg. The numbers of vaccine damaged children are much higher.[209]

Dr Buchwald concludes his book *Vaccination: A Business based on Fear* with:

> Vaccinations do not protect!
> Vaccinations are of no benefit!
> Vaccinations are harmful![210]

Children who are not vaccinated

All vaccines contain toxins and are therefore dangerous. There is no safe vaccine. The only safe vaccine is one that is never used. Autism does not only occur because of one vaccine only such as the MMR vaccine but can occur from any vaccine or the cumulative effect of all vaccines taken. The way to prove the truth of this statement is to examine communities where the children are not vaccinated and observe the rate of autism.

One control group (the majority of the US population) fully vaccinate their children. Two different control groups, the Amish and the patients of a Chicago medical practice do not vaccinate their children. The difference in autism rates between the vaccinated and the unvaccinated are staggering.

Journalist Dan Olmstead of UPI (United Press International) examined the autism rate of the Amish in Lancaster County Pennsylvania in April 2005. Given the US national rate of autism Dan Olmstead would have estimated about 130 Amish to have autism. He found only four cases of autism. One child had been exposed to high levels of mercury from a power plant. The other three—including one child adopted from outside the Amish community—had received their vaccines. Olmsted found a family MD in Lancaster County, Pennsylvania, who indicated that he had never seen an Amish person with autism.[211]

Dan Olmstead visited other Amish communities in the US. The Amish community around Middlefield, Ohio have an autism rate of one in 15,000, according to the medical director at a clinic for special needs children there. In contrast, the US national autism rate is estimated at one in 166.

Homefirst Health Services in Chicago have two things in common with Amish children, they have never been vaccinated and they don't have autism. The Homefirst medical practice has six MDs in Chicago

"We have about 30,000 or 35,000 children that we've taken care of over the years, and I don't think we have a single case of autism in children delivered by us who never received vaccines," said Dr Mayer Eisenstein, Homefirst's medical director who founded the practice in 1973.[212]

This is truly astonishing and is difficult for MDs to explain away. There is not a single case of autism in children who had never been vaccinated.

Let's extend this further: Are there any cases of Sudden Infant Death Syndrome (SIDS), Shaken Baby Syndrome (SBS), attention deficit disorders, dyslexia in the unvaccinated groups? I am certain that the results would mirror that for autism.

Vaccination: a business based on fear

Vaccinations are how we baptise our children into the Biomedical Paradigm. Vaccinations are big business: a business based on fear. Once we understand that there is no reason for this fear, that it is stoked up by the mass media with no attempt at any in-depth investigation; that the only reason we vaccinate our children is because of fear of these allegedly deadly diseases and phantom viruses; that ultimately there is nothing to be afraid of; that health and disease comes from within; only then will we realize that not only are vaccinations un-necessary, they are positively harmful. They need to be banned. The only people who will complain will be the MDs and other white-coats. After a few years of a complete ban and no epidemics and deaths, the MDs will be seen for what they really are: modern day witch-doctors, scaremongers and charlatans.

CHAPTER 21

Cancer Treatment

Cancer treatment is how many of us are terminated by the Biomedical Paradigm. Cancer treatment is the equivalent to the sacrament of the last rites in Christianity.

Once you receive cancer treatment you have been given notice that you have a 5% survival chance after 5 years and a 2% survival chance after 7 years. Modern Medicine has just given you notice of your impending death by its last rites.[213]

Modern Medicine relies on three main methods for cancer treatment: chemotherapy, surgery and radiation, otherwise known as poison, slash and burn.[214]

Chemotherapy – Poison

The first patient to undergo chemotherapy was treated with mustard gas in 1942. The advanced stage tumour did indeed shrink miraculously but the patient died three months later. And so began the age of chemotherapy.[215]

A true measure of a treatment's success is survival probability after a five year period, as well as quality of life. What is the point of allegedly extending a person's life by a few months if those few months are spent in terrible suffering from the side-effects?

The statistician, Ulrich Abel, after spending a year reviewing thousands of publications on chemotherapy, concluded that "for most organ cancers there exists no evidence that chemotherapeutic treatment—in particular the increasingly popular high-dose therapy—would prolong or improve the quality of a patient's life."[216]

Ulrich Abel studied the most common forms of adenocarcinoma: lung, breast, prostate and colon. The adenocarcinomas are all endodermal in origin with a tumour growing in the conflict-active phase and with it being destroyed in the reparation phase by the relevant microbes. At this stage, Ulrich Abel had spent ten years as a statistician in clinical oncology and was increasingly uneasy.[217]

"A sober and unprejudiced analysis of the literature has rarely revealed any therapeutic success by the regimens in question in treating advanced epithelial cancer." While chemotherapy is being used more and more extensively, more than a million people die worldwide of these cancers annually and a majority have received some form of chemotherapy before dying. Abel further concluded, after polling hundreds of cancer doctors, "The personal view of many oncologists seems to be in striking contrast to communications intended for the public." Abel cited studies that have shown "that many oncologists would not take chemotherapy themselves if they had cancer." "Even though toxic drugs often do effect a response, a partial or complete shrinkage of the tumour, this reduction does not prolong expected survival."[218]

What is interesting is the personal view of the oncologists. Many feel obliged to recommend and perform cancer treatments according to the dogmas of Modern Medicine but would not have chemotherapy themselves or for their family members. This is similar to the views of those MDs who vaccinate other peoples' children but would not vaccinate their own children. Surely if you would not have these treatments given to your own family, you could not, in good conscience, perform these same treatments on your patients who expect you to be responsible for their health?

Ulrich Abel further states that "Many oncologists take it for granted that response to therapy prolongs survival, an opinion which is based on a fallacy and which is not supported by clinical studies." A "response" to therapy is what the oncologists mean when they get a temporary shrinking of the tumour because of their chemotherapy. Taking comfort in a shrinking tumour at the cost of serious and often fatal destruction to the body is insanity. If treatments do not increase long-term survival, then why undertake them, especially as they have such awful side-effects?[219]

Epidemiologist Dieter Holzel also analysed survival rates from patients suffering the top four most frequently occurring cancers (breast, prostate, lung and colo-rectal) and found that despite alleged positive outcomes, patients do not live any longer. He admitted that no real progress had been made in the last 25 years. In fact he could potentially conceive of an Iatrogenic Effect, that the treatment itself is causing more cancer. In his words: "I am afraid that the systematic treatment with chemotherapy, particularly in patients suffering from breast cancer, might be responsible for decreased survival rates". He further complains that: “The big drawback with cancer medicine is the complete lack of any systematic documentation.”[220]

If this systematic documentation was completed on the real, horrifying results obtained from cancer treatment, even within the confines of the Biomedical Paradigm, these cancer treatments would be immediately terminated. This is not going to happen because of the enormous amounts of money to be made by the pharmaceutical industry and the MDs/oncologists providing these treatments.

Surgery – Slash

Radical surgery is used to cut away the tumour. If the tumour on a woman’s breast is deemed to be too big, the entire breast is surgically removed to prevent cancer spreading or metastasis. Radical surgery such as this can understandably cause further biological shocks and therefore further cancers - further proof of metastasis for the MDs but in reality proof of their Iatrogenic Effect.

When GNM is universally applied, the real need for such cancerous surgery will be drastically reduced. Surgery would only be needed, for example, if a tumour in the colon or large intestine became so big that the intestine was in danger of being blocked. This clearly would be a life-threatening situation. In this case the tumour would be cut back to allow nature further time to allow the necessary microbes do their work and decompose the tumour after the conflict has been definitively solved.

Radiation – Burn

The aim of radiation therapy is to burn away the tumour or the ulcer. Radiation damages human cells and radiation therapy harnesses this power to treat cancers. The principal use of radiotherapy is to tackle solid tumours found in just one location, for example skin, brain, breast or uterine cancers.

Once GNM is universally applied, radiation therapy will only be used for cosmetic reasons for those tumours that were not fully removed naturally at the end of the cancer or for impossible surgery at difficult areas close to a critical blood vessel in the body.[221]

Pain and morphine

In Modern Medicine all patients who have a cancer and have severe pain are given morphine or a morphine-derivative. One injection of morphine when the patient is already in the middle of the reparation phase, in deepest vagatonia, can be deadly. Morphine changes the brain waves and destroys the patient's morale. The stomach is paralysed and can no longer digest food. Although the patient is already in the middle of the reparation phase and suffering intense pain, he would be better again in few weeks time if nature was allowed to run its course.[222]

The MDs know rightly that once the patient takes morphine, their pain threshold is lowered or their feeling of pain is multiplied and higher doses of morphine are required to ease this pain. Their stomach doesn't function any more and they eventually die from hunger or thirst.[223]

The MDs, because of their absolute belief in the Biomedical Paradigm, believe that the onset of pain is the beginning of the end. Patients will willingly endure the intense pain that can occur in the reparation phase because it lasts for only a few weeks and does not continue indefinitely. Unfortunately the MDs do not know this.[224]

Morphine is used for "pain relief". It relives pain temporarily but quickly kills the patient. Morphine is probably the leading cause of iatrogenic death among cancer patients.

Cancerous treatment

The reality is that cancer survival rates have not improved since President Nixon launched the war on cancer in the 1970s. Cancer treatment by the MDs should be more accurately called cancerous treatment because their therapies cause further biological shocks and therefore secondary and tertiary cancers, which are further evidence of the Iatrogenic Effect.

We have continued with this cancerous treatment because the MD/oncologist is happy to offer the patient something and be handsomely paid for it; the patients are desperate to try anything and the pharmaceutical industry is very happy to supply these toxic agents for a hefty fee.

When we are told that we have cancer, most of us go into a blind panic and follow the treatments offered by the MDs like lambs to the slaughter, and will consider alternatives only as a last resort, but by then it is usually too late. The MDs will fill you with fear about the dire and deadly consequences if nothing is done immediately about your cancer. They will poison, slash or burn, but all with no proven benefit.

The only solution to prevent this awful cancerous treatment by the MDs is to learn about the German New Medicine while you are still healthy. If you get a cancer you will not be in a blind panic, you will have the German New Medicine to help you. Cancer is not a death sentence. There is hope. Krebs ist heilbar.[225] Cancer is curable.

CHAPTER 22

The Horror

If we do not understand the lessons of the past, we are condemned to continuously repeat the same mistakes. The practice of bloodletting, the salutary tale of Semmelweis, the Spanish flu pandemic of 1918 and the swine flu farce of 1976 were all medical horror stories inflicted upon mankind by orthodox medicine.[226] They serve to illustrate the continuing horror of Modern Medicine.

Bloodletting[227]

Bloodletting was one of the oldest medical practices, practiced by diverse ancient peoples, including the Mesopotamians, the Egyptians, the Greeks, the Mayans and the Aztecs. Bloodletting involved the withdrawal of often considerable quantities of blood from a patient in the hopeful belief that this would cure or prevent a great many illnesses and diseases. True stupidity is repeating the same thing over and over again in the hope of a different outcome. This is what happened with the practice of bloodletting for at least 3,000 years.

The popularity of bloodletting in Europe was reinforced by the ideas of a Greek physician, Galen (129–200 AD). There were two key concepts in his system of bloodletting. The first was that blood was created and then used up, it did not circulate and so it could 'stagnate' in the extremities. The second was that the humoral balance was the basis of illness or health, the four humours being blood, phlegm, black and yellow bile, which relate to the four Greek classical elements of air, water, earth and fire. Galen believed that blood was the dominant humour and the one in most need of control. In order to balance the humours, a physician would either remove 'excess' blood from the patient or give them an emetic to induce vomiting or a diuretic to induce urination.

Galen created a complex system of how much blood should be removed based on the patient's age, constitution, the season, the weather and the location. Symptoms of plethora or too much blood in the body were believed to include fever, apoplexy and headache. The blood to be let was of a specific nature determined by the disease: either arterial or venous, and distant or close to the area of the body affected. He linked different blood vessels with different organs, according to their supposed drainage. For example, the vein in the right hand would be let for liver problems and the vein in the left hand for problems with the spleen. The more severe the disease, the more blood would be let. Fevers required a lot of bloodletting.

This barbaric practice of bloodletting was even codified by the major religions. The Talmud (Jewish holy book) recommended a specific day of the week and days of the month for bloodletting. Christian writings advise which saints' days were favorable for bloodletting. The Hindus in India also had bloodletting as an integral part of Ayurvedic medicine, the ancient Hindu science of medicine.

Even after the medical dogma of the four humours fell into disuse, the practice was continued. Though the bloodletting was often recommended by physicians, it was carried out by barbers. This division of labour led to the distinction between physicians and surgeons. The barbershop's red-and-white-striped pole, still in use today, derives from this practice: the red represents the blood being drawn, the white represents the tourniquet used, and the pole itself represents the stick squeezed in the patient's hand to dilate the veins.

The practice continued throughout the Middle Ages but began to be questioned in the 16th century, particularly in northern Europe. In France, the Court and university physicians advocated frequent blood letting. In England, bloodletting declined throughout the 18th century, and briefly revived for treating tropical fevers in the 19th century.

Bloodletting was especially popular in the young United States of America. George Washington (1st US President) had about 1.7 litres of blood withdrawn by bloodletting, following a horseback riding accident which contributed to his premature death in 1799 by the Iatrogenic Effect.

So although bloodletting was initially carried out because of a medical dogma about plethora or too much blood in the body; it still continued long after this medical dogma had been discarded. Why?

One reason is that the key to curing disease remained elusive and the underlying belief was that it was better to give any treatment than nothing at all. It's better to "treat" or do something rather than do nothing at all.

Another reason, I'm certain, is that bloodletting was demanded by patients who had heard old-wives tales about various relatives and friends being cured from all sorts of ailments by bloodletting. The patients willingly allowed themselves to be treated in this barbaric manner.

So the MDs practiced bloodletting because they believed it was better to do something than do nothing at all, and most importantly because they were well paid for it. The patients demanded it, because by doing something the disease might go away, and they believed that other people had been cured using this vile practice.

Nothing has changed. The same mindset applies. The MDs believe it is better to do something than nothing at all, and get paid handsomely for it. We the patients want to be "treated", we demand outside intervention. We have learned nothing and have kept repeating the same mistakes as with bloodletting, hence our continued use of cancer treatment and vaccinations.

In the not too distant future, the current practices of cancer treatment and of vaccinations by Modern Medicine will be seen with the same horror as we currently regard the barbaric practice of bloodletting.

The salutary tale of Semmelweis[228]

Ignaz Semmelweis (1818–1865) was an obstetrician/gynaecologist. He worked in a maternity hospital in Vienna. There were two obstetrical clinics located there that used the same procedures for delivering babies. The second obstetrical clinic was staffed by midwives and was used for training them. The first obstetrical clinic was staffed by MDs and used for training them. The death rate of women giving birth from childbed fever or puerperal fever was about 2% in the clinic manned by the midwives. However in the ward managed by the MDs, the death rate was about 13%. The general public were aware of these death rates and some women preferred to give birth in the street rather than risk a visit to the Vienna maternity hospital.

In 1847, Dr Semmelweis's friend and colleague died from an infection contracted after his finger was accidentally punctured with a knife while performing an autopsy. The infection had all the symptoms of childbed fever. However, the victim was a male physician. Semmelweis guessed that there was something in the cadaver or dead body that had caused his friend's death. Semmelweis then deducted the reason for the disparity in death rates between the two wards. He proposed a connection between contamination from the dead bodies and childbed fever and made a detailed study of the mortality statistics of both obstetrical clinics. He concluded that he and the student doctors carried the infecting particles on their hands from the autopsy room to the patients they examined in the First Obstetrical Clinic, the clinic manned by the MDs.

Semmelweis instigated a policy of washing hands in a solution of chlorinated lime between autopsy work and the examination of patients. The mortality rate in the first clinic managed by MDs dropped to 2%, comparable with the clinic managed by the midwives.

Semmelweis observed the disparity between the death rates of both maternity clinics and came up with a hypothesis—pathogens on the dead bodies—and tested this hypothesis. It clearly worked as demonstrated by the reduction in the mortality rate of the first clinic manned by the MDs.

Was Semmelweis lauded by the medical profession for his discovery? No! Of course not! Firstly, if Semmelweis was correct, this would mean that the MDs had killed thousands of women giving birth in Vienna alone. Secondly, it was argued that an MD having to wash his hands before treating a pregnant woman involved too much work and wasn't practicable. Thirdly, Semmelweis's observations were believed by the MDs to give special significance to dead bodies, which was deemed to be religious or superstitious by the allegedly enlightened and of course scientific MDs. Fourthly, and most importantly, Semmelweis did not have a theory as to why the dead body was contaminated.

The theory of the time as to what caused disease, was a variation of the "four humours", simply some form of "bad blood", hence the general belief of the MDs was that there was nothing that the MDs could do about disease. Semmelweis had no theory as to what caused the dead body to harbour pathogenic organisms, but he knew by observation that they did. This lack of a scientific reason led to his observations being summarily rejected. Despite his empirical observations; despite the fact that his washing-protocols worked; he had no theory as to why they worked; all he had was his observation, his reasoning and the fact that his ideas worked in practice.

It has been scientifically proven for over a hundred years that bacteria work in dead bodies or cadavers in order to break down or decompose the dead body and produce toxins as a side-effect of this useful work. It is only under conditions of oxygen deprivation that bacteria produce toxins or dangerous poisons. It was these toxins that caused childbed fever and not the bacteria themselves, which produce these toxins as a side-effect of decomposing the cadaver.[229]

This point must be emphasised; bacteria do not cause disease. Bacteria working on a cadaver, under obvious conditions of oxygen deprivation, to decompose the body, to return it to dust, produce toxins as a side-effect of decomposing the body. The Germ Theory of Disease medical dogma still blames bacteria for causing childbed fever even though it is the toxins produced by the bacteria as a side-effect of decomposing a dead body that caused the childbed fever.

Semmelweis continued on with his work. During 1848, he had all the instruments coming in contact with the patients washed in a similar manner and virtually eliminated childbed fever. Despite this tremendous success, his work was not accepted in medical circles in Vienna. He left Vienna and returned to Budapest, where he was in charge of the maternity ward of St Rochus Hospital from 1851 to 1857. His washing protocols reduced the mortality rate to less than 1%.

Finally in 1861, with lots of fantastic statistics, thousands of mothers still alive who would have otherwise died, Semmelweis felt confident enough to publish his discoveries. He had unfavourable reviews and most MDs rejected his ideas.[230]

This rejection by the medical establishment caused his premature death. He deteriorated mentally over a number of years and was eventually committed to an asylum in 1865 and died there shortly after from injuries received in a fight with asylum personnel.

The Semmelweis Reflex

What happened to Semmelweis proves a common medical syndrome known to have affected orthodox medicine since the time of Hippocrates. It is called the Semmelweis Reflex. It is the automatic summary dismissal or rejection out of hand of any new information without thought, inspection or experiment by the medical profession even though it will save many lives.[231]

Dr Hamer and Dr Lanka are two victims of the Semmelweis Reflex. Dr Hamer has empirically proven by observation in thousands of cases the link between a biological shock, the effect on the psyche, the brain relay controlling the afflicted organ and the effect on the organ itself. It is an over-determined system. If you know what is happening on one level of the human trinity, you can predict what is happening on the other two levels. The theory is simple. A shock that has caught the patient unawares causes a particular disease, for example a biological shock concerning the loss of a loved one results in testicular/ovarian cancer. The affected brain relay can be observed on a CT scan. The MDs reject Hamer's German New Medicine out of hand—the Semmelweis Reflex—without bothering to test his five Biological Laws of Nature. There is, unfortunately, nothing new in this treatment of Dr Hamer.

Dr Lanka discovered a real virus in sea algae in 1988. The AIDS hysteria had started a few years earlier. He checked the literature and discovered that the virus that is supposed to cause AIDS, namely HIV, does not actually exist. He further discovered that no pathogenic or disease-inducing virus exists in any human, animal or plant. He told everybody. The white-coats would not listen because they were all devoted followers of the Biomedical Paradigm and scientists in name only.

The most infamous example of the Semmelweis Reflex is the verification by the University of Trnva of the five Biological Laws of Nature. Although three professors from the University of Trnva confirmed that the five Biological Laws of Nature applied in each and every case, the university refused to implement the German New Medicine because world medicine would be forced to admit the true nature of the horror that is Modern Medicine.

Spanish flu of 1918[232]

In relation to the current bird flu pandemic scare, all the experts refer to the Spanish flu of 1918. Apparently it is only a matter of time before we get a similar pandemic to the Spanish flu that killed, depending on the sources you read, from 20 million to 50 million people worldwide.

The Spanish flu was not caused by H5N1 (the bird flu virus), nor by any other flu virus, nor indeed by any virus at all, because viruses do not exist. The horrible truth is that the Spanish flu of 1918 was man-made: It was caused primarily by vaccines. The Spanish flu was the greatest iatrogenic epidemic ever in human history.

It is undoubtedly true that young soldiers, probably away from home for their first time, and living in terrible conditions, would have also had biological shocks of separation, Fear of Death, etc and that these biological shocks alone without any vaccinations would have caused many deaths. However the vast majority of deaths from the Spanish flu would have been caused by vaccines.[233]

Spain did not participate in WW1 (1914–1918) and therefore had no need for propaganda to its own people and the Spanish press openly reported the terrible flu that was afflicting Spain and Europe. Because of this open reporting, the flu was called the Spanish flu by the British and American allies, implying by its name that it originated in Spain. Interestingly, the Spanish press called it the "French flu".

The Spanish flu was unusual in that it struck down the young and healthy with greater intensity than the usual victims of flu, the new-born, the old and the infirm.

It was a common expression during the First World War among American soldiers that *"more soldiers were killed by vaccine shots than by shots from enemy guns."* The worst recorded outbreaks of the flu were among soldiers both at the front line and in camps, mostly young and very healthy men.[234]

The reason why the outbreaks were worse in the army is because they rigorously enforced vaccinations and the soldiers were the first to suffer from the terrible Iatrogenic Effect of vaccinations.

A report from US Secretary of War, Henry L Stimson, confirmed that seven soldiers had dropped dead in an army camp after being vaccinated and that there had been 63 deaths and 28,585 cases of hepatitis as a direct result of the yellow fever vaccine during 6 months of WW1. This yellow fever vaccine was one of 14 to 25 shots given to US soldiers.[235]

It is quite evident from a number of accounts of conditions for the soldiers in WW1 that they were given clean water, good food and had relatively good sanitary conditions. The lessons from previous wars had been learned in relation to hygienic practices. Many of the returning soldiers from WW1 were insane not from "shell-shock" but from post-vaccination encephalitis. Many were permanently disabled by vaccines.

The vaccine manufacturers wanted to continue selling their vaccines to the general public after WW1 and their advertising campaign concerned the dangers posed by "infected" soldiers returning from far-away lands. The general public needed to be vaccinated in order to prevent an epidemic. The soldiers were sick from vaccine-induced diseases and the general public were encouraged to get more of these vaccines, to prevent the spread of these "infectious diseases".

The family of Eleanora McBean, author of *The Swine Flu Expose*, refused all vaccinations and remained healthy during the medically created Spanish flu. She states that the flu only affected those that had been vaccinated. Because her parents weren't vaccinated and were therefore healthy, they helped look after the sick. If a pathogenic virus had been the cause of the Spanish flu they would surely have been affected. But of course the answer will be that they had a "strong immune system". One medical dogma explaining another, explaining another, to explain the impossible within the pattern of thinking called the Biomedical Paradigm.

People were weakened by the cocktail effect from the many different vaccines they had been given. The Spanish flu was not caused by viruses, because viruses do not exist. Eleanora McBean provides a convincing alternative explanation for the true cause of the Spanish flu. The name "Spanish flu", did indeed cover up the real cause of the 1918 flu pandemic: vaccines.

Until the true cause of the Spanish flu is recognised, we are all in mortal danger from another catastrophic medically induced epidemic.

The US swine flu panic[236]

In February 1976, an army recruit at Fort Dix, New Jersey, died from so-called swine flu. Two weeks after he died, the MDs declared that swine flu was the cause of his death. The US was in the midst of a swine flu pandemic. Back in 1976, the MDs and other white-coats speculated that swine flu was the cause of the Spanish flu pandemic of 1918 and in 2007 they speculated that bird flu was the cause of the 1918 pandemic. Which was it then, the swine flu, or the bird flu?

Swine flu was about to infect the entire US with millions of people dying. Action had to be taken to head off a major pandemic. Health officials urged that every person in the US be vaccinated for swine flu. Twenty four per cent of the US population was vaccinated by the time the program was cancelled.

The swine flu vaccine was at least responsible for at least 25 deaths and thousands of cases of paralysis.

The mundane reality was of course that swine flu was an iatrogenic disease caused by vaccinations. All the soldiers at Fort Dix, New Jersey, had been inoculated with the Port Chalmers flu vaccine, which allegedly protected against all strains of flu. Shortly after having been vaccinated, over 500 men got sick with the flu. At the very least the flu vaccine did not work and was a total failure. It was worse than that. The flu vaccine caused the men to get ill and caused at least one of them to die from it. The trick is for the MDs to certify the death as being from pneumonia, hepatitis, meningitis, swine flu, anything but the true cause: vaccine damage.

Although the swine flu vaccine luckily didn't kill many people, it can be regarded as a dry-run for a potential bird flu catastrophe, killing more people than the infamous Spanish flu.

The AIDS horror story in Africa

Our well-educated MDs and scientists (white-coats, all), by labelling poor Africans living south of the Sahara as being HIV-positive, means that we can avoid dealing with the underlying cause of these diseases. These people mostly give up hope and die once they are told by a white-coat that they have AIDS.

These poor unfortunate people are told that AIDS is incurable. Infected people risk passing on AIDS to their husbands, wives, to their babies and by their blood. It is not too hard to image what can happen in Africa, if a woman just after giving birth is diagnosed with AIDS. Her husband doesn't want to risk getting AIDS; he doesn't want his other children to be infected, let alone himself; he is fearful; he believes his wife got AIDS from somebody else because he tests negative for HIV. He kicks her out of her home.

The AIDS-diagnosed people living in Africa are told to take some drugs once or twice a day. These drugs weaken them further and with poor living conditions, lack of food, dirty water and with being ostracised from their family, friends and community, it is not too difficult to imagine what the likely outcome is: premature, painful, lonely and unnecessary death.

We could give them hope and tell them the truth. They do not have AIDS. They do not have the HIV virus. The HIV virus does not exist. The white-coat is just a modern sophisticated version of an old charlatan, the witch-doctor. The Africans do not need to be condemned to Hell on Earth. We could help them with low-cost, workable solutions for sanitation, clean water and adequate nutritious food.

The AIDS diagnosis for sub-Saharan Africa is absolutely horrendous. It is a crime against humanity; it is the greatest such crime ever in world history. The Africans do not need our pity; they do not need our HIV drugs; they do not need our vaccinations; they need help in ensuring that they have clean water, effective sanitation and enough food. The real solution to the African HIV-AIDS catastrophe is simple. Let's just do it!

The South African President Thabo Mbeki is the only senior politician worldwide that I know of to have openly questioned the HIV-AIDS medical myth.

President Mbeki has strongly reacted against the Western characterisation of Africans as being promiscuous, and Africa as a continent of disease and hopelessness because of AIDS. Speaking to a group of university students in 2001: "Convinced that we are but natural-born, promiscuous carriers of germs, unique in the world, they proclaim that our continent is doomed to an inevitable mortal end because of our unconquerable devotion to the sin of lust."[237]

President Mbeki stated in an interview that he was concerned about the AIDS drug AZT being given to pregnant women because of its toxicity.[238] He was asked the question, "shouldn't he trust the relevant experts?" He wisely replied that a head of government is not necessarily a soldier, nor an economist, nor a teacher but that doesn't mean he cannot make an informed decision about defence, the economy or education. The argument that you leave specialist matters to the experts is absurd. Our health is much too important to be delegated to the MDs and other white-coats.

President Mbeki is absolutely correct in his statement. Anybody is entitled to form an opinion based on their personal experience and common sense without being an expert.

President Mbeki, although not fully aware of the full horror that is the Biomedical Paradigm, is most definitely aware that the prevailing medical orthodoxy brooks no dissent, and will fanatically condemn these dissenters, even though they may have very valid scientific viewpoints.

The AIDS horror story in the First World

We have already condemned two major sub-groups with the AIDS diagnosis: drug users and homosexuals. Current guidelines call for people considered at high risk to be tested for the virus. They are now extending the net to diagnose more people, usually poorer people, with the AIDS diagnosis.

In December 2006, the US CDC issued proposals that everyone from 13 to 64 would be screened. Pregnant women would get extra screening to help ensure they do not pass the virus on to their baby.

They want to help the 250,000 people in the US who are allegedly HIV-positive but are not aware of it. They do this with the altruistic purpose of helping them so that they don't infect their partners and get treatment for themselves.[239]

One must ask oneself, what has been the effect of the diagnosis of being HIV-positive on a young homosexual man, or a poor refugee/emigrant, or a poorly educated citizen in the First World? It has been an absolute horror story with millions killed by the drugs they have taken to destroy this putative HIV virus. Faced with an AIDS diagnosis alone, I am sure that most people would just give up the will to live and die prematurely. Their death is speeded by the toxic drugs they have taken to destroy this putative HIV virus.

A possible bird flu pandemic?[240]

The white-coats have been planning this pandemic for many years. They have created huge stock-piles of anti-viral drugs in every country in the First World, which by definition must be used when they declare a bird flu pandemic. I do not know when the potential bird flu pandemic will happen. It could happen any winter now from 2007 onwards. It will happen if we do not recognize the true cause of the Spanish flu and that the bird flu virus H5N1 simply does not exist. It will happen if we do not wake up.

On a beautiful summer's day, thousands of geese are found dead beside a lake in a remote region of Northern China. They are tested by Chinese white-coats and by international white-coats from WHO. Both the Chinese and the WHO white-coats confirm that these birds died from H5N1. The great fear is that the H5N1 virus could now spread to humans, causing a pandemic similar to the Spanish flu of 1918. The death of these birds is given tremendous publicity. Fear is deliberately stoked up worldwide.

The real reason for the geese dying was because they were poisoned by chicken faeces accidentally released into a river from an intensive poultry farm a few kilometres up-stream of the lake. The plant manager is positive about this, but the explanation of the phantom H5N1 virus suits the officials and other managers at the plant. Ironically the poultry farm was sponsored under a technology-transfer programme by the FAO. The FAO official in charge of the program also agrees privately with the plant manager. Both of them do not publicly voice their opinions primarily because the WHO white-coats, along with their Chinese counterparts, are vehemently positive that the H5N1 virus caused these deaths.

The path of these migratory birds is reported widely in the media. The WHO white-coats are geared up and ready for action.

A Burmese man returns home to his village in a remote part of the country for a wedding. He is feeling bad, run-down. He carries on as normal for a few more days at home but finally takes to bed. He has a bad flu. His home village is about 100 km away from the path of these migratory birds. As bad luck would have it, there are two local poultry farmers who raise thousands of caged hens in appalling conditions. Simultaneously a number of hens in these farms get flu-like symptoms and die. This is noticed by a local official who reports it up the chain.

The white-coats from the WHO are informed. They test these dead hens for H5N1. This gets international media attention almost immediately. The media want the birds to have died from H5N1. They want a story. Nobody from the press investigates the fact that these caged hens are in a village 100 km from the known flight-route of these migratory birds. The fact that they are incarcerated in cages indoors with no natural light at all meant that it would have been impossible for the migratory birds to have infected these caged hens even if they were only a few meters away from them.

The Burmese man is in bed with a bad flu. His mother also gets a flu and has taken to bed. This is noticed by the local MD who informs the WHO white-coats. The white-coats immediately quarantine the man and his mother and the extended family.

They initially had a bad cold or a flu. Now they are isolated in plastic tents, not allowed to have their friends or relatives visit them, surrounded by white-coats from the WHO and elsewhere dressed in space-suits breathing in purified air. They are injected with anti-viral drugs and other drugs in order to suppress the phantom H5N1 virus. They die within two weeks from multiple organ failure.

The results of the tests on the poultry have come back. Positive. All the poultry are destroyed. The village is quarantined. The results of the tests on the man and his mother come back. Positive. The nightly news in every country in the world devotes most of the bulletin to the nascent pandemic.

The villagers and the WHO white-coats are given anti-viral drugs. Many get sick. Six weeks later, they are given more anti-viral drugs. After a few weeks, almost every day one or two villagers die. One of the white-coats also gets severely ill and dies.

A similar scenario happens in a small village in Thailand about 300 km away from the path of these migratory birds. More white-coats and the international media descend on that village.

The Government of Thailand orders all medical and other front-line personnel to take these anti-viral drugs. Many people in Bangkok, particularly medical personnel, come down with flu-like symptoms. We are told by the white-coats and the media that the containment measures have failed, and that we are now entering the first-stage of a global pandemic.

Front-line medical personnel worldwide take the anti-viral dugs. It is a particularly cold winter in the northern hemisphere. More people than normal get the flu that December. The pandemic has definitely spread. These people are given anti-viral drugs and the standard flu vaccine that might help. These anti-viral drugs only work for six weeks, so some people end up getting multiple doses. Many die, officially because of the deadly H5N1 virus, but in reality from repeated doses of the anti-viral drugs.

The race was on for a vaccine. A small research company in Ireland developed a vaccine for H5N1. It was given the seal of approval from the WHO, European white-coats and a large pharmaceutical company. The big pharmaceutical companies set about manufacturing large quantities of this vaccine.

The vaccine is given to soldiers, politicians, medical and other front-line personnel. Many more people come down with the flu. Nobody links the flu with repeated doses of anti-viral drugs nor with the so-called vaccine. It is the deadly pandemic that the experts have been predicting for years.

The BBC re-runs its "Pandemic" program that was originally broadcast in November 2006. They congratulate themselves on how prescient they were. This show is translated into many languages and shown worldwide. This show is a key part of the fear and panic that is being propagated worldwide.

Some hospitals in the US and other countries have armed security staff, so desperate are people for these drugs. Many people do not go to work for fear of catching the virus. Schools are closed. Martial law is declared in many countries. The stock market collapses. Many companies are forced out of business. The unemployment rate increases dramatically. The world economy is in melt-down. Dawn-to-dusk curfews are common in many cities worldwide. There has been an international break-down of law and order.

The winter is severe in the northern hemisphere, with January and February being the coldest months for many decades in a number of countries. It is now estimated that 8% of the population in Europe have the bird flu. People are increasingly desperate for the anti-viral drugs and for the new vaccines.

As a beautiful summer begins in the northern hemisphere, the global pandemic is declared to be over by the WHO. It has claimed an estimated hundred million lives, with the young and affluent, particularly health care personnel, being badly affected. It has been such an enormous shock that people cannot listen to the medical dissidents, who say that this bird flu pandemic was vaccine-related.

The vaccination program continues apace. Without vaccinations, the white-coats tell us that it is only a matter of time before the next pandemic that will wipe out the planet. Stoked by fear, 99% of us comply. We are now in the end-time.

How to prevent the end-time

The HIV-AIDS myth is a real life horror story that happens every day. The MDs and other white-coats propagate the myth about the phantom HIV virus. Many of us take AIDS tests that measure so-called antibodies against a non-existent virus. We believe the MDs and take the drugs that are supposed to help us live with AIDS. However bad the out-working of this medical myth is in rich countries and it is bad and is likely to get much worse, the HIV-AIDS diagnosis for sub-Saharan Africa is an absolute catastrophe.

The bird flu pandemic is a re-run of the Spanish flu pandemic of 1918. Unless we wake up, the white-coats will get their way in the next few years and will be proven correct with the unnecessary deaths of 50–100 million people and maybe more.

The only hope for a safe virus-free world is for most of us to wake up before it is too late. Where is the proof for the existence of the HIV virus, bird flu virus, measles, mumps and rubella viruses? Ask for the direct proof, for the scientific paper that proves the existence of these viruses. When shown a photograph of a virus, ask if it is a direct photograph of this virus?

Learn about and understand the German New Medicine. All cancers and other diseases are caused by a biological shock. You just need to understand this simple concept, this first Biological Law of the German New Medicine.

Wake up! Ask questions. Think for yourself. Do not be intimidated. Do not be afraid. Do not allow others, the experts, the MDs, the white-coats to do your thinking for you. The white-coats will not succeed in creating the end-time if enough of us manage to wake up.

Just wake up!

For God's sake, wake up!

4

THE PROOF

Believe nothing just because a so-called wise person said it. Believe nothing just because a belief is generally held. Believe nothing just because it is said in ancient books. Believe nothing just because it is said to be of divine origin. Believe nothing just because someone else believes it. Believe only what you yourself test and judge to be true.
Buddha (Siddhartha Gautama, 563–483 BC)

A good scientist has freed himself of concepts and keeps his mind open to what is.
Lao Tse (Chinese philosopher, 570–490 BC)

Most of the fundamental ideas of science are essentially simple, and may, as a rule be expressed in a language comprehensible to everyone.
Albert Einstein (American physicist, 1879-1955)

Facts do not cease to exist because they are ignored.
Aldous Huxley (English writer, 1894–1963)

An error can never become true however many times you repeat it. The truth can never be wrong, even if no one ever hears about it.
Mahatma Gandhi (Indian Prime Minister, 1869–1948)

In a time of universal deceit, telling the truth is a revolutionary act.
George Orwell (English writer, 1903–1950)

Nothing is more difficult to overcome than the problems we thought were already overcome.
Alexis de Tocqueville (French political scientist, historian, 1805–1859)

The reasonable man adapts himself to the world. The unreasonable man persists in trying to adapt the world to himself. All progress, therefore, depends upon the unreasonable man.
George Bernard Shaw (Irish playwright, 1856–1950)

It is impossible to understand disease without considering the experience of the diseased.
Dr RG Hamer (German physician, 1935–)

The doctor of the future will give no medicine but will interest his patients in the care of the human frame, in diet and in the cause and prevention of disease.
Thomas Alva Edison (American inventor,businessman, 1847–1931)

CHAPTER 23

The Missing Evidence for the Existence of Viruses

My image of a virus

Before I discovered the Ultimate Conspiracy, my image of a virus was of microscopic entities that invade a host cell in the human body, multiply uncontrollably in the host cell and which can ultimately destroy the host cell and possibly even the person in the case of HIV-AIDS and bird flu-H5N1.

Diagnosis of a virus by an MD[241]

A living organism is something that performs three tasks in succession: taking in stuff (eating, breathing), metabolising stuff (digesting, absorbing) and excreting waste. A fourth necessary task is reproduction. No alleged virus performs any of these tasks.

The current identification of viruses is done in laboratories by measuring the level of antibodies against specific viruses, not by measuring or demonstrating the virus itself. Thus viruses are currently detected by indirect means.

Viruses are impossible to directly prove because they do not exist in humans, animals or plants.

The diagnosis of viral infection by MDs is mostly made on clinical symptoms alone and the assumption that it fits into a known disease pattern for which there is no known causative factor. Summarising this scientific knowledge, we can say that viral infections are not diagnosed by finding the specific virus, but by guessing that a virus is the cause of the symptoms.

A diagnosis of a viral infection means that the MD doesn't know why you are sick and diagnoses a viral infection which is completely meaningless particularly since viruses do not exist. This happens quite a bit, doesn't it?

Dr Lanka's definition of a virus[242]

Structures which can be characterised as viruses are detected in many species of bacteria and in simple life forms similar to bacteria. The viruses are component parts of cells, similar to the bacteria in all our cells, which assist the transfer of oxygen (the mitochondria), or the bacteria in all plants which produce oxygen (the chloroplasts).

Bacteria in plants or humans cannot leave the host cell because they have been created by the metabolism of the host cell. Whereas viruses can leave the host cell because they are not carrying out any important survival tasks within the host cell. Thus viruses are component parts of the cell which have given their entire metabolism over to the host cell and they can also leave the host cell. Outside the host cell, they help other cells, in that they transfer building and energy substances. Nothing else has ever been observed. The actual scientifically proven viruses perform a helpful and a supportive function in the highly complex interactions of the cells. These viruses do not perform a destructive function.

It is extremely important to note that viruses are component parts of very simple organisms. It is worthwhile to re-emphasize this point: viruses do not and cannot exist in humans, animals or plants; they only exist in simple life forms.

The viruses that allegedly cause AIDS, bird flu, flu, measles, mumps and rubella simply do not exist. In so-called viral diseases affecting humans, one has never been able to isolate a virus. One has never been able to isolate a structure which one could characterise as a virus neither from an infected person nor from a body fluid. This image of a virus as being a dangerous external entity, a foreign invader is false. It is much worse than being a simple lie: Millions of people are killed each year by the MDs because of this image and belief.

The burden of proof for the existence of a virus

In science if you make an assertion, then you are duty-bound to prove it by the rules of science. The burden of proof is on the person who makes the assertion. The burden of proof is not on the people who are listening to this scientist to disprove his assertion. Science can only effectively work when the scientist makes an assertion and can then publicly prove his assertion. Any experiment to prove his assertion must be repeatable by other people. Once this is done, one can accept the assertion as being true.

I served as a juror on a case concerning grievous bodily harm (GBH) with intent in December 2006. The defendant pleaded guilty to GBH but was charged by the prosecution with intent to cause GBH, that is, the defendant deliberately set out to cause GBH, which is a much more serious offence. It was made very clear to the jury that the burden of proof lay with the prosecution. The defense did not have to prove the defendant innocent. The prosecution had to prove beyond a reasonable doubt that the defendant was guilty. The prosecution made an assertion that the defendant is guilty of GBH with intent and it had to prove its case beyond a reasonable doubt.

The general principle is that whoever makes an assertion whether a scientist or a prosecutor is duty bound to prove his assertion. I do not have to prove that viruses do not exist. The white-coats and MDs who state that viruses exist and poison us with vaccines and other drugs on this basis are duty-bound to prove the existence of these viruses.

Corn-circles (flattened corn in the shape of a circle) in a large corn-field could provide indirect evidence of the landing of a UFO. A piece of metal in the middle of this corn-circle could be from the alleged UFO that landed the night before. To prove that the piece of metal came from the UFO you would have to know the composition of the metal from a UFO and at the very least have a picture of the same UFO. Unless you have direct evidence for the existence of the UFO, indirect evidence such as corn-circles does not prove the existence of any UFO, no matter if there are thousands of such corn-circles. If you have direct evidence for the existence of an UFO, then indirect evidence could be legitimately used to prove the existence of UFOs in other parts of the world.[243]

Although the case has been made for over a hundred years that viruses exist, and cause diseases such as measles, mumps, rubella and now more recently bird flu-H5N1 and HIV-AIDS, the burden of proof is on the scientist or MD who makes this assertion to provide the evidence.

To prove the existence of a virus it must be firstly proven to exist directly. Indirect evidence for the existence of any virus is not sufficient to prove the existence of the virus. Before we rely on any putative indirect evidence for the existence of viruses we have to have directly proven that they exist in the first place.

Proof for the existence of a virus[244]

There are three steps involved in proving the existence of a virus. It must be:

1. Isolated from the host cell.
2. Photographed.
3. Biochemically characterised.

In order to definitively identify a virus, one would have to firstly isolate the virus from the host cell. In the isolation of a virus, the virus must be isolated from the cells, body fluids or cell culture and above all must be freed from contaminants. This is the first step in the virus isolation and is very simple for two important reasons:

1. In contrast with living cells, viruses always exhibit, according to type, the same size and form. They can be easily separated from other cellular components because of their weight and/or sedimentation characteristics.
2. For a long time suitable fluids have existed such as silicon-globules, which don't emit any osmotic energy and which allow the virus particles to remain intact in the solution.

It doesn't matter what the virus was isolated from, whether from body-fluids, cell cultures, plasma or serum: Once isolated, a pure virus is seen regardless of where it came from.

Secondly, the isolated viruses should be photographed through an electron microscope. These isolated particles must look like the viral particles observed in cells, body fluids or cell cultures to distinguish them from other cellular particles which look like viruses, but are not. One can observe particles which appear similar to viruses but are no such thing, especially in placenta tissue and cancer tissue but often and spontaneously in cell cultures.

Thirdly, the proteins making up the viral coat must then be separated from each other and photographed. They are separated in an electrical field according to their size. This produces a pattern, which is characteristic of the species of virus. A similar separation and identification procedure must be gone through for the DNA or RNA of the virus. It is legitimate to speak of a new virus only after the viral proteins and nucleic acid components have been properly identified. This process is called the biochemical characterisation of the virus.

One can only speak of a new virus when these three steps are documented and the analysed virus can be differentiated in the composition of its protein and its genetic substance.

The electron microscope was discovered in the early 1930s. Biochemical characterisation has been only possible since the early 1970s. Thus only scientific papers from the 1970s on are relevant in proving the existence of a virus.

The fibre algae virus discovered by Dr Lanka[245]

Viruses only exist in simple life forms such as fibre algae, a particular type of a unicellular chlorella algae and of very many bacteria. In these simple life forms the viruses are not poisonous but perform a useful and necessary function. They are not harmful in any way to the host organism.

In the course of his studies, Dr Lanka succeeded in demonstrating the existence of the first virus from sea algae. This proof was first published in a scientific publication in 1990. This virus reproduces itself in the algae, can leave the algae and reproduce itself again in other algae of this kind, without having any negative effects. The sea algae continue to bloom and flourish in the presence of this virus. This virus in the sea algae has no connection whatsoever with any disease.

Dr Lanka and the missing viruses

Dr Lanka had discovered a real virus in the late 1980s. The AIDS hysteria had started a few years previously. Dr Lanka read the scientific literature concerning the HIV virus. He was astonished to discover that nobody had claimed to have proven the HIV virus to exist. He told everybody, but nobody listened. He had proven the existence of a real virus in seawater. But despite the expenditure of enormous amounts of money, billions of euros, dollars, pounds, yen and Swiss francs nobody has ever proven the existence of the HIV virus.

Having discovered that the HIV virus did not exist, this led him to investigate the existence of other pathogenic viruses said to affect humans such as the measles, mumps and rubella viruses. One must remember that these viruses were first postulated or suggested to exist in the late 19th century before it was technically possible to prove their existence. Despite their existence being taken for granted by the MDs and virologists for over a hundred years, there was no scientific paper proving the existence of these viruses.

These viruses that were postulated by the MDs to exist were blamed by MDs of the time for vaccine damage. If a patient had a terrible disease caused by a vaccine such as encephalitis, it was convenient to blame it on a phantom virus and not on the vaccine the patient had been given a short time earlier. The evidence from Dr Lanka is quite explicit. Viruses do not exist in humans, animals or plants. Viruses only exist in simple life forms such as sea algae. If a child has measles then it should be possible to isolate the measles virus from the child, photograph it and biochemically characterise it. Unfortunately for Modern Medicine, this cannot be done.

It was impossible for Dr Lanka to engage the scientific community, the MDs and the virologists about the complete absence of proof for the existence of these so-called pathogenic viruses. The white-coats were scientists in name only. They were devoted followers of the Biomedical Paradigm. Dr Lanka eventually realised that it was impossible to convince them that viruses do not exist, that the Germ Theory of Disease is a complete fallacy, despite the empirical scientific evidence, because he was competing with a set of beliefs and dogmas known as the Biomedical Paradigm. The only way to succeed in this was to engage the general public, but how?

Klein-Klein-Aktion (Small-Small-Actions)

Karl Krafeld and Stefan Lanka initiated this concept of "citizen enquiry" in late 2000 after requesting their audience in Austria and Germany not to believe them (because this is emphatically not a faith or a new religion), but to query the authorities themselves for proof of the existence of viruses. Most people at these meetings expected the authorities to swiftly provide this evidence. The authorities didn't provide any evidence and Klein-Klein-Aktion developed from this successful action: ordinary citizens asking the authorities for proof that viruses such as measles, mumps and rubella, against which we vaccinate our children actually do exist. This is how ordinary citizens with no training in virology or medicine can expose this criminal fraud: the Germ Theory of Disease medical myth.

In Germany (and I'm sure, in every country worldwide), the legal basis for vaccination does not rely upon "accepted practice" or "dominant medical opinion" nor on medical hypotheses and dogmas but on the perceived “real” threat from these viruses. If these viruses cannot be proven to exist, then there is no basis for vaccination regardless of the dominant opinion of Modern Medicine. It is impossible to vaccinate against a phantom virus that simply does not exist.

Once we accept that we cannot vaccinate against so-called viruses, we also have to realise that vaccinations against bacterial diseases like tuberculosis and tetanus are ineffective because these bacteria do not cause the respective diseases but are merely present when the disease is present in the host organism. There is no scientific basis for vaccination what-so-ever.

The virus fraud (as part of the Germ Theory of Disease medical myth) has deadly consequences; children are poisoned and permanently damaged or killed by vaccines because of phantom viruses; millions of people are condemned to a premature death because of a HIV-diagnosis and the drugs they are subsequently prescribed; many more millions of people could be potentially poisoned and killed because of the phantom bird flu virus.

Questioning the authorities

When you question the authorities about the existence of viruses, they refer you to three sources for the criminal lie that viruses exist:

1. Medical text books.
2. Photographs of viruses.
3. Scientific publications.

Medical text books

When you initially question the authorities for proof of the existence of viruses, they usually refer you to a medical text-book as definitive proof for the existence of a virus. A text-book is not a scientific work, but a book for teaching alleged facts that are proved elsewhere in scientific journals. A text-book is called a secondary source in technical language. A primary source such as a scientific journal provides direct proof for a scientific assertion. One can then legitimately refer to these primary sources in a secondary source such as a text-book.

These medical text-books contain no bibliographical data that list scientific publications that prove the existence of these viruses. They cannot list any scientific publication proving the existence of any virus because none exist.

Photographs of viruses

Sometimes the authorities produce photographs of viruses as evidence that they exist. That seems to be a slam-dunk, a clincher; a photograph of the virus! These photographs are sometimes also shown on TV and claim to be true representations of the measles, mumps, rubella, bird flu and HIV virus. However, these photographs are not of isolated viruses, but of what the authorities believe to be viruses in wafer-thin tissue slices. They believe the image to be a virus because of their unconditional belief in the Germ Theory of Disease medical myth. But these images are not direct photographs of an isolated virus. The scientists who produced these photographs cannot claim that they are direct photographs of a virus because the virus has not been isolated from the host cells. Despite all this, the responsible authorities and virologists allege the contrary to the general public. Certainly my understanding as a layman (prior to learning about the Ultimate Conspiracy) was that these were direct photographs of viruses as one would normally understand a photograph to be.

How to detect a fraudulent photograph of a virus

There are two easy ways to detect a fraudulent picture of a virus:

1. By reading the caption under the photograph
2. By examining the photograph of the virus

1. Read the caption of a virus photograph

The caption under most of these photographs states that it concerns cells which allegedly contain viruses. The captions do not even claim to have isolated the virus yet they are being fraudulently and criminally misrepresented to the general public as being direct pictures of viruses.

These photographs show cells and contained in the cells are typical cellular substances of all types. These structures are well known and serve functions such as transport inside and outside the cells. These are fraudulently claimed to be viruses by the white-coats.[246]

2. Examine the photograph of the virus

All viruses of a particular type always have the same size and shape. If the pictures show a particular type of virus but with the virus particles having different shapes, you then immediately know that they are fraudulent.

The white-coats believe that these viruses exist because they believe in the Biomedical Paradigm. The virus photographs that they are showing are what they believe to be viruses contained in a tissue sample. This is quite simply a quasi-religious belief or dogma with no basis in scientific fact. They are not photographs of isolated viruses.

When the authorities, the scientists and the MDs say that these photographs are direct photographs (as we would normally understand a photograph to be) of viruses, they are deliberately lying. There is no other way to put this; they are being criminally negligent because they are supporting a huge lie that viruses actually do exist.

Scientific publications

On rare occasions the authorities cite original scientific publications. These have been examined by the Klein-Klein-Aktion team and specifically by Dr Lanka. Again these scientific publications invariably describe how a photograph of a wafer-thin size tissue was produced which allegedly contains a virus. However the putative virus has not been isolated from the tissue sample. The scientific publication does not even attempt to fraudulently state that it has isolated any of these viruses.

The Emperor's New Clothes[247]

This is all very reminiscent of the morality tale by Hans Christian Anderson called The Emperor's New Clothes.

A long time ago there lived an Emperor who had a passion for clothes. One day he heard about two tailors who could make the finest suit of clothes from the most beautiful cloth. This cloth had the special characteristic that it was invisible to anyone who was either stupid or not fit for his position.

The Emperor first sent two of his trusted men to see it. Of course, neither would admit that they could not see the cloth and so praised it. One was afraid to admit to the other that he couldn't see the cloth because he might appear to the other to be stupid or inferior.

The Emperor persuaded by the assurances of his trusted lieutenants put on his beautiful clothes for a procession through the town. He too couldn't see any clothes but was too afraid to admit it – after all his trusted lieutenants assured him that they were beautiful!

Initially the townspeople praised the magnificent clothes of the Emperor: they were also afraid to admit that they couldn't see the Emperor's new suit for fear of being called stupid. Finally a little boy unburdened by adult illusions said "but he has nothing on". The adults standing beside the boy had their illusions punctured and were able to see the reality and realised that the little boy was right and that the Emperor indeed had no clothes on. Eventually everybody in the crowd was shouting that the Emperor had nothing on.

The point of this fable is that just because everybody believes something to be true doesn't necessarily mean that it is true. Just because the white-coats all believe in phantom viruses does not mean that they actually exist.

The missing viruses: Proof of collective scientific delusion

As a young researcher, Dr Lanka is like that little boy who could clearly see that the Emperor had no clothes on and was stark naked. Dr Lanka discovered a real virus in sea algae. According to strict scientific standards he isolated the virus, photographed it and biochemically characterised it. He has scientifically proven that this virus existed.

The AIDS hysteria was at its peak in the mid to late 1980s. Dr Lanka searched all the scientific journals for proof that the HIV virus which allegedly causes AIDS actually does exist. Nowhere could he find an article in any scientific journal that described how the HIV virus has been isolated, photographed and biochemically characterised. Nowhere! Astounded, Dr Lanka also searched the scientific literature for proof of the existence of viruses like measles, mumps and rubella. There was no proof!

Unlike the little boy who whispers "But he has no clothes on", and who manages to wake the townspeople from their illusions, Dr Lanka has repeatedly given lectures and written articles and co-founded Klein-Klein-Aktion with a view to trying to get the general public to see the truth, but most of us haven't woken up yet.

The only hope we have is that enough people wake up and question the relevant authorities for the proof of the existence of these viruses that allegedly cause so-called infectious diseases and that finally some brave and honourable scientist in a major scientific organisation does the right thing, examines his conscience and confesses the truth that there is no evidence for the existence of any pathogenic virus. Viruses are only said to exist because of an infamous dogma from Modern Medicine called the Germ Theory of Disease.

The Emperor has no clothes. The Germ Theory of Disease is a moral and scientific fraud; germs do not cause disease and viruses do not exist.

CHAPTER 24

Measles, Mumps, Rubella and Chickenpox

The four diseases, measles, mumps, rubella and chickenpox all occur in the reparation phase of various conflicts. The original Meaningful Biological Program of Nature (MBP) is caused by a biological shock in all cases and is not caused by a phantom virus.

Mumps

Mumps is caused by not being able to eat or insalivate a bit of food or a morsel of food that one had already mentally tasted. To prove this hypothesis in a live case of mumps, one would have to talk to the child/person with mumps and determine exactly what had caused the biological shock, but in each and every case the theme of the conflict would be that of not being able to eat or insalivate the morsel of food in order to swallow it or even to spit it out.

The parotid salivary glands produce saliva for the mouth and are found toward the back of each cheek in the area between the ear and jaw. In symptoms of mumps, these glands typically swell and become painful. These symptoms of mumps are not controversial for the MDs. However, MDs believe mumps is caused by a phantom virus. The following illustrative story about a little girl called Lisa Strong will demonstrate the true cause of mumps.

Case study 1: Lisa's mumps[248]

Lisa Strong is a happy four-year-old girl. She has a loving family. It is nearly lunch-time and she is feeling a little hungry. Her Mammy[249] tells her that lunch will be ready in about twenty minutes or so. Mrs Strong is very strict about eating sweets, biscuits, or chocolates before meals. But Mrs Strong is not in the kitchen and Lisa knows that her favourite biscuits are hidden at the back of the cupboard. She climbs up onto a chair and opens the cupboard. She reaches in and takes a biscuit out of the packet. She is just about to eat the biscuit, and her mouth is watering with anticipation of this yummy biscuit when her Mammy walks into the kitchen. "Lisa, what are you doing! Put that biscuit back! You know you are not allowed biscuits before meals." The punishment is that Lisa is not allowed any sweets and definitely not her favourite biscuits for a whole week.

Lisa gets a biological shock, a DHS, from not being allowed to eat her favourite biscuit. Unbeknownst to Lisa, the squamous epithelial cells in her parotid glands are being broken down. Lisa was not able to digest the biscuit or to insalivate the biscuit quickly enough. The biological purpose of this "not being able to eat/insalivate" the biscuit is a breakdown of the squamous epithelial cells in her parotid gland in order to produce a better and faster flow of saliva. In the conflict-active phase, this cellular breakdown is not painful and usually goes unnoticed as it did in Lisa's case. Sometimes it can cause a mild ache but nothing severe.

Mrs Strong is very strict. Lisa has to wait for a week before she can eat her sweets. Lisa has a very sweet tooth so this is a major punishment for her; the worst ever! The week is up and Mammy invites Lisa into the kitchen for a few of her favourite biscuits and some cidona.[250] Yummy! What a treat!

Later that day, just before bed-time, Lisa had a terrible pain under her ear, around her cheeks and in her neck. The pain was so bad she started to cry. Mammy and Daddy rushed into the bedroom. They saw that Lisa was in pain. Her face was so swollen, it looked like a full moon. Her neck was also swollen.

Fortunately though, Daddy and Mammy knew about GNM. They immediately diagnosed mumps and they both knew why it had happened. Mammy Strong was sad because she knew that Lisa had gotten mumps as a consequence of her catching Lisa just about to eat a biscuit. Daddy Strong assures Mammy Strong that there is nothing to be sad about; it is a good thing that Lisa has gotten mumps now. She'll get over it in a week or so and is unlikely ever to get it again. Mumps is caught when you really want to eat something, you have mentally eaten it, but then unexpectedly you are unable to eat it.

Mammy and Daddy Strong are confident about their diagnosis. They wouldn't go anywhere near an MD, but they do not feel it necessary to call their GNM therapist for an expert opinion. Mammy Strong wraps some ice in a damp cloth and puts it on the painful and swollen areas, mostly between the ear and jaw. The ice-pack is tied at the top of Lisa's head. The ice-pack eases the pain and makes the swelling go down more quickly. It gets a bit messy when the ice melts but that is OK.

Some kids prefer to have something warm wrapped around their face but most kids prefer something cold. One should always listen to the children and do what they are most comfortable with.

Mumps and the five Biological Laws of Nature

First Biological Law: The DHS

The biological shock causing mumps is one of not being able to swallow/spit out or insalivate a morsel of food quickly enough.

Second, third and fourth Biological Laws

In the conflict-active phase the squamous epithelial cells of the excretory ducts of the parotid gland break down or ulcerate. In the reparation phase, the ulcers in the parotid glands refill or replenish and can become blocked causing the condition known as mumps.

Fifth Biological Law: the quintessence

The biological purpose is in the conflict-active phase with the goal of producing enough saliva (a better and faster flow of saliva) in order to more rapidly swallow/spit out or insalivate the morsel of food.

Measles, rubella and chickenpox

Measles, rubella and chickenpox are caused by a separation-conflict. To prove this for a live case of measles/rubella/chickenpox, one would have to take each individual case and perform an anamnesis and determine exactly what had caused the biological shock. But in each and every case the theme of the biological shock would be that of a separation-conflict. All diseases affecting the epidermis are separation-conflicts; either wanting someone to go away or wanting someone to come back.

Measles causes a full-body skin rash and flu-like symptoms, including a fever, cough and runny nose. Rubella is a milder version of measles, but both of these "diseases" occur in the reparation phase of a separation-conflict. The story that follows is based on measles but it could equally apply to rubella or chickenpox.

Case study 2: Lisa's measles[251]

Lisa Strong wakes up one morning. She feels good. She reaches over and picks up her teddy, the big brown one, her favourite one, gets out of bed and walks over to the door.

As she opens the door, she hears Mammy and Daddy having a row. There is some mention of Granny Strong. She doesn't know what the argument is about, but she knows that both Daddy and Mammy are shouting at each other.

Her Daddy is really mad with Mammy. He shouts, "Well then, I'll just have to move out", and Daddy storms out. Lisa hears the front door banging. Lisa quietly shuts her bedroom door and goes back to her snuggly bed with her favourite teddy and hugs it and kisses it. She feels very alone and very sad. She feels that it must be her fault that Mammy and Daddy had a fight.

A few minutes later, Mammy knocks at the bedroom door and calls her down for breakfast. Mammy looks very sad and does not say very much. Lisa is also very sad and is not able to eat very much for breakfast. Mammy is annoyed. All Lisa can think about is what life would be like without Daddy, with no more bed-time stories, no more bear-hugs; it would be awful.

Mammy drops Lisa off at the nursery school. Lisa doesn't want to play with the other kids. She just sits down on her own and talks to her teddy. Even though the heat is on, and the room is very warm, Lisa feels very cold.

Lisa has suffered a DHS, a "separation-conflict", because her father has walked out of the family home after a terrible row with her mother over an impending visit by her grandmother, her father's mother.

Mammy Strong picks Lisa up from the nursery school later that day. Lisa is normally very chatty after coming out of nursery school, but today she is very quiet. Mammy Strong talks to Lisa and discovers that she overheard the row earlier that morning and is very upset by it.

Mammy Strong is very clever and realizes that the row with Daddy Strong is stupid and has badly affected Lisa. Mammy Strong likes Granny Strong but doesn't like her enough for a three-week visit! She phones up Daddy Strong and they talk and talk, make up and finally come to a compromise.

That evening when Daddy Strong returns home from work, he gives Mammy Strong a big hug and a kiss and they quickly make up and are friends again. Daddy Strong goes out to the garden and finds Lisa in the sand-pit. She was very sad and was moping and crying, but as soon as she sees Daddy she is really happy. Daddy gives her a big kiss and a bear-hug. All is well with Lisa, or so it seems.

Lisa had a separation-conflict from her father after he walked out of the house this morning. She thought he would never come home again like what happened to her best friend, Clodagh. Now that her father is back home again, Lisa's separation-conflict from her father has been resolved. She is now in the reparation phase of this separation-conflict.

The next morning Lisa woke up feeling groggy with a bad headache. She doesn't feel right. She goes to the bathroom to wash her face. She gets a shock because her face is covered with hundreds of ugly little red spots. Not just on her face, the red spots are all over her body. She shouts "Mammy, Mammy", starts to cry and runs out of the bathroom downstairs crying and shouting for her mother.

Daddy and Mammy Strong both give Lisa a lot of kisses and a big hug. They feel bad because their row had caused Lisa to get the measles. But they know that measles is not dangerous and it is normal for a child to get it. It's all part of growing up. They have studied the GNM for many years and know exactly what to do. They do not bother to contact their GNM therapist. It's only measles and they know what to do.

They explain to Lisa the reason why she got measles. Lisa must have gotten a "separation-conflict" when she overheard the terrible row between her mother and father. They explain to Lisa that in the conflict-active phase you feel cold, don't feel like eating and generally feel miserable. This only happened the previous day so Lisa remembers it very well. During this conflict-active phase the squamous epithelial cells of the skin are broken down. Neither Lisa nor Mammy nor Daddy noticed this at all. They explain this to Lisa by saying that "squamy", a builder breaks down the cells in her skin when she has a separation-conflict of this type. In the reparation phase, squamy rebuilds the skin cells that were broken down in the conflict-active phase. Squamy did an extremely good job and rebuilt the necessary cells but under conditions of swelling and heat because Lisa is in the reparation phase. This is called measles.

The measles were itchy and Lisa felt tired and had a fever. She was very hungry. The tiredness, fever and hunger are vegetative symptoms that the conflict has been solved in the psyche. The fever is not something to be feared. It is a good thing because it helps the body to get rid of the measles quickly and efficiently. The itchiness on the measles spots can be treated with a little vinegar. Lisa has to stay at home and take it easy until her fever has gone. This happens when the measles spots have finally disappeared.

Measles/rubella/chickenpox and the five Biological Laws of Nature

First Biological Law: The DHS

The biological shock causing measles/rubella/chicken pox is a separation-conflict.

Second, third and fourth Biological Laws

During this conflict-active phase, the squamous epithelial cells of the skin are broken down. In the reparation phase, squamous epithelial cells of the skin are rebuilt or replenished, which creates the "disease" known as measles or rubella or chickenpox.

Fifth Biological Law: The quintessence

The biological purpose of measles/rubella/chickenpox in the conflict-active phase is to strip away excess epidermis skin layers so that the sensitivity of the skin decreases; the skin looses feeling and thereby "forgets" or "eliminates" contact with the person or object they feel separated from. The touch-sensitive parts of the skin can no longer touch the person or object they feel separated from.[252]

Measles and rubella scare-stories

The white-coats stir up fears that rubella is very dangerous for a pregnant woman. There is some truth in this. For example if a pregnant woman gets a huge separation-conflict (which fulfills the conditions of a DHS) from her husband, this separation-conflict could be passed onto her unborn child. The child could be born with what the MDs currently call congenital rubella syndrome. However the child has not been infected by a phantom virus.

The white-coats stir up fear by stating that measles is dangerous because one can get other diseases such as a middle-ear infection, laryngitis and more serious diseases such as encephalitis and meningitis.[253]

Laryngitis occurs in the reparation phase of a panic attack conflict. A middle-ear infection occurs in the reparation phase of a particular "hearing-morsel" conflict because the child didn't hear what he/she wanted to hear, "Yes, you can have it", or heard something such as, "No you can't have it", which he/she didn't want to hear. Meningitis and encephalitis are more complicated, but in essence they are diseases that occur in the reparation phase of other conflicts and are emphatically not the result of measles in an unvaccinated or vaccinated child.[254]

These alleged complications of measles are repeated ad nauseum by the white-coats in order to terrorize us into vaccinating our children. These scare-stories are repeated endlessly by a completely supine media and stoked by the fear of these alleged complications from the phantom measles virus so that we willingly allow our children to be poisoned through vaccinations by the MDs.

Counter-arguments to the GNM explanation for mumps, measles, rubella and chickenpox

How can GNM explain the enormous reduction in the incidence of measles, mumps and rubella in the last forty years, which are now vaccinated against? How can GNM explain the continuing prevalence of chicken pox in Ireland where there is currently no vaccine used against chickenpox? How can GNM explain the phenomenon of contagion?

Chickenpox

In Ireland, my children and my friends' children have all gotten chickenpox but have not gotten mumps, measles or rubella. This fact would seem to prove that the MMR vaccine is effective and prevents the occurrence of these diseases in the first place.

Chickenpox also occurs in the reparation phase of a separation-conflict just like measles and rubella. The strange thing is that Irish children still get chickenpox, but do not get measles or rubella. I currently have no definitive explanation for this phenomenon. I am certain that a correct explanation will emerge once vaccines are banned and there is a general acceptance of the truth of the German New Medicine.

Decline in the incidence of measles, mumps and rubella

The more interesting observation in the official figures from Ireland is that the incidence of measles, mumps and rubella has declined dramatically in the last forty to fifty years, and naturally enough, the vaccination industry claims credit for this. They claim that the vaccines are working: hence the death rates from measles, mumps and rubella have declined dramatically as well as the incidence of these diseases.

According to the Irish official figures, the current death rate from measles, mumps and rubella is extremely low.[255] A proper, scientifically conducted risk benefit analysis would conclude that the risk of suffering iatrogenic diseases like SIDS, (Sudden Infant Death Syndrome), or autism from the MMR vaccine would far outweigh the benefits of this vaccine even within the straitjacket of thinking called the Biomedical Paradigm.

We know that vaccines had nothing to do with the decline in mortality from these diseases. Mortality rates had almost reached negligible proportions by the time the vaccines were introduced. Mortality rates merely continued their decline after the introduction of these vaccines.

What is also certain is that the incidence of measles, mumps and rubella has declined dramatically in the last forty years. The white-coats believe that this is because of the efficacy of vaccines. The vaccines cannot be effective because these viruses do not exist.

There are a number of theories about the real reduction in the incidence of these diseases. One theory I have repeatedly heard from a number of different sources is the retagging or re-labelling of diseases. For example, if a child has measles, and has received all its vaccinations, the MD calls it chickenpox instead of measles because there is no vaccination currently against chickenpox and the child has received the measles vaccine.

When I initially heard this, I was sceptical because I believed that the symptoms of measles, rubella and chickenpox were quite distinct. However this is not the case. A simple experiment to prove this would be to give a number of MDs pictures of kids with these three diseases and ask them to diagnose the condition from the photographs alone. The MDs would not know the vaccination status of the children. The results of the experiment would prove or disprove the retagging theory of disease classification by the MDs.

The only way to verify any theories on the real reduction in the incidence of measles, mumps and rubella will be to observe what happens after all vaccines are banned. Will the incidence remain the same or will the incidence rise? If the incidence continues to remain low after the banning of all vaccines we will need an alternative explanation such as the changes in the last forty years in how children are raised in the First World and what biological shocks modern kids are exposed to. If the incidence rises, we will need an explanation from the MDs and other white-coats.

Contagion

The Germ Theory of Disease medical dogmatic belief in phantom viruses does seem to be confirmed when twenty kids in one class get measles or chickenpox at the same time. It is certainly much easier to explain an occurrence of measles contagion in a school with the Germ Theory of Disease and blame it on the fictitious measles virus. The reality of contagion or the simultaneous occurrence of the same disease does seem to confirm the idea that there is a deadly virus about. There must be an alternative explanation because the measles virus does not exist.

Many other diseases were previously explained by the phenomenon of contagion. At one point cholera, yellow fever and typhoid were all deemed to be contagious by the medical profession of the day. People infected with these diseases were isolated in order to contain the alleged epidemic. But it is now accepted that these diseases are caused by contaminated water and are not contagious from one person to another. The common denominator was that they were all drinking the same contaminated water. But one can understand how MDs and, more importantly, ordinary people got the idea of contagion from person to person as an explanation for these diseases.

In time when GNM is accepted, we will understand clearly that measles, mumps, chickenpox and rubella are also not contagious.

An explanation for the outbreak of measles among a large number of classmates can be achieved, but it will require an individual explanation from each pupil. There is no contagion, but merely the simultaneous occurrence of the same disease among a number of individuals belonging to a particular group or class.

A possible reason for a mass outbreak of measles in a particular class could be, for example, if a much-loved teacher is ill for a few weeks and many pupils in the class get a separation-conflict from their great teacher. When the teacher returns and the conditions of the DHS are met, then it is possible that a number of pupils will simultaneously get measles. It could also happen if a classmate is injured in an accident and is off school for a few weeks or months and then returns.[256]

When the knowledge of GNM is universally accepted, we will eventually understand the true reason for the occurrence of these "outbreaks" or epidemics just like we now know that contaminated water supplies in the past caused diseases like cholera, typhoid and yellow fever, and that these diseases were not contagious.

MMR – Nothing to Fear

Measles, mumps and rubella are relatively harmless diseases of themselves. They do not kill and do not cause any permanent damage. They are not infectious because none of these respective viruses exist and there is therefore no virus to transmit.

Measles, mumps and rubella are not to be feared. We have been conditioned to believe that these diseases are dangerous. It is this fear that makes us believe the MDs and other white-coats who terrorize us through the mass media in order to get our children vaccinated. Once we see through it all and are not afraid of measles nor of a fever, nor of any other disease, we will have overcome the Biomedical Paradigm, which is the Ultimate Conspiracy.

Vaccination is a business based on fear.[257] We vaccinate our children against the measles, mumps and rubella viruses on the basis of advice from the MDs and other white-coats. These diseases in themselves are harmless to a well-nourished child, well-cared for and well-loved baby in the First World. Love and care and attention are what babies need, what all of us adults also need, not vaccines.

What causes disease and is sometimes deadly is the MMR vaccine, which allegedly prevents these so-called viral diseases. Measles, mumps and rubella are not caused by phantom viruses. You cannot vaccinate against diseases like mumps, measles or rubella because they are all caused by biological shocks and you obviously cannot vaccinate against biological shocks. The MMR vaccine is therefore not necessary. The MMR vaccine is only necessary if you want to poison, permanently damage or kill children.

CHAPTER 25

Liver Cancer

The first cancer I had to fully understand was liver cancer because my father died from it. The shock causing liver cancer has a starvation/existence theme.[258]

The biological purpose of liver cancer (like all organs comprised from the endodermal germ layer) is in the conflict-active phase. The parenchyma of the liver grows or expands with the biological purpose that the person can extract as much nutrition from the limited food they are eating in order to enable them to survive for longer in a famine situation.

The statistics on worldwide liver cancer death rates are revealing. Liver cancer is rare in Western Europe and North America accounting for 2%–3% of all cancers. Primary liver cancer accounts for between 50%-70% of all cancers in sub-Saharan Africa according to a study cited by Dr Hamer in his book *Summary of the New Medicine*.[259]

Cancer of the liver parenchyma is the most prevalent cancer in countries suffering from famine. In the case of sub-Saharan Africa, the reason is simple, there is a real fear of starvation because famines still occur and consequently primary liver cancer is many times more prevalent than in the First World. In the case of Japan and Korea, the higher rate of liver cancer than Europe and the US is more existential and would require a more elaborate explanation.

When one sees pictures of starving children, they invariably have a swollen stomach. I remember seeing these photographs as a child and thinking that these kids looked fat and I didn't believe that they were actually starving to death. In the case of starving children, there are other possible reasons for a swollen belly but in the vast majority of cases it would be because they have liver cancer. Liver cancer causes the liver parenchyma to expand, which causes the swollen belly. Once the famine is over, and more importantly, once the person knows this and knows that they will survive the famine, their conflict is naturally solved and the liver tumour reduced in size.[260]

Liver cancer symptoms

In the conflict-active phase, one has all the usual symptoms such as weight loss or sleeplessness. Specific symptoms are a pain in the belly in the location where the liver is and a swollen belly.

My father's liver cancer

In my father's case, the MDs said he had liver cancer and a suspected colonic primary or primary cancer in the colon/bowel. Statistically, this makes sense in the First World. A primary cancer in the colon can be followed by a secondary shock/DHS where the patient gets liver cancer because they have a biological shock that they will starve to death as a result of having had colon cancer. They fear that the food will not get through their stomach because of the growing tumour and then they get liver cancer. The MDs treat this as proof that the cancer has spread because of the medical myth called metastasis. In reality, it is a second biological shock, a DHS.

In my father's case, the general surgeon couldn't find a primary cancer in his colon because there wasn't any. Instead he had a DHS or biological shock with the theme of a starvation conflict, which resulted in his liver cancer.

My father's CT scans

In May 2007, I visited the radiography department at Wexford General Hospital and requested the CT scans that were performed on my father in August 2002. I dealt with a secretary who conferred with an MD. The MD did not want me to have copies of my father's CT scans even though he was dead for over four years. I made a formal request for two copies of the CT scans under the Freedom of Information Act. The FOI Officer at the hospital was very nice. She never asked me why I wanted the CT scans and dealt with my request in a professional manner.

I was slightly apprehensive because I had clear expectations of what I should see on the CT scans. Would I see what I expected to see? I was almost certain that my father had primary liver cancer only. I therefore expected to see a HH (concentric circular rings) around the brain relay for his liver located in the brain-stem. I also expected to see a similar HH on his liver. I didn't expect to see a HH around the brain relay controlling his colon because the general surgeon in Wexford was not able to find any evidence of a primary cancer in my father's colon, presumably because he did not have colon cancer at all.

Would I, a complete novice (with regard to CT scans if not GNM itself), be able to see something that the MD or a radiologist had completely missed or ignored? I received the CT scans on Friday, 22nd June 2007. It was like opening the envelope containing your exam results, I was that nervous about it. I had great expectations.[261] Would they be met, or would I be disappointed?

I was being excessively naive. There were no brain CT scans. According to the FOI officer, there were none performed. They had sent me CT scans of his lungs and of his abdomen. There was one CT sheet with eleven CT scans of his lungs. There were three CT sheets with CT scans/photographs of his abdomen. Each of the three sheets had twenty-photographs; four photographs per row and five rows. Thus there were sixty sequential photographs in total on three sheets. The first CT scan was taken at a distance of 139.00 mm. The second photograph was 6.5 mm further away at a distance of 145.5mm. The final photograph was at a distance of 522.5mm.

I saw circular rings on what I assumed was his liver in a number of these photographs, but I wasn't sure if I was seeing what I expected to see. I mailed a copy of the CT scans to Harald Baumann in late June and we discussed them a few weeks later on Sunday 9th July 2007.

Harald told me that my father must have had a large number of repeated starvation conflicts that were in the reparation phase and that had become oedematic. They were clearly viewable on the CT scan as darker patches on the liver. Harald said there were also a number of active HHs, with concentric rings. Where, I asked? When it was pointed out, I could clearly see one active HH on slide 18 taken at 233.50 mm.

It appeared that my father must have had multiple starvation conflicts over a period of years, most of which were in the reparation phase but some of which were active. The shock would occur, it would be solved again, probably a few days later, and then it would reoccur again. I had expected a single active biological shock with a giant HH on his liver. But clearly it was more complicated in my father's case as it probably is in most cases.

Harald also explained that it was difficult to be absolutely certain from the CT scans but he was almost 100% positive that my father did not have colon cancer. The MDs had suspected that the colon cancer was the primary cancer and that liver cancer was the secondary cancer having "spread" to the liver from the colon.

There were also eleven photographs of his lungs on another sheet, beginning at 139.00 mm up to 204.00 mm. His lungs were clear. On the 21st August 2002, he did not have a Fear of Death biological shock. If the same CT scans had been taken a few weeks prior to his death he would almost certainly have had lung cancer.

Primary liver cancer in the First World

How can one explain primary liver cancer in a man who had been a highly successful civil engineer, was recently retired and was financially secure? He could afford to eat out every day for the rest of his life in the finest restaurants if he so desired. However in the First World, the starvation conflict is clearly in a transposed sense. Even if the person is unemployed they clearly will not die from starvation but for some reason they believe that they could starve to death.

The only way for me to try and understand why my father had gotten liver cancer was to examine various case stories of biological shocks or DHSs that had caused liver cancer occurring in people living in rich countries with no actual real threat of starvation.

Liver cancer case study 1: The hairdresser[262]

Armando worked with his partner Sarah as a hairdresser in Zurich, Switzerland. It was her business and he worked there ostensibly as an equal business partner, but in reality Sarah ran the business. They had lived together for almost fifteen years in an apartment that Sarah owned. They had no children. The relationship went fine for the first ten years, but Armando never really showed much initiative in the business. It was in effect run by Sarah and she was the boss both in the business and in their personal relationship.

After about ten happy years of living together, Armando started drinking heavily. This went on for about three to four years. The drinking bothered Sarah, but she did nothing about it. One day he quit work early and abandoned some customers. Sarah was left on her own to deal with the situation. He came home blind drunk that night. He found a suitcase packed with his clothes outside the apartment. There was a note telling him that he was no longer welcome in Sarah's apartment.

This was an enormous shock for Armando. Sarah owned and managed the business and although ostensibly a business-partner Armando was effectively an employee. Sarah owned the apartment. They were not married and he had no legal rights to the apartment nor to the business. Moreover and most important of all, Sarah cooked their meals and Armando liked the way she cooked the food for him. Nobody cooked food as well as did Sarah. His first thoughts on reading her note was that he would starve to death. He remembers the DHS very clearly: He would not be able to survive on his own and he would literally starve to death if he was on his own.

He lived in a hotel for a few weeks and continued to work with Sarah in the hair-dressing salon. He stopped drinking. Sarah would not take him back. She had had enough.

Armando noticed that he had a pain in his stomach in the lower right side where the liver is located. His stomach was also slightly bloated and tender at this spot. He went to the MD in August 1999 and got a diagnosis of parenchymal liver cancer with six months to live at most. Fortunately Sarah was friendly with another hairdresser who knew about the German New Medicine and had informed her about it on a number of occasions. Her friend had attended a seminar given by Harald.

Sarah told Armando about the German New Medicine and they both went to Harald for one 90-minute consultation in early October 1999. They had the organic diagnosis from the MD: liver cancer. They found the cause of the DHS in one session. The solution was obvious: If Sarah would take him back, Armando's liver cancer would reverse and become normal again.

Sarah did take Armando back. His liver cancer reversed and disappeared. Armando was understandably terrified to go back to the MD and get him to confirm that the liver cancer had disappeared. The fact that he still lives despite his liver cancer diagnosis in August 1999 is proof that liver cancer and all other cancers do reverse once the conflict is solved.

Liver cancer case study 2: Grandparents diagnosed with liver cancer[263]

A couple named Vreni and Clemens in their 60s were grandparents living in the canton of Zurich. Their son, Frank, had two children. Frank lost his job and was unemployed on and off for a few years.

Every time they visited Frank during his periods of unemployment, they both strongly felt that their grandchildren looked badly dressed and seemed to be very hungry. They both got a shock or DHS on seeing their grandchildren in this wretched condition: They both felt that if this situation continued, their beautiful grandchildren would starve to death. They couldn't talk about this situation even with each other. It was too painful for them. The conditions for the DHS were met; this shock was acute and isolative for both of them.

Both were diagnosed with liver cancer by the MDs within a few weeks of each other in August 2000. Fortunately the grand-mother Vreni had previously been to one of Harald's seminars. They endured no medical treatment by the MDs. They both visited Harald and understood their DHS within a few minutes. The solution to their liver cancer was to bring their grandchildren to their own house and feed them and provide Frank with some money to buy clothes and food for the children.

Frank eventually found a well-paid job. His family now had enough money and the conflict was naturally solved for the grandparents. They were understandably too afraid of all white-coats to go back to the MD for an official all-clear. As of June 2007, they are both fine almost seven years after the original terminal diagnosis.

Liver cancer case study 3: Self-employed mechanic[264]

Tommy Kuza is a highly competent self-employed mechanic. Tommy's partner Daniela Amstutz has two surviving children from a previous marriage. Tommy was the sole breadwinner at the beginning of their relationship. He was happy; his life had a purpose because after many years of searching he now had a goal in life to provide for his family.

Tommy had had a number of minor accidents with his car and motorbike and had been banned from driving for an earlier offence dating back to August 1995. Despite this ban, he infrequently continued to drive his motorbike when he felt it was absolutely essential for an important errand.

In May 2002, he was illegally driving along a country road on his motorbike when the car in front of him braked suddenly and he crashed into the back of it. Tommy was not injured. He was so angry because he believed that the man in the car had deliberately hit the brakes to cause Tommy to crash into him. He had an altercation with the car driver and ended up slapping him in the face. He regrets this now and is ashamed of himself. He was arrested and given the alternative of a heavy fine or prison. He didn't have the financial resources to pay the fine so he had to go to jail for 47 days in November and December 2003.

In jail, Daniela told him about all the business they were losing, of the customers who came by but nothing could be done for them. Tommy mentally worked out all the money he was losing and the fact that he could no longer provide financially for his family. Daniela was not a mechanic. She couldn't run the business; they were totally dependent on him and he got a biological shock or DHS that his family would starve to death because he was in jail and could not provide for them.

By the time he was released from prison, Tommy had a bloated and sore stomach. Fortunately Daniela knew about the GNM because of the tragic death of her son Angelo caused by the MDs. They discussed what the problem could be and figured it was a starvation conflict and therefore liver cancer. Tommy got a CT scan of his liver in January 2004, which confirmed their original guess. Daniela showed it subsequently to Harald and he agreed that it was clearly liver cancer.

The solution was obvious. Tommy had to work hard, keep out of jail and provide for his family. The tumour receded and was normal again a few months later.

Daniela Amstutz has wonderfully illustrated the booklets that she and Harald Baumann have both written. These illustrated booklets are designed for both children and adults and explain the German New Medicine for specific diseases such as mumps, measles or glandular breast cancer. My nine-year-old son has a clear understanding of the causes of cancers and other diseases from these booklets. The booklets are part of the ongoing campaign to spread the good news of German New Medicine.

Liver cancer case study 4: The cigarette vendor[265]

A cigarette vendor named Freddy was in his late fifties and had an area franchise in the Eastern part of Switzerland from a cigarette company. Sales are dropping in the current climate of hysteria over cigarette smoking because of the alleged threat from lung cancer and other diseases. His company blamed him for the reduction in sales and reduced the size of his territory in half. They gave him the worst half of his franchise-area. His first thoughts on getting this news was that he would not be able to provide for his children's education and that they would starve to death. His liver cancer was a starvation conflict on behalf of his children.

He visited Harald once in June 1998 and phoned a few times. Harald was certain that he understood the German New Medicine. However he was unable to solve his conflict. He was coming to the end of his working life in cigarette sales; he understood his business; he couldn't do another line of work; and his company would not give him the full franchise back. He couldn't solve his biological conflict. He didn't want to be unemployed because he was too proud. He remained in the conflict-active mode with an increasing tumour and in the end died from cachexia just like my father.

I included this story as a possible failure of GNM, but it does not demonstrate that GNM is not successful, not at all. The patient is solely in charge of solving his biological shock. If he cannot solve it, then in the case of liver cancer, the outcome is certain painful death. This case proves that the tumour, with its brain relays located in the old-brain, keeps growing in the conflict-active phase until the DHS has been solved. If the patient solves the conflict in time, before enough conflict mass has built up, the tumour will recede and eventually disappear.

Experimental proof that liver cancer is caused by a Fear of Starvation biological shock

Unfortunately we live in a world where famine still occurs. A simple experiment to prove that liver cancer is caused by a Fear of Starvation biological shock would be to go to a famine zone. One would take a group of starving people, who include children with clearly distended bellies, and assure them that they will not starve from death, and feed them, clothe them, house them, look after them and give them the means for long-term survival. Tests made on the first day would prove that, as well as suffering from a host of other diseases caused by famine, they would all have liver cancer on the first day of the experiment. The parenchyma of the liver would be much larger than normal and this would be particularly apparent with young babies who cannot get any breast-milk from their starving mothers.

Three months later, these people would have gone through the reparation phase of a starvation conflict and would now be fine with no ongoing Fear of Starvation Meaningful Biological Program of

Nature. Most of them will be fine: Some will obviously die from the preceding effects of the famine. Now let the white-coats test them for liver cancer. In each and every case the liver parenchyma will have reduced in size, which proves a direct link between a Fear of Starvation biological shock and liver cancer, with the liver growing in the conflict-active phase to enable survival for a longer time with the meagre food supplies available and then shrinking in the reparation phase once the Fear of Starvation biological shock is definitively over.

One could also observe the HH or brain-relay on these people using a CT scan. On the first day, the brain-relay for the liver, (which is located in the brain-stem) would be in target configuration. The liver itself would also display a HH in target configuration. Brain and liver CT scans could be performed every week or two-weeks to determine the progress of the HHs. Once the patients realised that their famine was over and their Fear of Starvation biological conflict had been solved the reparation phase would begin. In the reparation phase, one would observe the HH for the brain relay become oedematic in the PCL-A phase and then fill up with excess glia cells in the PCL-B phase.

We do not need to perform cruel and unnecessary animal experiments by deliberately starving animals to death to induce a Fear of Starvation biological shock. We unfortunately have a real-life laboratory where this hypothesis can be definitively proved for humans who are suffering from famine.

As well as helping these people survive in both the short-term and long-term, which is obviously the most important aspect of this experiment, it would also determine the cause of cancer in the parenchyma of the liver as a Fear of Starvation biological shock. This experiment would also conclusively prove the five Biological Laws of Nature of the German New Medicine.

Liver cancer and the five Biological Laws of Nature

First Biological Law: The DHS

The biological shock or DHS causing liver cancer is that of a Fear of Starvation conflict in a famine area. In most cases in the First World, liver cancer is an existence conflict with a starvation theme. The person has a Fear of Starvation biological shock in their psyche manifesting itself by the brain-relay for the liver located in the brain-stem being in the target configuration in the conflict-active phase.

Second, third and fourth Biological Laws

The parenchyma of the liver is endodermal in origin, which causes a growing tumour in the conflict-active phase and tumour decomposition in the reparation phase. Fungi microbes are used for decomposing all endodermal tumours.

Fifth Biological Law: The quintessence

The biological benefit of liver cancer, as for all organs that are comprised of endodermal tissue, is in the conflict-active phase of the Fear of Starvation Meaningful Biological Program of Nature. The liver cancer occurs in order to aid survival in conditions where there is very limited food. The liver grows in size or becomes cancerous so that as much nutrition can be absorbed from the limited food available to enable survival over the famine period. Liver cancer is therefore not a meaningless breakdown of the normal functioning of the liver, but is a meaningful biological event.

Liver cancer and me

I can speculate about my father's case, but I do not definitively know the nature of the shock that caused his liver cancer. I do know that the shock could have been pin-pointed with the knowledge of GNM, and he would in all probability have been able to solve the DHS that caused his liver cancer and would have survived. He was a goal-oriented and driven man. I am certain that if he had understood the GNM, he would have solved his biological shock.

In 1981, Dr Hamer had discovered the first Biological Law, the IRC, over twenty-years prior to my father getting liver cancer. GNM has been ruthlessly suppressed by the MDs because of their irrational belief in the Biomedical Paradigm. GNM should have been universally available by the time my father got his liver cancer. My father should be alive today. My father's unnecessary death has motivated me to spread the word of the good news of German New Medicine.

Liver cancer does not have to be terminal. Liver cancer is reversible once the patient has solved the biological shock or DHS. Liver cancer is curable: Nobody should die from it.

CHAPTER 26

Laterality

The meaning of laterality

By laterality, all that is meant is whether one is right-handed or left-handed. Some people write with their right hand, but do other things more naturally with their left hand. There is a fool-proof way of determining laterality. The patient claps his hands, as in applause after a concert and the hand that is doing the clapping (and this must feel very comfortable or normal), the leading hand, determines the laterality. For example, if the leading hand is the right hand, and the right hand is clapping the left hand, then one can definitively say that the patient is right-handed.

Importance of laterality

When a GNM therapist treats a patient, one of the most important things to know about the patient is their laterality. The incredible thing about laterality is that it can inform you about the person involved in the biological shock that causes your cancer or disease.

If you are right-handed, then you will respond on the right-side of your body to any shocks concerning a person you consider to be your partner such as a friend, spouse or even your adult children - no longer considered by you to be children, but considered by you to be grown-up, to be equal adult partners and even a beloved pet that you might treat as an equal, as a partner.

If you are right-handed, then you will respond on the left-side of your body to any shocks concerning your own mother, your own children or other children that you might care deeply about and even a beloved pet that you might consider to be your child.

This is all reversed for people who are left-handed. The left-side of your body will be for shocks concerning a partner and the right-side of the body will be for shocks concerning your mother or children.

Laterality and testicular cancer

Dr Hamer first discovered the IRC after he got a biological shock when his son Dirk died. Dr Hamer got a teratoma in his right-testicle. Dr Hamer is right-handed. This meant that Dr Hamer considered his nineteen-year old son Dirk to be a partner, to be grown-up, to be an adult and hence the teratoma in the right testicle and not the left testicle.

The testicular cancer was a meaningful event in that it occurred because of the loss or disappearance of a loved one. The fact that it occurred on his right testicle was also meaningful because it indicated that he considered his nineteen-year old son to be a partner, an equal.

As Dr Hamer had been healthy all his life, and being a questioning man, a true man of science, as well as an MD, he suspected that there was a link between his testicular cancer and the terrible shock he experienced because of the death of his son. The five Biological Laws of Nature and German New Medicine are the incredible result of his investigations.

Laterality and breast cancer

Laterality can be vividly demonstrated by breast cancer. Let's take the example of glandular breast cancer. The tissue in the mammary glands belongs to the mesodermal layer, whose brain relays are all in the cerebellum, which is part of the old-brain. This means, that according to the third Biological Law, the tumour grows in the conflict-active phase, and the tumour is decomposed in the reparation phase.

I gave the example earlier of the woman who has seen her child knocked down by a car. She got a biological shock or DHS because of her child's injury. If she is right-handed, she will get a tumour on her left breast because the biological purpose is to provide more milk to enable a more rapid recovery of the stricken child. This is an archaic biological program and even though she is probably not breast-feeding the child, she nonetheless gets a tumour growth on the left breast in order to provide more milk for the stricken child.

Once the woman understands that a tumour growth is not because of some uncontrollable cell multiplication for some unknown reason, but because of a particular event that occurred in her life, which caused her a biological shock, she will not panic.

The great benefit of the German New Medicine is that it frees us from fear. Once you understand something you do not fear it. Once the woman knows that the tumour on her breast has occurred for a specific reason she will no longer be in a blind panic. Breast cancer is curable: No woman should die from it.

Laterality and bone cancer

Bone cancer is commonly called osteolysis or osteoporosis by the MDs. It is more common in older people and is always caused by a self-devaluation conflict. The self-devaluation conflict is a Meaningful Biological Program of Nature (MBP), which causes bone cancer/osteolysis/osteoporosis or holes in the bone in the conflict-active phase and leukaemia or the refilling of these holes in the reparation phase.

Bone cancer also works according to the laws of laterality. A hip replacement operation is common-place. It occurs because of a self-devaluation conflict; or a conflict of tremendous effort. The patients ask themselves when will this end, how long will I have to hold out, and how much longer will it last?

Bone problems with the shoulder or osteolysis of the shoulder indicate a conflict of self-devaluation, that you feel that you are an unworthy partner or an unworthy son to your mother, etc.

Again, if the person is right-handed, they will get bone cancer in their right hip/right shoulder for a partner conflict and in their left hip for a mother/child conflict.

Laterality and eczema

Laterality is also vividly demonstrated with rashes and eczema. Imagine a person wrapped up tightly in a foetal position. The problems on the skin facing out concerns a desire for people to go away; whereas skin problems on the skin facing in concerns a desire for people to stay.

The outer layer of skin is the epidermis. Any skin complaints concerning the epidermis are always separation-type conflicts of either wanting the person to stay or alternatively wanting the person to go away.

If a right-handed man has had a severe rash/eczema on his right-hand for many years, what kind of shock does this signify? Clearly this concerns a "partner" conflict. A conversation with him reveals that he has enormous problems with his wife and mostly wants her to leave him alone, not to bother him, thereby causing the rash on his right-hand.[266]

Sun and skin cancer

If the skin is badly burnt by the sun you can get skin cancer but it will be deemed non-malignant because it will stop growing because you are no longer directly under the sun. This skin cancer can be easily removed for cosmetic reasons if the patient wants it. It causes no harm. In cases of skin cancer caused directly by the sun laterality clearly plays no role, the only significant factor is which part of the body was over-exposed to the sun.

Strokes

Strokes are similar to heart attacks because they also occur in the EC (Epileptic Crisis) during the middle point of the reparation phase. Strokes are caused by either blocked or burst blood vessels in the brain. Strokes normally occur because of territorial conflicts just like heart attacks. A stroke is a milder form of a brain haemorrhage.

Laterality case study 1: The anticipated promotion[267]

A Swiss police officer called Hans thought that he should be next in line to command a municipal region of Switzerland. In Switzerland, the position of Police Commander is a political appointment, and it is therefore necessary to get the support of the politicians. Hans believed initially he had the support of his colleagues and the politicians.

However a number of colleagues that he thought were backing him ended up applying for the same job. This was an acute and isolative shock for Hans. Hans had to struggle hard to convince his colleagues and the politicians to support him. In the summer of 1982, he succeeded and got the job of Police Commander, which would mark the high-point of his professional career. This hard-earned promotion marked the solution of a territorial conflict that had lasted a total of eight months.

Three weeks later in July 1982, when Hans was hiking up in the mountains, he had a massive stroke. Although he had succeeded in getting the job that he had long desired, the struggle was too intense a territorial conflict for him, and he died from it.

Hans was right-handed, and the stroke occurred on the right brain hemisphere. The importance of laterality in this case is that it determines where the stroke occurs. In the case of a right-handed male, this conflict was going to hit his right brain hemisphere first. If he was a left-handed male, the affected brain hemisphere would have been his left brain hemisphere. The situation is reversed for women.

This case study indicates one aspect of laterality, which brain hemisphere will be affected first by a stroke.

Laterality case study 2: The anticipated wedding[268]

An Italian man named Giuliano living in London was in love with an English girl. He had been asking her for over two years to get married but she kept putting him off. She announced that she was pregnant in October 1998. Giuliano was delighted. They would now get married quickly and he would finally have the wife and family which he had longed for. Two days later she told him that he was not the father of the baby. He was shattered. He had lost his territory; his girlfriend and future wife and his child. He immediately broke off his relationship with this girl. He returned to live in Italy three months later in January 1999.

Back home in Rome, he fell in love with an Italian girl, and they decided to live together. She got pregnant in October 2000 and gave birth to a boy in June 2001.

He had a stroke three months later in August 2001. He was left-handed so according to the laws of laterality the stroke affected the left-side of his cerebral cortex, which caused the right-side of his body to be paralysed.

Giuliano had lost his territory, his girlfriend, his unborn child, his family, the entire life he had constructed for himself in England. This conflict was definitively resolved for him when he had a new family, a girlfriend and a newborn son.

Laterality can be confusing. It has two aspects to it; it can indicate who the conflict was with; alternatively it can determine which brain hemisphere is affected by the first conflict.

Giuliano was paralysed on the right-side of his body. He was left handed. Therefore this paralysis could have indicated a problem with his mother or with a child. In this case, it was the first such territorial conflict he had experienced and had affected his left brain hemisphere first because he is left-handed causing the right-side of his body to be affected.

Laterality and the DHS/biological shock

Laterality is important for two reasons:

1. It can determine who the conflict was with, whether it is a partner conflict or a mother/child conflict.
2. It determines which brain hemisphere is first affected by a biological shock.

The importance of laterality is critical in helping a GNM therapist determine who the person was in conflict with when they had a biological shock or DHS. If the person is right-handed, all physical manifestation on the right-side of the body are to do with a partner. All physical manifestations on the left-side of the body are to do with your own mother or children. This aspect of laterality is most vividly represented by breast cancer. For a right-handed woman, the left breast is affected by a mother/child conflict and the right breast by a partner conflict.

There are two important caveats to this. Obviously an accident or physical injury can affect any side of the body and is not indicative of any conflict. A second important caveat is that the side of the body affected could be purely because of which brain hemisphere was affected.

Laterality also determines which side of the brain is affected by the first, second and subsequent conflicts. A right-handed male will respond to his first DHS on his right brain hemisphere and a left-handed male to the first DHS on his left brain hemisphere. The situation is reversed for women.

In the two stroke cases given above, laterality determined which brain hemisphere was first affected; the right brain hemisphere for a right-handed male and the left brain hemisphere for a left-handed male. The affected body side is the opposite side to the affected brain hemisphere.

Further proof for this empirical observation by Dr Hamer is for you to test it on people you know with any physical manifestation. You will be amazed!

CHAPTER 27

Brain Relays and Brain Tumours

Brain tumours

Modern Medicine defines a brain tumour as any intra-cranial tumour created by abnormal and uncontrolled cell division. The problem with the term, "brain tumour", is that it is inaccurate. The brain cells do not multiply after birth. What is multiplying or engaging in an allegedly uncontrolled cell division is the interconnecting cells or binding tissue or glia cells in the brain.[269]

In 2000, it was estimated that there were 16,500 new cases of brain tumours in the United States, which accounted for 1.4 % of all cancers, 2.4% percent of all cancer deaths, and 20%–25% of paediatric or childhood cancers. Ultimately, it is estimated that there are 13,000 deaths per annum in the US as a result of brain tumours.[270]

The statistic that up to 25% of all childhood cancers are brain tumours is truly shocking. I met an Irish family on vacation that had lost one of their two sons to a brain tumour. The boy died at around ten-years of age. He had been "treated" for a few years. No parent can ever get over the loss of a child, particularly one so young. However this boy wasn't killed by the brain tumour. He was killed by the Iatrogenic Effect. There is no need for anybody to die from a so-called brain tumour, particularly a child, especially if the conflict is definitively solved and the preceding conflict mass was not too big. If the conflict was intense, it is possible for a person to die in the reparation phase. However the deaths from so-called brain tumours will be greatly reduced once GNM is universally applied.

Brain relays

The brain relays are observable on a CT scan when the conflict is ongoing. In the conflict-active phase, the affected brain relay is surrounded by concentric circles. These concentric circles are similar to a stone being thrown into a lake, with the brain relay at the centre and circular rings emanating out from the brain relay at the centre. Dr Hamer's opponents stated that these concentric rings are "artefacts" or imperfections caused by the CT equipment. They contemptuously named these concentric rings "die komischen Hamerschen Herde" or "Hamer's strange focii" because they were trying to ridicule him by using this term. Dr Hamer now proudly uses this term "Hamerscher Herd" (HH) to describe affected brain relays, which can be observed on a CT scan in the conflict-active and reparation phases.

The term, HH, originally applied to the concentric rings around the brain relay, which exist in the conflict-active phase. It now also applies to those same concentric rings that become oedematic (or fill up with fluid) in the reparation phase.

The brain relays are only observable on a CT scan in the conflict-active phase or in the reparation phase. With no conflict ongoing, the brain relays are not viewable on a CT scan. A HH is strictly a brain-relay in the conflict-active phase or in the reparation phase.

Experimental proof for the existence of the HH[271]

In May 1990, Dr Hamer set up an experiment with Mr Feindor, the head of the CT division of Siemens (manufacturers of the CT equipment) to establish whether HHs could be viewed. Dr Hamer wanted to specifically establish that the HHs in the conflict-active mode, which present a target configuration on the CT scan were not artefacts but were real and were correctly represented on the CT scan.

The Siemens engineers agreed to these testing protocols with Dr Hamer in December 1989. The experiment would examine a patient with an active biological conflict and thus with a HH in the conflict-active phase. The patient would be moved 2 cm to the left and then 2 cm to the right of centre. The CT equipment remained fixed in place. If the HH moved with the patient and remained in the exact same place on the brain, this would prove at the very least that the HH is linked with the patient. If the HH remained fixed, even when the patient moved, this would prove that the HH was an imperfection in the CT equipment.

Dr Hamer performed these experiments in 1990 with his fellow MDs and radiologists. However, the radiologists present disputed these findings and continued to treat the HHs in target configuration (conflict-active phase) as being "artefacts" or imperfections caused by the CT equipment.

One of the radiologists present still argued that they must indeed be artefacts because he had noticed similar "artefacts" around organs. This was astonishing news for Dr Hamer at that time. This target configuration can only be observed on the compact organs on which CT scans can be performed. These organs are the liver, spleen, kidneys and bones. However, it can only be observed on those compact organs at the beginning of the conflict.

Therefore, the HH is viewable on the CT scan at the start of a conflict and similar concentric rings are also viewable on the body organ. This revealed the astonishing fact that both the brain relay or HH and the organ have the target configuration in tandem. We do not yet know the exact mechanics of this manifestation, but we do know that we can observe these ring formations around certain organs at the start of the conflict.

When the conflict is solved, the circular rings around the HHs become oedematous, which means that they fill up with fluid in the PCL-A phase. The oedema or excess fluid develops to provide protection of the recovering neural tissue. This is similar to what occurs with a wound on the human body. These changes are clearly noticeable on a brain CT scan: the sharp target rings submerge in the oedema and appear now as blurry, indistinct and dark.[272]

This oedematous behaviour occurs during the first half of the reparation phase (PCL-A). At the height of the reparation phase, when the brain oedema has reached its maximum size, the brain triggers a brief, strong push that expels the oedema. This is called the epileptic or epileptoid (EC) crisis in the terminology of the GNM. It marks the turning point to normality.[273]

In the second half of the reparation phase (PCL-B), the brain's harmless connective tissue, the glia multiply and fill the circular rings of the HH to repair it. The glia cells are at the site of the HH in order to restore the function of the nerve cells that were affected by the DHS. The biological purpose of the extra glia cells is to repair the brain relay and enable it to operate more efficiently.

Modern Medicine calls this excess glia cells in the reparation phase "brain tumours". But brain tumours do not exist. Brain cells cannot divide after birth. What can and does indeed multiply is the glia or the connective tissue of the brain. The glia cells multiply to fill the space formerly filled by oedematous tissue.

Having observed thousands of patients, Dr Hamer has determined a topography of the brain, which lists all the brain relays and the respective organs that they control. Each brain relay is activated or switched on because of a specific psycho-biological conflict theme. The result of this scientific work is the creation of a *Psyche-Brain-Organ Disease Chart* that outlines the disease; the theme of the biological conflict that caused it; the location of the corresponding brain relay; and how the disease manifests itself in the conflict-active and reparation phases.

I believe that the fact that one can observe the HHs (when a disease is ongoing) on a CT scan is the scientific proof needed to convince people that there is something to these discoveries of Dr Hamer.

Experimental proof for the non-existence of brain-tumours

A simple addition to the above experiment performed by Dr Hamer would be to observe a patient in the conflict-active phase of a particular MBP. The HH would be in target configuration. The next part of the experiment would be to get the patient to solve the conflict. A CT scan would then be done on the patient's brain, which would prove that the so-called brain tumour is in the exact same location as the HH in the conflict-active mode and that this "brain tumour" is nothing more than the same HH in the reparation phase. It would prove that brain tumours do not exist and are another insane dogma from Modern Medicine.

This simple experiment performed on a few patients would bring an end to the sheer lunacy and mass murder that is performed daily by the cancerous treatment of these HHs in the reparation phase of so-called brain tumours.

Blinding headache – Symptom of a HH in the reparation phase

If a patient presents with a blinding headache to a GNM therapist, a CT scan might be performed to confirm that the headache is caused by a HH in the reparation phase. Once the patient understands what the shock was, and that he had solved the DHS and that he deserves to be congratulated on solving his problem, and that the blinding headache is a consequence of the brain relay or HH being healed, the patient will no longer be afraid. There is no need for radiation therapy, chemotherapy or brain surgery. There is no reason for a secondary cancer or metastasis caused by the original diagnosis of a brain tumour. There is no need for the Iatrogenic Effect.

The solutions are simple; stay at home, indoors and avoid direct sunlight and drink coffee, tea or coke. These are great diuretics and cause the body to lose fluid. It is also better not to go outdoors because the direct sunlight can heat the head, which causes the HH with the oedematic fluid to expand thereby putting pressure on other parts of the brain and causing severe headaches and, depending on the conflict mass, a possible brain haemorrhage.

Brain tumour case study 1: A terrible phone-call[274]

Adelheid, whose husband Leo worked for Swiss railways, received a terrible phone call around lunchtime in October 2001. The caller told her that her husband had fallen down on the railway lines and had just been run over by a train. He had lost both legs and was on his way to the hospital. The woman was in a blind panic. Fifteen minutes later her husband Leo phoned her. He told her he couldn't meet her for lunch because he had to cover for a colleague at work. Adelheid was stunned: She asked him if he was in hospital? He replied that he was at work and definitely not at hospital. Adelheid told him about the nasty phone call. She was clearly in a distressed state. He rushed home to her and comforted her.

A few days later, while out shopping, she fainted and remained unconscious. She was brought to hospital. When she woke up, she was immediately told that there was no hope because she had had thirteen separate brain tumours. Adelheid had heard from a friend about GNM and immediately arranged an appointment with Harald. Harald read the CT scan and was able to reassure her that everything was fine. She had been living with them for many years. The thirteen so-called brain tumours were the excess glia cells that remained after the reparation phase of the thirteen separate conflicts. Harald was able to describe the nature of each and every conflict from the CT scan and the woman confirmed that yes all these shocks had occurred and were now resolved. The final brain tumour which had occurred while she was out shopping had happened in the EC point where the brain is pressing out the excess fluid of the HH. She was outside in direct sunlight and would have been better off at home taking it easy after such a terrible shock.

Nevertheless, despite Harald's warnings, the white-coats frightened her into traditional radiation and chemotherapy treatment, from which she died on the 24th June 2003. She was only forty-four years old.

Brain haemorrhage

A brain haemorrhage occurs in the EC (Epileptic Crisis) in the midpoint of the reparation phase. It occurs because the brain is trying to squeeze out the excess oedema around the affected brain relay. The pressure exerted by this squeezing can be so great (depending on the conflict mass) that it could potentially cause a burst blood vessel in the brain. The brain interprets the blood as excess fluid and continues to squeeze out the excess blood thereby potentially killing the person.

When a brain haemorrhage occurs, there are no more signals or heavily impaired signals from the brain to the organ(s). Depending on the intensity of the conflict it can be fatal.

Brain haemorrhage case study 1: The proud father and his three daughters[275]

Hans was the proud father of three daughters. He always had a feeling that he did not have as strong an influence on his three daughters as he would have liked. He was closest to his youngest daughter. She caused the most problems for him for years as a teenager and young woman. She ended up being jailed for minor offences on a few occasions.

In December 2006, at a family meal, a number of his relations remarked on how well all three daughters had turned out, particularly the youngest daughter who had caused him many a sleepless night. Hans took this personally as a great compliment: He had been a good father. His territorial concern for his daughters was now definitively over. He was particularly proud that his youngest daughter was doing so well and was married with two children. He had fulfilled his role as a father.

Three weeks later, in January 2007, he had a massive brain haemorrhage and died on the same day in hospital. There was too much conflict mass built up from his territorial concerns for his daughters and he died from his brain haemorrhage. Harald Baumann examined the brain CT scan, which confirmed the cause of death given by the MDs.

Brain relays and the five Biological Laws of Nature

First Biological Law: the DHS

Every time a person gets a biological shock, a particular brain relay or HH is affected. As long as the conflict is active, the HH is said to be in target configuration. The HH will have concentric rings around it in the conflict-active phase when observed on a CT scan.

Second Biological Law

The HH remains in target configuration for as long as the conflict is active. To rephrase this, the affected brain relay has concentric rings around it for as long as the conflict is active. The brain relay in this conflict-active mode is called a HH because it is viewable on a brain CT scan.

Once the conflict is solved, the HH becomes oedematic or fills up with fluid. This occurs during the first half of the reparation phase PCL-A. The Epileptoid Crisis (EC) occurs at the middle point of the reparation phase.

Third Biological Law

The HH in the conflict-active phase is not noticeable by the patient at all. The patient only notices the physical symptoms of their cancer/disease in the conflict-active phase.

In the reparation phase, the person can get very bad headaches depending on the conflict mass. This happens in the reparation phase, either when the HH becomes oedematic in the first half of the reparation phase, or in the second half of the reparation phase, when excess glia cells are inserted to repair the HH.

Fourth Biological Law

The respective microbes operate in the reparation phase on the organs controlled by the controlling brain relay or HH.

Fifth Biological Law: The quintessence

When a biological shock occurs, an archaic emergency programme in the body is switched on to solve this biological shock. The affected brain relay is switched on; it is now in target-configuration, and it controls the affected organ and orders a tumour to grow in the conflict active phase of an old-brain HH, or a necrosis/loss of functionality in the conflict active phase of a new-brain HH. In the reparation phase, it orders the reverse to occur; necrosis for an old brain HH, or a tumour/return of functionality for a new brain HH.

Sometimes the symptoms on the organs can go unnoticed by the patient, but they can notice the effect of the HH in the brain by persistent and severe headaches.

In the conflict active phase, the HH is in target-configuration with concentric circles around the affected brain-relay. There are no specific symptoms associated with a HH in the target-configuration in the brain. In the reparation phase, the HH becomes oedematic in the PCL-A phase in order to facilitate the extra glia cells produced in the PCL-B phase. These glia cells are produced in order to aid the repair of the tissue in the brain relay/HH. Once the reparation phase is over the brain relay can operate almost as effectively as before.

In the reparation phase, with the HH becoming oedematic (PCL-A) or filling up with extra glia cells (PCL-B), this clearly causes pressure on other areas of the brain (because the brain cannot expand beyond the skull) and can cause severe headaches and fainting.

Once you understand that the blinding headaches are caused by a HH in the reparation phase; once you understand that they are the result of a biological shock that you have solved and you understand what caused this DHS; you will know that the HH will be repaired very soon; you will know that you do not have a brain tumour nor brain cancer; you will rest up until the headaches are gone and you feel better; you will not be afraid because you have nothing to fear.

CHAPTER 28

Experimental Proof of the Fear of Death Biological Shock

Fear of Death biological shock

The alveoli in the lungs are made up of tissue from the endodermal germ layer. The brain relay controlling the alveoli is part of the old brain in the brain-stem. They consequently exhibit tumour/alveoli growth in the conflict-active phase.

We can survive for weeks without food, days without water, but only minutes without oxygen. The alveoli in the lungs are where the exchange occurs of oxygen into our blood stream. It makes biological sense that such a critical "Fear of Death" biological shock would cause the alveoli in the lungs to multiply to increase the amount of oxygen that can be absorbed into the blood for a fixed amount of air, which increases the possibility of survival in such a conflict situation. The biological purpose of this Fear of Death biological shock is therefore in the conflict-active phase.

Experimental proof of the true cause of alveolar lung cancer

With the knowledge of the five Biological Laws of Nature, one could construct a number of experiments that would conclusively prove that lung cancer is caused by a Fear of Death biological shock and not by smoking.

1. One possible experiment would be to expose laboratory/house mice (the mice that have lived beside humans for generations, usually in barns or near farms) to cigarette smoke.[276] Many of them will get alveolar lung cancer; thus according to the biomedical paradigm, cigarette smoke is carcinogenic. I say "many" because it is possible that many generations of laboratory mice have lost their fear of smoke, but certainly, if the experiment was performed on barn mice, they would all get alveolar lung cancer.

2. Hamsters have never lived symbiotically or together with humans. Their natural habitat is underground burrows. If hamsters are exposed to cigarette smoke, they will not get alveolar lung cancer. All things being equal, they would be fine. This experiment was actually carried out and the hamsters exposed to cigarette smoke lived longer than the control hamsters exposed to clean air; not because smoking increased their life expectancy but because the hamsters exposed to cigarette smoke were certainly better looked after.[277]
3. Another experiment would be to expose laboratory/house mice to smoke from burning wood. They will all get lung cancer in the same proportion as those that get lung cancer from cigarette smoke. This would prove that smoke in general induces lung cancer in mice and not just cigarette smoke.
4. Another experiment would be to expose laboratory mice to smoke from burning hay. They would all get lung cancer in the same proportion as those who get lung cancer from cigarette smoke, which proves that smoke in general causes lung cancer in mice.
5. A particularly cruel experiment would be to expose laboratory mice in a glass cage to full view of a cage with a large mouse-eating snake. The snake would be fed live field mice (from another control group not in contact with the snake) and the effect on the laboratory mice in full view of the snake would be observed. They would all get alveolar lung cancer because there is a real genuine Fear of Death.

   If some laboratory mice developed lung cancer, and are removed from full view of the snake and returned to the control group before they die of lung cancer, they will develop TB and cough out the excess alveoli or sputum and will normally recover fully unless the conflict mass is too large. None of the other mice in the control group will contract TB, which proves that TB is not contagious.
6. Another variant of the snake/mice experiment would be the boa constrictor/squirrel monkey experiment. In the wild, the boa constrictor is a natural predator of the squirrel monkey.

   It is an extremely cruel experiment. One would feed the boa constrictor a live squirrel monkey from a control group (not in view of the snake) and observe the effect on a cage full of squirrel monkeys in full view. The squirrel monkeys would naturally enough be in fear of their lives. They would all get alveolar lung cancer, which would conclusively prove that lung cancer is caused by a Fear of Death biological shock.

If, after a period of time, the squirrel monkeys observing these gruesome events were removed from such a situation into an environment with no such ongoing bestiality, they would fully recover and display symptoms of tuberculosis; They would cough out the excess alveoli or sputum, but would recover fully unless the conflict mass is too large. None of the other squirrel monkeys in the control group would contract TB, which proves that TB is not contagious.

Experimental conclusions

Do experiments 1, 3 and 4 mean that cigarettes, wood and hay are carcinogenic? Or if smoke from wood, hay and cigarettes causes lung cancer, is any kind of smoke (whether caused by cigarettes, hay or wood) carcinogenic? But then why do hamsters not get lung cancer from cigarette smoke or indeed smoke of any kind?

According to GNM, laboratory mice (and specifically, their house mice ancestors) that have lived symbiotically with humans in barns or farm-houses for thousands of years have an in-built fear of smoke. They inherently "know" that smoke means fire and that they had better run out of the barn to safety. Thus they will understandably get lung cancer from any kind of smoke including cigarette-smoke because alveolar lung cancer is caused by a Fear of Death biological shock. Hamsters live underground in burrows and consequently have no inherent fear of smoke and thus will not get lung cancer from smoke of any kind.

These sets of experiments would also conclusively prove that there is no such thing as carcinogens.

The result of Experiment 5 and 6 will be that the group of animals (mice or squirrel monkeys) observing the snake killing and eating members of their own species every day will have a Fear of Death biological shock and will all develop alveolar lung cancer as a result. This group of animals will eat less, and not sleep very well, all because they are in the conflict-active phase initiated by lung cancer.

The control group that has a laboratory mouse or squirrel monkey taken away from their midst several times a day will do fine because they have no knowledge of what happened to their fellow member, who was eaten alive by a snake not too far away. However, they will collectively be aware, that one of them is being removed every day or so. In order to minimize the effect on the control group of one squirrel monkey being taken away from them, one could introduce two new squirrel monkeys for every one taken away.

The results of Experiment 5 and Experiment 6 would be to prove that TB is the reparation phase of lung cancer. These experiments would vividly demonstrate the second Biological Law, namely, that all cancers have two phases: a conflict-active phase when the conflict is ongoing and a reparation phase when the conflict is resolved.

The fact that TB and lung cancer are the reparation and conflict-active phases of the same "Fear of Death" biological shock would be astounding news for the MDs and white-coats.

Other animal experiments

With the knowledge of GNM, there are a whole series of animal experiments that one could perform to prove that lung cancer is caused by a "Fear of Death" biological shock and that tuberculosis occurs in the reparation phase of lung cancer.

How about incarcerating a Golden Eagle in a moving car or van for a day or two? The moving vehicle would disorientate the eagle by giving it the sensation of movement without actually flying. It would be certain to suffer a Fear of Death biological shock and get lung cancer and upon release from captivity, a definite solution to the Fear of Death biological shock and tuberculosis.

I do not suggest these animal experiments because I hate animals or consider them inferior beings. I don't. They are our fellow creatures that we share this planet with. I am not a vegetarian, I am still pondering that question, but I would consider all animals and plants to be God's creatures and to be treated with absolute respect. They all have a psyche and a soul.

These cruel animal experiments to prove that lung cancer is caused by a Fear of Death biological shock would be also entirely beneficial to the animal rights lobby. It would prove them to be absolutely correct, that animal experiments prove nothing and are cruel and inhumane. These suggested animal experiments would hopefully be the last such animal experiments and would bring to an end all the pointless, cruel and unnecessary experiments that are performed to allegedly prove that a particular substance is carcinogenic, all because of an insane belief in the Biomedical Paradigm.

End of animal experimentation

The knowledge of GNM and the fact that there is no such thing as a carcinogenic substance will finally bring to an end all the cruel and totally misguided animal-experimentation in the name of so-called medical-science.

There are two key-points in all these animal experiments:

1) Firstly one must take the psyche of the animal into account. For example, mice have an in-born fear of smoke, whereas hamsters don't.
2) Substances like cigarette smoke do not work locally. Instead one must take the psyche of the individual animal into account.

In determining that smoking causes cancer, the white-coats initially assumed in performing their experiments that smoking would cause bronchial carcinoma. This is entirely logical from the Biomedical Paradigm view-point because they assume that all so-called carcinogenic substances work locally, and that the psyche of the animal does not have to be taken into account. From the viewpoint of Modern Medicine, it is entirely logical that when one breathes in cigarette smoke, it stays for a small amount of time in the throat and is then inhaled into the bronchial tubes for a much longer period of time and then finally into the alveoli of the lungs, where the air is exchanged into the blood. The really interesting thing here is that most of the smoke is filtered out in the bronchial tubes before it enters the alveoli of the lung. This is why the MDs originally expected cigarette smoke to cause bronchial cancer and not to cause alveolar lung cancer.

Incentive for carrying out these experiments

There are three major interest-groups that should be strongly interested in carrying out these suggested experiments that would prove that lung cancer is indeed caused by a Fear of Death biological shock, and also the five Biological Laws of Nature of the New Medicine. These sets of experiments would only cost several million euros to perform. These three major interest-groups are the tobacco industry, the animal rights lobby and all major employers outside of the biomedical paradigm.

The tobacco industry has been forced by most governments worldwide to state on cigarette packs that lung cancers and other cancers are caused by smoking. This alleged fact has indeed become generally accepted wisdom. I certainly believed it to be true for most of my life. The tobacco industry would be able to recover billions of euros in lawsuits against various governments worldwide.

The animal rights lobby would be vindicated in their belief that all animal experiments are cruel, unnecessary and pointless. A major reason for animal experiments is the medical myth that carcinogens exist. These experiments would conclusively prove that there is no such thing as carcinogens and that all cancers are directed from the psyche via the brain. Animal experiments would therefore be pointless.

Major employers, unconnected with the Biomedical Paradigm, who are burdened by ever-rising health care costs, particularly in the US, would have a strong financial incentive in proving these five Biological Laws of Nature and therefore in significantly reducing their health care costs.

An open challenge to real scientists and the tobacco industry

These experiments would be entirely beneficial to the tobacco industry because they would definitively prove the true cause of alveolar lung cancer: a Fear of Death biological shock.

We know from the work done by Lauren Colby that there is no evidence from animal experimentation to prove that lung cancer is caused by smoking. The only evidence is from epidemiological studies. The scientists and MDs who fabricated this evidence refused to present it to an independent third party, Lord Nimmo-Smith, a judge who could make up his own mind about this putative evidence. The reason why they refused to present it was because it was completely flawed.

The tobacco industry has a huge financial incentive to carry out these suggested experiments and conclusively prove that alveolar lung cancer is not caused by smoking but is caused by a Fear of Death biological shock.

Lung cancer and tuberculosis and the five Biological Laws of Nature

If these experiments are actually carried out they will conclusively prove the five Biological Laws of Nature. In relation to the boa constrictor/squirrel monkey experiment, the five Biological Laws of Nature are fulfilled as follows:

First Biological Law: The DHS

The Fear of Death biological shock would be induced by exposing a number of squirrel monkeys to a boa constrictor fed daily with a live squirrel monkey. This would result in a biological shock or DHS resulting in alveolar lung cancer.

Second Biological Law: The law of two-phases of an MBP

The Fear of Death biological shock would be resolved by removing the squirrel monkeys from the presence of the boa constrictor. This would result in the squirrel monkey getting tuberculosis, but surviving if the conflict hasn't lasted too long.

Third Biological Law: The symptoms of the MBP

The symptoms of the Fear of Death biological shock are observable in the conflict-active phase and in the reparation phase as lung cancer and tuberculosis, respectively.

Fourth Biological Law: The ontogenetic system of microbes

The tuberculosis microbes observed in the reparation phase of this biological shock are tubercular bacteria which are specific to the germ layer that the alveoli are made from, the endodermal layer.

Fifth Biological Law: The quintessence

The purpose of a Fear of Death biological shock is to cause the alveoli of the lung to multiply in the conflict-active phase. The biological meaning is in the conflict-active phase to enable a longer survival time if air was in short supply. A Fear of Death biological shock is the most existential of DHSs. This is why it is one of the most common cancers.

Alveolar lung cancer is not caused by smoking. Alveolar lung cancer is caused by a Fear of Death biological shock.

CHAPTER 29

Lung Cancer and Tuberculosis

Fear of Death biological shock – Lung cancer and tuberculosis

A Fear of Death biological shock causes a Meaningful Biological Program of Nature with the clinical symptoms of lung cancer in the conflict-active phase and tuberculosis in the reparation phase.

If you have a Fear of Death biological shock for another person, usually a spouse but clearly a loved one, you will get a single cluster of excess alveoli growth in the lung. A Fear of Death biological shock for yourself results in excess alveoli growth all over the lungs.

Lung cancer and tuberculosis symptoms

The key symptom of lung cancer is a persistent cough that gradually gets worse. One can also have a shortness of breath, persistent chest pain and a drop in the ability to exercise. Other general symptoms of a conflict-active phase include loss of appetite, weight loss and general fatigue.

The key symptom of tuberculosis is a persistent cough accompanied by the ejection of the excess alveoli by coughing out sputum, blood and pus. Naturally, when one coughs out blood and excess tissue with the diagnosis of tuberculosis, it is not too surprising that one can believe that one is about to die, which causes the lung cancer to recur, and this causes a vicious cycle which results in death.

Lung cancer case study 1: A grandfather's Fear of Death shock on behalf of his granddaughter[278]

A grandfather had a horse-riding school in Lucerne, Switzerland. As part of his business he led groups of people on horse-treks around the countryside. His young seven-to-eight year old granddaughter desperately wanted to go on a trek with him and had been pleading with him for many months.

Finally he agreed to allow her come and they went for a cross-country trek in August 1998. They crossed a river at a shallow point. Unfortunately his granddaughter lost control of her horse and they both fell into the river. She was swept downstream. Understandably, the grandfather had a Fear of Death biological shock on behalf of his granddaughter. He leapt off his horse and swam downstream looking desperately for her. A minute or two later he saw her and pulled her out of the river and revived her. He brought her to hospital and she was given the all-clear. Once he knew that she was fine, his Fear of Death biological shock had been naturally solved.

He had a routine medical check-up with his MD a few weeks later. The MD discovered a single cluster of excess alveoli growth of about 3 cm in diameter in his left lung. The diagnosis was lung cancer. Because the grandfather was a heavy smoker, the MD emphatically stated that cigarette smoking was the cause of lung cancer and that he must immediately give up smoking. However he couldn't give up smoking and had a bad conscience as a result.

It is not too hard to imagine what could have happened. The MD had correctly observed a cluster of excess alveoli in the grandfather's lungs. He was already in the reparation phase and a few weeks later the excess alveoli would have completely disappeared. But he had been told that he had lung cancer. Because of this diagnosis and because he couldn't give up smoking, he might have gotten another DHS, a Fear of Death conflict on behalf of himself and gotten full-blown lung cancer.

Fortunately his wife had heard about the German New Medicine and sent her husband to visit Harald.

In one session lasting 90 minutes in December 1998, they discovered the cause of the DHS (biological shock), the fact that it had been naturally solved because his granddaughter was well and that he was already in the reparation phase and that he had nothing to worry about.

He was relieved and told Harald that he understood everything. He was dying for a cigarette and could now enjoy it with a clear conscience. He certainly had earned it and he deserved it.

He had one more test with the MD to monitor the progress of the lung cancer after his talk with Harald. The cluster of excess alveoli growth was not increasing but neither was it decreasing. He must not have gotten a Fear of Death biological shock for himself because the cancer had not spread throughout the lung. He was absolutely relieved and felt that Harald had been vindicated. He hasn't been to an MD since.

Lung cancer case study 2: Misdiagnosis of a bronchial carcinoma[279]

Christina, a German lady in her mid fifties, had been incorrectly diagnosed with terminal lung cancer by an MD. She was a non-smoker. But you should now know that cigarette smoking has nothing to do with either alveolar lung cancer, bronchial cancer or any other type of cancer or disease.

She was given six months to live if even that. She sold all her worldly possessions and travelled to her friends and relations in America and Germany to say goodbye to them. Somehow she heard about the German New Medicine and at the end of her travels on her way back from her relations in Munich, Germany to die in Bern, Switzerland, she stopped off in Harald's village to visit him. She was ready to die. But when given an imminent death sentence, you clutch at straws, you will try anything and this is what she was doing.

The symptoms of her so-called lung cancer were persistent coughing and difficulties in breathing. She didn't have lung cancer; she really had a bronchial carcinoma in the reparation phase.

Christina met her husband a Swiss man in the US. There, she had a successful career as a journalist, and had a close circle of friends. Her husband wanted to return to his hometown of Bern, Switzerland. She reluctantly agreed to follow him. She had difficulties in getting a suitable job in Switzerland, and she missed her friends in the US and had tremendous difficulties with her hostile mother-in-law. After a few years living there, her husband wanted a separation. He moved out of the apartment and eventually emigrated.

She had lost her good job in the US, her friends in the US, had been afraid of losing her husband and now had eventually lost him and was in dire straits. She had been afraid of losing her territory; her husband. This type of DHS is a Fear of Loss of Territory conflict. The tissue in the walls of the bronchial tubes ulcerates so that she can breathe in more air and have more energy in order to fight for her territory that she fears she will lose.

Dr Hamer explains this very simply using an example from the animal kingdom. A stag has been in charge of his territory for a long time. Along comes a younger stag to challenge him for his territory. The older stag gets a DHS because he is in danger of losing his territory. He must mobilise all his resources to fight back. His bronchial tubes ulcerate so that he has more energy for the battle.

This lady knew she had to get a job in order to survive and she succeeded. She got a good job as a journalist with a newspaper in Bern. She solved her DHS. She had now re-established her territory that she now fully controls without her husband.

But in the reparation phase, the bronchial tubes that had ulcerated (unknown to her) in the conflict-active phase had to be repaired. The tissue of the bronchial tubes as of all ducts in the body is ectodermal in origin. The biological benefit of an ectodermal cancer is in the conflict-active phase. In the case of a bronchial carcinoma, the ulceration of the bronchial tubes allows more air to enter the body, which enabled her to mobilise the resources necessary to win back her territory.

In the reparation phase, the ulcers in the bronchial tubes are replenished. This causes swelling of the bronchial tubes, causing them to be narrowed, with consequent difficulties in breathing and persistent coughing.

She had one session lasting 90 minutes with Harald in 2005. She understood her MBP, returned to Bern, reorganised her life and recovered over a period of a few months.

Lung-cancer case study 3: A Scuba-diver's Fear of Death biological shock[280]

A non-smoking scuba-diver named Paolo had recently completed a scuba-diving course. He had completed a handful of dives with his diving-partner. On one particular dive in May 1999, he was about 30 m depth below water when he realised with a tremendous shock that:

1. He had lost track of his diving-partner;
2. The battery on his torch did not work;
3. He did not have enough air in his tank to make it back safely to the surface, bearing in mind that one must stop at intervals on the way back to the surface if one wants to stop the lungs from being damaged. If one goes immediately to the surface from a 30 m depth, the lungs can become damaged and cause death.

Paolo was clearly in a panic. He was in imminent danger of death. What should he do? Luckily his diving partner found him and they shared air all the way up to the surface. They came up a little too quickly and suffered some complications, but Paolo was now safe on the boat. His DHS was over; he was safe; he was alive; and he was now in the reparation phase of this Meaningful Biological Program of Nature.

However as he had just taken up diving and had a circle of friends who were divers, he continued to dive. Although he had survived the original DHS and was in the reparation phase of it, he was now afraid of diving and each time he put on his wetsuit, he thought that he would die. This is what is called a "track" in the German New Medicine. Each time he put on his wetsuit and went scuba diving he thought he was going to die because he went back onto the "track" of his original biological shock. The DHS or biological shock that he had originally suffered was reactivated for as long as he was scuba-diving and he was back in the reparation phase once the dive was over. So he was mostly in the reparation phase but occasionally in the conflict-active phase. This would be termed a "hanging-healing conflict" (in the terminology of GNM) because he kept going scuba-diving and got back onto the "track" of his original DHS.

He had a persistent bad cough and had difficulty in breathing. He went to the MD who stated that he had a number of clusters of excess alveoli growth in his lungs. He had terminal lung cancer and had a few months to live if even that. Obviously he was in a blind panic, but he found out about GNM through a friend and made his way to Harald.

One session with Harald was enough for Paolo to understand his cancer. Because he reactivated his Fear of Death biological shock every time he went diving, he was back on the track of the original DHS and was reliving this horrible experience with every single dive. The solution was simple. He sold all his scuba-diving equipment: He would never scuba-dive again. It took him a short time to make up his mind and sell the equipment. He phoned Harald a few days later and told him about his decision.

He now had a definitive solution to his Fear of Death biological shock. He was in the reparation phase and the conflict-active phase was not being reactivated with his dives. In the reparation phase he got tuberculosis and was coughing out the sputum or spitting out blood and excess tissue. He was also sweating a lot at night. He was well prepared for these symptoms and did not consult an MD.

Lung cancer case study 4: The case of Superman's wife, Dana Reeve[281]

Christopher Reeve was an actor who played the title role of Superman in the movies. He was paralysed in March 1995 in a horse-riding accident. His actress wife Dana Reeve had never been away from her husband and their only son for an extended period since his accident. In October 2004, she was working thousands of miles away in a theatre in Los Angeles.

A few days before he died, Christopher Reeve was being treated for a pressure wound. This is a common complication for people with paralysis that he had experienced many times before. The wound had become severely infected but was no unusual cause for concern. On Saturday, October 9th, Christopher Reeve attended a hockey game their son was playing in. That night he suffered a cardiac arrest after taking an antibiotic. His wife Dana made it back home just before he died the next day on the 10th October 2004.

This is clearly speculation, but one can certainly speculate that on hearing the news that her husband that she had lovingly looked after for nearly ten years since his accident and had never been far away from him for any length of time, that she must have suffered a Fear of Death biological shock for him on hearing the news of his heart attack.

She would have had a single cluster or nodule of additional alveoli cells produced because of her shock on hearing the news of her husband's heart attack. This Fear of Death biological shock would have only lasted for a few days at most and would have been naturally resolved by the sudden death of her husband.

However to further complicate her story, her seventy-one-year-old mother was diagnosed with ovarian cancer in January 2005 and died in February 2005 from an operation for her ovarian cancer. She lost her mother four months after the death of her husband.

Again one is speculating but she probably was in the reparation phase of lung cancer for her husband when she heard the news about her mother's ovarian cancer three months after the death of her husband. She was now immediately back on the tracks of a Fear of Death biological shock on behalf of her mother this time.

Again this Fear of Death biological shock would have been solved a month later by the death of her mother in February 2005. We know that she eventually attended her MD after having had a persistent cough for a few weeks. She officially announced her diagnosis of lung cancer in August 2005 and died in March 2006. She had lived a healthy life. She had never smoked but had still gotten lung cancer. Cigarette smoking has nothing to do with alveolar lung cancer, but this fact is included to drive home the point that lung cancer is not caused by smoking, but is caused by a Fear of Death biological shock.

Presumably she had been diagnosed a few months earlier prior to her public announcement. However, in reality she was suffering from tuberculosis and not from lung cancer. In the reparation phase of this MBP, she had a persistent cough because her body was getting rid of these excess alveoli cells.

It is not too difficult to imagine what happens to the individual that is told that she has lung cancer. She now probably got a further shock or DHS that she herself would die. The cancer now spread all over her lungs instead of in just one or two clusters. The MDs probably told her that the cancer was "aggressive" and was spreading rapidly in her lungs. Together with being poisoned by chemotherapy this diagnosis would have crushed her and one can be assured that she died a painful, premature and unnecessary death at the young age of 44.

Her father was an MD, a retired cardiologist. We can therefore presume she had the best possible treatment that Modern Medicine could provide. Modern Medicine killed her. All that she had to know was that her persistent cough was because she was in the reparation phase of a Fear of Death biological shock for both her husband and her mother, that she was suffering from the disease called tuberculosis in the reparation phase of this MBP and that in a few weeks time the excess alveoli would have disappeared and that she would have been healthy again.

The contrast with the story about the scuba-diver, Paolo, is instructive. Paolo had the good fortune to have heard about the German New Medicine prior to his diagnosis with terminal lung cancer and then to have contacted Harald Baumann. Paolo immediately understood the German New Medicine and came up with a real solution to his DHS. Dana Reeve instead relied on Modern Medicine and was killed by it.

The only moral in this story is to learn about and fully understand the German New Medicine while you are still healthy. Once you are diagnosed with any cancer and follow the usual remedies of poison, slash or burn[282] you are in a certain game of death, where death is guaranteed but the only variable is the length of time and the pain you have to go through before you die prematurely.

Further proof of the Fear of Death MBP[283]

To prove that lung-cancer and tuberculosis are the conflict-active and the reparation phase of a Fear of Death MBP, one could conduct an experiment on a large number of patients diagnosed with lung cancer either a primary or a secondary lung cancer caused by a Fear of Death biological shock. Once it would be determined that the original diagnosis had been correct, namely alveolar lung cancer in each and every case, it could be experimentally proven that the real cause of lung cancer was a Fear of Death biological shock for each and every patient. The patients that can solve their shock will get tuberculosis in the reparation phase and will recover fully. Those that can't will die from cachexia or waste away because of their lung cancer. The five Biological Laws of Nature will apply in each and every case of a patient with alveolar lung cancer.

The result of this experiment would be to conclusively prove that lung cancer is not caused by smoking, but by a Fear of Death biological shock. There would be no need to perform cruel experiments on animals, and try and induce a Fear of Death biological shock in them, so as to prove or disprove this hypothesis. One would also conclude that tuberculosis occurs in the reparation phase and that lung cancer occurs in the conflict-active phase of the same Meaningful Biological Program of Nature – a Fear of Death biological shock.

Lung cancer and tuberculosis and the five Biological Laws of Nature

First Biological Law: The DHS

The DHS is a Fear of Death biological shock. It causes lung cancer in the conflict-active phase and tuberculosis in the reparation phase.

Second, third and fourth Biological Laws

This biological shock causes a lung cancer in the conflict-active phase and tuberculosis in the reparation phase. The reparation phase occurs when there is a resolution of the Fear of Death biological shock. The lung cancer will cause excess alveoli growth everywhere in the lung if it is a Fear of Death biological shock on behalf of yourself. If it is a Fear of Death biological shock on behalf of someone else it will cause a single cluster of excess alveoli growth to occur. These excess growths are removed in the reparation phase by tubercular bacteria.

Fifth Biological Law: The quintessence

The biological benefit of the excess alveoli growth is in the conflict-active phase to enable longer survival times in cases of perceived oxygen deprivation or a Fear of Death biological shock. Alveolar lung cancer is not caused by smoking. It is caused by a Fear of Death biological shock. Alveolar lung cancer does not have to be terminal. Lung cancer is curable. Nobody should die from it.

CHAPTER 30

Breast Cancer

There are two major types of breast cancer: Intra-ductal breast cancer and glandular breast cancer. Glandular breast cancer causes the classic tumour or lump on the breast. Intra-ductal breast cancer causes the affected breast to shrink in the conflict-active phase and to swell up in the reparation phase.

How to detect breast cancer[284]

Breast cancer can be detected when physical changes are noticed in the breasts such as:

1. A change in outline, shape or size of the breast.
2. Puckering or dimpling of the skin.
3. Any lump or thickening in the breast or armpit.
4. Any flaking skin or discharge from the nipple.
5. Unusual pain or discomfort.

Laterality

We have to understand the rules of laterality in relation to breast cancer. To summarise, a right-handed woman will respond to a DHS concerning her mother or a child with her left-breast. She will respond to a DHS concerning her partner, her husband or anyone she considers to be her partner with her right breast. The situation is reversed for a left-handed woman.

Glandular breast cancer

The mammary glands are made up of mesodermal tissue. The brain relay controlling the mammary glands is in the cerebellum. The cerebellum is part of the old-brain. The symptoms of all old-brain conflicts are tumour growth in the conflict-active phase and tumour degradation in the reparation phase.

Breast cancer case study 1: mother-child worry conflict[285]

Mrs Strong is walking on the pavement with her daughter Lisa holding her hand. They are on their way to the summer fun-fair. After what seemed like a long walk to Lisa she suddenly saw a gigantic Ferris wheel. Lisa wanted to get to the fun-fair as quickly as possible. Lisa tore her hand away from her Mammy's firm grip and darted across the road. Mrs Strong could do nothing but look on in horror. She saw a red car bearing down on Lisa and braking loudly. Mrs Strong screamed. The red car hit Lisa and she was flung into the air. When Mrs Strong saw Lisa flung through the air by the red car it was as if she had been hit by a bolt of lightning. She had a biological shock; a mother-child worry conflict and in that split second the Meaningful Biological Program (MBP) for this particular conflict is switched on.

In biological terms, an injured offspring recovers faster when it receives more milk; extra milk production is immediately stimulated by increasing the number of breast gland cells. Even if the woman is not breast feeding, the event still triggers the onset of this response as it has done over millions of years. As long as a woman is in the conflict-active phase (because her child is still in hospital), the breast cells will keep dividing and multiplying to form a glandular breast tumour. The biological benefit is in the conflict-active phase of increased milk production to feed an injured offspring in order to speed up the healing of the injured child.

As soon as the conflict is resolved in a meaningful way for the mother (when Lisa is well again and released from hospital), the tumour immediately stops growing. Since Lisa is out of danger, there is no longer a need to produce extra breast gland cells. During the reparation phase the now superfluous cells are broken down with the help of mycobacteria. The tumour will be completely removed by these microbes with the completion of the healing process.

Breast cancer case study 2: Worry/caring conflict for her own mother[286]

The mother of a Swedish woman called Agnete fainted in Hong Kong in 2002. She had had a stroke and could not speak. Agnete was back home in Sweden and did not hear about this until a few days later. Agnete immediately had a worry conflict for her mother and because she is right-handed she got a tumour growth on her left breast. Agnete was in the conflict-active phase of glandular breast cancer.

Agnete didn't know exactly what was wrong with her mother. She had two young children and could not just leave them. It took her about a week to arrange for the care of her children so that she could fly to Hong Kong. Agnete was in Hong Kong for a week and was able to bring her mother home to Sweden. Her mother recuperated rapidly at home and began to talk again. Agnete's worry or caring conflict for her mother was now over.

A few days after her DHS had been naturally resolved by the recuperation of her mother, Agnete discovered a warm lump in her left breast. Agnete visited the MD and had a mammogram. Agnete was diagnosed with breast cancer and would require immediate chemotherapy. At this time her friend was attending a course given by Harald in Norway. Agnete visited Harald one evening on 25th October 2002 and explained her problem. Harald told her to do nothing; that her lymph nodes might swell in the reparation phase because of the increased metabolism to decompose the tumour but that otherwise she would be ok. Agnete understood the GNM and did nothing. She didn't feel like going to see any MD afterwards to prove the breast cancer had gone away.

Breast cancer case study 3: Death of a sister through chemotherapy[287]

Britt had a younger sister called Anne that she was very close to. Her younger sister had had marriage problems for a number of years. Her husband initiated divorce proceedings against her wishes and divorced her in 2000. Her sister was also diagnosed with breast cancer two months later. Harald did not make case-notes of what type of breast cancer her sister had but deduced that it probably was intraductal breast cancer, in her right breast if she was right-handed caused by the unwanted divorce from her husband. Britt watched her sister deteriorate and eventually die over a six-month period from the chemotherapy administered by the MDs.

Her sister seemed to deteriorate almost every day, both physically and mentally. Britt's conflict was not one of separation from her sister but a conflict of caring for her dying sister hence her glandular breast cancer as opposed to intra-ductal breast cancer.

Britt was 54 years old in 2003. She was right-handed, with a big lump approximately 2–3 cm in her right breast. She had a 90-minute session with Harald in February 2003. She understood her conflict. Her caring conflict was definitively over because her sister was dead. The lump was in her right-breast, and this indicated a partner conflict because she was right-handed.

Britt did nothing. Her caring conflict was over and her lump degraded naturally over a few months.

How Modern Medicine deals with glandular breast cancer

If the lump is large relative to the breast, a mastectomy or removal of the breast may be recommended. If the lump is small relative to the breast, the cancerous lump is removed. After both kinds of operation, as a standard procedure, radiotherapy or chemotherapy is given in order to prevent the reoccurrence of cancer.

The surgeon also removes the lymph nodes from under the woman's arms because there is a medical dogma that cancer is spread to other parts of the body by the lymphatic system.

The lymph nodes located near the breast do swell up when the woman has a tumour in her breast, but this is because of the heightened metabolism and not because the lymph nodes are "spreading cancer" according to the metastasis dogma of Modern Medicine.

Glandular breast cancer and the five Biological Laws of Nature

First Biological Law: The DHS

The biological shock or DHS causing glandular breast cancer is a worry/quarreling/caring conflict.

Second, third and fourth Biological Laws

The glandular tissue in the breast is mesodermal in origin controlled by brain relays in the cerebellum. Consequently, one gets tissue growth in the conflict-active phase and tissue degradation in the reparation phase. The tissue degradation is carried out by bacterial microbes in the reparation phase.

Fifth Biological Law: The quintessence

The biological purpose of the increased tissue growth is to produce extra milk to help the injured partner or child. The lump is a good thing; it proves the woman got a DHS because she really loved the person she was worried about.

She will no longer be afraid of the lump on her breast. Once the conflict is over the tumour will degrade naturally. There is no need for any panic or fear of metastasis or of cancer spreading. She will not be afraid because she understands the reason why she got the lump on her breast. Breast cancer is curable: No woman should die from it.

Intra-ductal breast cancer

The other type of breast cancer is called milk duct or intra-ductal breast cancer. The breast milk ducts have their brain relays in the cerebral cortex and the milk ducts are comprised of tissue from the ectodermal germ layer. They ulcerate in the conflict-active phase.

This type of cancer has to do with a "separation" conflict, if the woman loses her child or her husband. Again, the rules of laterality apply. If the woman is right-handed, a mother-child separation-conflict will result in intra-ductal breast cancer on the left breast. A partner separation-conflict will affect the right breast.

The biological benefit of such a conflict is to cause ulcers in the milk ducts so that the milk ducts become wider in order to aid the discharge of milk that is no longer required biologically speaking for the person that is no longer present. The biological benefit is in the conflict-active phase. Intra-ductal breast cancer causes minor pain in this phase. It is unnoticed by the MDs because they are only looking for tumours or excess growth.

As soon as the separation-conflict is resolved the ulcerated tissue will be replaced. This cell proliferation during the reparation phase is currently termed an "intra-ductal carcinoma". One gets swelling of the pavement-epithelium mucous membrane in the milk duct around the area of the ulcer. Secretion build-up occurs which is unable to move freely because the milk ducts are swollen and blocked.

Intra-ductal breast cancer: Example of the reparation phase[288]

A young, attractive woman with an excellent figure presented to a GNM therapist with her left breast significantly swollen in comparison with the right breast. The oncologists stated that this breast should be removed. In reality, she had solved her separation-conflict and was in the reparation phase. The milk ducts were swollen causing the fluid build-up and hence the swollen appearance of the breast. Dr Hamer suggested that she "milk" the breast regularly, and help it to discharge the excess fluids that had built up in the reparation phase because the milk ducts were swollen and blocked. She got her partner to help and her left breast returned to normal.

Intra-ductal breast cancer: Example of the conflict-active phase[289]

A middle aged woman presented to a GNM therapist with her right breast much smaller than her left breast. The nipple was also inverted on the smaller breast. She had suffered a massive and ongoing separation-conflict on the death of her father seven years earlier. She was clearly still in the conflict-active phase and had not resolved it: Consequently she had a shrinking breast. However disturbing this was to her (and it must have been), she was still alive because she had not suffered any iatrogenic or cancerous treatment.

In this case, if she managed to solve her conflict the shrunken breast would swell up enormously. The reparation phase could potentially cause her worse problems than the shrinking breast in the conflict-active phase. Alternatively, without her solving the separation-conflict, one could with her full consent, carry out surgery and remove the shrunken breast and replace it with an artificial breast. This would be an example where surgery by an MD might still be necessary for aesthetic reasons and because the woman cannot solve this separation-conflict. However, the need for surgery is much reduced once GNM is universally applied.

Breast cancer case study 5: The office manager and the redundant employee[290]

Marianne had worked as an office manager in the same company (a concrete manufacturer and construction company) for over 20 years. She got along well with the man who started the business and was now working well with his son who took over the business in 1992. When the son took over, the business experienced a major downturn and about twenty employees were put onto a short working week and sometimes were unemployed for a few weeks or months at a time.

This grieved her deeply. She regarded all these men as her friends. She gave them their pay-check every month and had a great rapport with all of them. It hurt her deeply that these men had been made redundant. She met some of them while out and about in the town. Many of these men had spent their entire working career with this company and were still working part-time or were unemployed several years later.

The DHS for the office manger was the last conversation she had with these men as they left the company. It hurt her deeply every time and she couldn't talk about it with anybody. The conditions for the DHS were met. She had an intra-ductal breast cancer diagnosed in 1998. She was right-handed and the separation-conflict from the laid-off employees she considered to be her partners had affected her right breast. The breast shrank somewhat and she had a slight pull in the breast.

Her intraductal breast cancer resolved itself when the company experienced an upturn and most of the men were re-hired. Her separation-conflict from these men she considered to be her partners was now definitely over. Her right breast swelled up and became inflamed for a few days.

Marianne met up with Harald initially at a seminar and later at a 90-minute session and understood what had happened. She knew to "milk" her right breast to rid it of the excess milk and that it would normalize within a few days. This she did and she is fine as of June 2007.

Intra-ductal breast cancer and the five Biological Laws of Nature

First Biological Law: The DHS

The biological shock or DHS causing intra-ductal breast cancer is a separation-conflict from a loved one who is torn away from the breast or bosom. If the woman is right-handed, the right breast concerns partner conflicts and the left breast concerns conflicts with her mother or children.

Second, third and fourth Biological Laws

The intra-ductal tissue in the breast is ectodermal in origin as are all ductal tissue. The brain relay controlling breast ducts are in the cerebral cortex. The stricken breast shrinks in the conflict-active phase and swells up in the reparation phase.

Fifth Biological Law: The quintessence

The biological purpose of the widening ducts is in the conflict-active phase to enable the flow of milk that is not required because of separation from the partner or mother/child.

Once the woman understands GNM and, more importantly, that her breast cancer occurred because of an event that had occurred in her life, which she can deal with and solve herself, she will have nothing to fear.

No woman will fear breast cancer once she understands it. Breast cancer is curable. No woman should die from it.

CHAPTER 31

Prostate Cancer

The prostate is a small gland situated behind the bladder in men. It produces an alkaline liquid. This liquid is alkaline and it allows the semen to survive better the acidic path to the woman's ovaries.

Symptoms of prostate cancer[291]

The first sign of prostate cancer is difficulty in urinating, either increased frequency or difficulty maintaining a full stream.

The symptoms are caused by a growth of cells pushing against the urethra, the thin tube which links the bladder to the penis.

Other symptoms of prostate cancer include:

1. Painful urination or ejaculation.
2. Blood in urine or semen.
3. Pain in lower back, hips or thighs.

Detection of prostate cancer[292]

There are three main methods of detecting prostate cancer.

1. A digital rectal examination, in which a gloved finger is inserted into the rectum, through which an enlarged prostate can be felt.
2. Blood tests will detect the levels of certain chemicals in the blood which are known to increase because of prostate cancer. These are known as tumour-markers by the MDs.
3. More sophisticated techniques like ultrasound scans and X-rays.

Prostate cancer case study 1: The French colonel and his granddaughter[293]

A French colonel called AD was diagnosed by an MD in Marseilles with prostate cancer. His daughter had heard about GNM and phoned

Harald Baumann in 1997 and asked him what caused prostate cancer. Harald explained that prostate cancer was always caused by an ugly-sexual conflict with a strong territorial aspect. He enquired about relations with the colonel's wife, the mother of this woman. She reported that relations were fine, that her father had never had an affair nor had he ever been with a prostitute. She took real offence at this type of question as one could imagine. But Harald was just trying to ascertain the nature of the ugly-sexual conflict. After a few phone calls and further explanations of the causes of prostate cancer, the daughter herself had a possible idea of the cause of this ugly-sexual conflict.

The colonel had served in the French army fighting against the Algerian freedom fighters during their war of independence from 1955–1962. The colonel deeply resented the defeat of the French by the Arabs in Algeria. The woman's daughter got along extremely well with her grandfather. They were very close. One day she arrived at his house with her husband-to-be. He was a French-Arab of Algerian decent. The colonel was horrified. He couldn't accept that his beloved granddaughter would be sleeping with, marrying and having children with the enemy that he had a terrible time fighting for many years. He couldn't talk with the granddaughter nor with his own daughter about this. The conditions of the DHS were met, particularly the isolative aspect of the DHS, which is an important characteristic of the DHS.

The mother talked with her daughter and explained to her the conflict that had caused the prostate cancer for her grandfather. Harald does not know how much the granddaughter really loved this French-Arab guy, but in any event she visited her grandfather, and assured her grandfather that she would not marry him. This greatly pleased her grandfather. His ugly-sexual conflict had reached a definite solution: He was now in the reparation phase. The granddaughter ended up marrying a man her grandfather approved of, so there would be no repeat of this particular ugly-sexual conflict. The colonel's prostate cancer disappeared once the ugly-sexual conflict had been solved.

Prostate cancer case study 2: Rolf and his young girlfriend[294]

Rolf was a man in his mid-60s. His wife had died a few months earlier. He met a woman twenty years younger than him in 1989. They fell in love and moved in together. Two years later she left him for another man a couple of years older than her. Rolf got an ugly-sexual conflict because this other man was having sex with the woman he still counted as his partner. He did not like this: It was an ugly-sexual conflict.

Rolf had already taken an interest in GNM prior to getting prostate cancer. He had attended two or three seminars given by Harald. He understood the cause of his cancer very quickly. The solution for Rolf was to get another girlfriend, thereby forgetting about his previous girlfriend and thus not really caring about whom she was sleeping with. This might sound callous and pragmatic but it was a real solution for Rolf's prostate cancer.

This he managed to do and his prostate returned to normal health and he has no further problems with his prostate.

Ugly-Sexual conflict MBP

The Ugly-Sexual MBP results in prostate cancer in the conflict-active phase. The reparation phase of an ugly-sexual conflict results in a condition called prostatitis, which is simply an inflamed prostate.The man has probably been suffering quietly for a while and, although having solved the biological shock, eventually visits the MD because he is still having problems. He is usually told that he has got an inflamed prostate caused by some phantom virus. All he has to do is wait a while more and the prostate will go back to its normal size and all will be well.

The grandfather did not like a person he considered to be his enemy being his beautiful granddaughter's husband. Rolf did not like another man sleeping with his ex-partner. The ugly-sexual conflict almost always has a territorial aspect. Somebody I don't like is sleeping with my wife, ex-wife, ex-partner, daughter, granddaughter, or niece.

Prostate Cancer and the five Biological Laws of Nature

First Biological Law: The DHS

The DHS or biological shock causing prostate cancer is always an ugly-sexual conflict with a strong territorial aspect. To put it bluntly, someone I don't like is having sex with my ex-girlfriend, ex-wife, daughter, niece or granddaughter and I don't like it. Another possibility would be for an older man married to a younger woman to get a DHS concerning his ability to father children and get prostate cancer because this would be an ugly-sexual conflict.

Second, third and fourth Biological Laws

The prostate gland expands in the conflict-active phase and contracts in the reparation phase. The symptoms are prostate cancer in the conflict-active phase and prostatitis in the reparation phase.

Fifth Biological Law: The quintessence

The biological purpose of prostate cancer is in the conflict-active phase. The biological purpose is to produce more of the alkaline liquid so that the semen can survive the acidic path toward the fallopian tube and the ovaries. The man is now more capable of having children, because his sperm can better survive in the acidic surroundings of the womb.

No man will fear prostate cancer once he understands it. He can solve the biological conflict that caused it. Prostate cancer is curable: No man should die from it.

CHAPTER 32

Colon Cancer

Colon cancer may also be called bowel cancer, rectal or colorectal cancer.

Symptoms of colon cancer[295]

The symptoms of colon cancer include:

1. Rectal bleeding.
2. A persistent feeling of needing to empty your bowels even after a visit to the bathroom.
3. Abdominal pain.

If these symptoms persist for a few weeks most people would visit their local MD.

Detection of colon cancer[296]

There are three methods of detecting colon cancer:

1. A "rectal examination" is carried out by the MD to check for any abnormal changes by inserting a gloved finger in the rectum.
2. A colonoscopy is performed in order to further investigate these symptoms. This involves inserting a probe into the bowel. It has a tiny camera on the end which allows the MD to look for cancerous areas on the bowel wall.
3. Sometimes a dye which shows up on X-rays is injected into the lower bowel to help MDs spot signs of cancers.

Colon cancer case study 1: Right-of-way dispute – colon cancer[297]

A woman lived with her husband in her parent's house in a rural area of Switzerland. Their neighbour for many decades was an old woman with whom they got along very well. They bought a parcel of land from the old lady on the other side of her house so that they could build a new house. However they needed to pave a small dirt-track that she owned, so they could have a proper paved driveway into their house. This was verbally agreed to, but there was nothing legally agreed.

The old woman kept a handful of geese around the house. The husband of the woman who was building this new house complained out-loud one day about the smell of the geese that belonged to their neighbour. The neighbour overheard this complaint and took huge offense at it. She refused to allow them to have access to her right-of-way. In order to annoy them she bought many more geese and the resultant smell was significantly worse.

Built to her exact specifications, the new house was the dream home for the woman. The fact that she couldn't properly access the house became an ugly-indigestible anger conflict for her. It's an archaic program. The colon is the large intestine. She couldn't digest this morsel of indigestible anger: Anger with the old woman; anger with the authorities; anger with her lawyer; anger because she couldn't have her dream home the way she wanted it.

She couldn't absorb this indigestible anger because the neighbour would not give her a proper paved access to the house. Every time she thought about this house, she got angry because she couldn't reach it comfortably by car. They initiated legal action to gain legal access to this right-of-way but this took a long time to achieve.

In the meantime she was diagnosed with colon cancer. The tumour grew in the large intestine/colon with the biological purpose of producing more intestinal digestive juices so as to be able to digest this large morsel of indigestible anger.

Anger is in the transposed sense like a morsel of indigestible food, from a biological viewpoint. An area for genuine medical research would be to establish which part of the colon is responsible for an indigestible anger conflict with family members, enemies, government, or other authorities.

She had an operation to remove part of the tumour and went to recuperate at her brother's home in Canada. While there she was fine and was recovering nicely. As soon as she returned home to Switzerland, she got back on to the track of the morsel that she could not digest; her indigestible anger at not being able to digest the fact that she had no proper paved access to her newly-built dream home. She was back on the tracks of the metaphorical morsel that she had swallowed but could not digest, and the tumour continued to grow in her colon. She had another round of chemotherapy and another operation.

At this stage, she visited Harald and explained her story. Harald advised her to immediately sell the house and forget the entire business of her dream home. She died because she couldn't solve her problem; she couldn't get the right-of-way legally established to her new house. This was achieved about a year after she died, but she was now dead and for what?

I tell this story as possibly another failure of GNM, but it is not at all a failure. She couldn't solve her biological conflict and she died. The tumour kept growing to enable her to solve this biological shock of an indigestible morsel, which in a transposed sense is an ugly-indigestible-anger morsel. She couldn't digest this morsel and she died.

Colon cancer case study 2: The gambling son[298]

A father was comfortably off with three grown-up sons and he loved them all equally. Two of them were independent and caused no concern to their father. The third son, Willi, was a gambler and spendthrift and everyone in the village in which they lived in Switzerland knew this, and knew that his wealthy father would pay off his debts. He paid off his debts once and then again and again.

This caused him a DHS; an ugly-indigestible-anger conflict. Why should he pay off his son's gambling debts? They were his son's problems. He never told his other two sons about this issue because this would have created a problem with them. He didn't tell anybody and the conditions for the DHS were met.

He had the usual symptoms of a colon cancer and went to the MD. The diagnosis was colon cancer with a recommended course of chemotherapy to decrease the size of the tumour. Fortunately he had heard about Harald from his seminars and came for a consultation. Harald explained why he got the tumour and the man understood immediately.

He solved his conflict very simply. Willi would have to survive financially on his own. He had had a bad conscience about helping out the errant son at the expense of the other two worthy sons. He would give his other two sons the same amount of money that he had given to his spendthrift son.

The father's tumour regressed after he had solved his ugly-indigestible-anger conflict and stayed off the tracks of it repeating again. He was healthy again. In the meantime and coincidentally, Willi learned his lesson, got a good job, stopped gambling and was able to survive independently.

Colon cancer case study 3: The complaining husband[299]

A married couple in their 80s had lived happily together for many, many years. However, in the last few years the husband had taken to constantly criticizing his wife, Annie. Annie had forgotten to do something or didn't do it right. She was an excellent housewife and in effect mothered her husband so in reality he had nothing much to complain about. However in his eyes, she always did something wrong and he criticized her in front of their adult children and other visitors to the house. It was an embarrassing and uncomfortable spectacle. At some point, this had become an ugly-indigestible-anger conflict for Annie. She must have gotten a shock or DHS from some remark of her husband complaining about something or other.

She was in the conflict-active phase and the cancer in the colon was growing but she hadn't noticed it. In the meantime her husband of 54 years had died. This was naturally a sad time for her and she grieved deeply for her husband. However her ugly-indigestible-anger conflict was now over. She did not have to listen to any more unwarranted criticism from him; she was not drawn back onto the tracks of this conflict on a daily basis.

A few weeks after he died, she noticed something strange with her stool. Her daughter, an expert in the New Medicine, immediately knew that she had flushed out the remains of her colon cancer tumour. She told her mother not to worry about anything. The old lady is hale and hearty in her 80s and continues to live a contented life unaware that she had ever had colon cancer.

Colon Cancer and the five Biological Laws of Nature

First Biological Law: The DHS

The DHS for a cancer in the colon is an ugly-indigestible-anger. Something has happened that you just can't take in; you cannot accept it; you cannot digest this morsel because it is from an ugly-indigestible-anger conflict.

Second, third and fourth Biological Laws

The colon is endodermal in origin, which means that there is tumour growth in the conflict-active phase and there is tumour degradation in the reparation phase. The microbes involved in the reparation phase are fungi and bacteria.

Fifth Biological Law: The quintessence

The biological purpose of the growing tumour for all organs comprised of endodermal tissue such as the lining of the colon or the large intestine is in the conflict-active phase. The biological purpose of the growing tumour inside the colon is to produce more digestive juices in order to better digest this large morsel of food. This archaic program lasting for millions of years is now transposed into an ugly-indigestible-anger tumour that we must mentally and spiritually digest.

This fifth Biological Law reassures us that you didn't get colon cancer for no particular reason but because of a particular type of biological shock with the theme of an ugly-indigestible-anger conflict. Once we solve this conflict, and can mentally and spiritually digest this morsel of ugly-indigestible-anger, our tumour will start to decrease.

You no longer fear colon cancer because you understand it. You can solve the conflict that caused it and reverse the tumour growth. Colon cancer is curable: Nobody should die from it.

CHAPTER 33

Heart attacks

There are two types of heart attacks, a myocardial heart attack and a normal regular heart attack. They have distinct causes.

Myocardial heart attack

The type of conflict causing a myocardial heart attack is when the person feels himself to be overwhelmed, under constant and intense pressure and has a feeling of being completely over-burdened.

In the conflict-active phase, the striated heart muscle or myocardium undergoes necrosis or it weakens. In the reparation phase of such a feeling of being completely over-burdened, the striated heart-muscle strengthens. A myocardial heart infarction or myocardial heart attack is initiated in the EC (Epileptoid Crisis), or the mid-point of the reparation phase, when the striated heart muscle suddenly weakens and beats much slower than normal. You don't seem to get enough air, and you are constantly short of breath, and you feel completely exhausted. A myocardial infarction is directed by the brain (specifically the cerebral medulla), in a similar manner to all cancers and other diseases.

Athletes and myocardial heart attacks

There have been a number of cases of athletes dying while running. Invariably when the white-coats do a post-mortem they say that it was a case of "faulty heart-valves" and then ask for money for "research" into the cause of the faulty heart-valves.

In reality, these athletes must have suffered a myocardial infarction, and because they were in the middle of a football match or a run, they felt obliged to keep on going, and felt they were capable for it, but they died from the myocardial infarction and not from a faulty valve.

Normal heart attack

The biological shock causing a heart attack is one of a territorial-loss conflict. The brain relays controlling the heart's arteries and veins are located in the cerebral cortex. The normal rules of laterality apply for all cerebral cortex conflicts. If a right-handed male has no ongoing MBPs (Meaningful Biological Programs) and gets a territorial conflict, it would impact the brain relay on the right-side of the cerebral cortex that controls the coronary arteries. He also becomes immediately depressed and undergoes a personality change.

In the case of a left-handed male, the exact same territorial conflict will impact the brain relay on the left-side of the cerebral cortex that controls the coronary veins, which results in the individual becoming manic or restless. The biological purpose of having this excess energy is to enable the left-handed male to solve his territorial conflict by constant action and activity whereas the right-handed male will become depressed, dull, sad and dejected.

The situation is reversed for women, with a right-handed female responding to the same territorial conflict like a left-handed man and a left-handed woman responding like a right-handed man. This is complex but this is how all cerebral cortex biological shocks work.

I will illustrate a territorial-loss conflict MBP for a right-handed male in order to keep it as simple as possible. A right-handed male with no ongoing biological shocks gets a biological shock concerning his territory. The right-side of his cerebral cortex is affected and the brain relay controlling his coronary arteries is now in the conflict-active phase: the brain relay is viewable on a CT scan and is in the target configuration. The right-handed male's arteries widen by ulceration in the conflict-active phase of a territorial conflict, so that more blood flows through the arteries, providing his heart muscle with more blood, giving him more energy, so that he has the ability to win back his territory. If the territorial conflict is intense enough he will get angina pectoris in the conflict-active phase.

In the reparation phase, the ulcers in the coronary arteries are replenished. In doing this replenishment, or refilling of the ulcers, the organism overcompensates for the ulcers that occurred in the conflict-active phase. This is called arterio-sclerosis by the MDs. The critical point for all territorial conflicts is in the middle of the reparation phase; the Epileptic Crisis (EC). This is when the heart attack or the stroke occurs.

The severity of the heart attack depends on its conflict mass. If the conflict mass has been built up sufficiently the person will die of a heart attack in the middle of the reparation phase.

Heart attack case study 1: Harald Baumann's myocardial heart infarction[300]

All Swiss males have to do compulsory military service. Harald Baumann was a Captain in the Swiss Army in charge of a company of 240 men in 1980–1981.

Harald spent 9 months full-time with the Swiss Army over a one-year period in 1980–1981 at the age of 31. He returned home every Saturday night and was back on duty on Sunday night. He did not sleep more than four hours any night while on duty. He only got the normal eight hours sleep every Saturday night at home.

On his last day of military service on the 4th July 1981, Harald was absolutely relieved that it was all over. The crushing burden of military service had been removed from him. Life could go back to normal. He was driving home to St Gallen, a drive of about 240 km, when he pulled over because of tiredness. He had done this before and had intended to cat-nap for fifteen minutes so that he could complete the journey safely.

Harald slept for six hours instead of fifteen minutes. Harald arrived home very late. His wife and children had already eaten. Harald sat down at the kitchen table and prepared to eat his dinner. He started trembling; it felt as if ants were crawling all over his body. He had cold extremities: cold hands and cold feet. Harald thought he had had it. He couldn't eat his dinner. Harald had had a myocardial heart infarction. Harald drank a glass of water and went to bed. He slept almost non-stop for thirty-six hours.

Harald left with his family two days later than planned for their vacation in Nice, France. While on vacation, Harald still felt bad and was short of breath. He flew home less than a week into their three-week vacation to Switzerland for an appointment with an MD.

The MD luckily misdiagnosed a nervous breakdown, and told Harald to take it easy for the next few months and he would be fine. If the MD had correctly diagnosed a myocardial heart infarction, Harald would have probably had an operation to insert a pacemaker.

Harald took no medication for his heart nor for his "nervous breakdown". He was still able to work but he had absolutely no energy at all. It took him a year to get back to his normal physical abilities. It took a year for his heart muscle to return to its full strength and for his heart beat to return to normal.

Heart attack case study 2: The Dutch cook/acupuncturist[301]

A Dutch chef called Hans is married to a Swiss woman Melanie. He worked as a chef during the week. Now in his forties, he wasn't happy with his career as a chef. He studied acupuncture and shiatsu in the evenings with a view to becoming a registered therapist. To pay for his studies, he also had to work Saturdays in a supermarket, where he dished out hot lunches to customers.

Hans felt himself to be under tremendous pressure. He didn't enjoy his work during the weeks as a chef, but he didn't find it a tremendous burden either. He found his night classes to be a tremendous burden, particularly the upcoming examination in December 2006 to become a registered therapist. He also found his Saturday job to be extremely difficult. It was a tremendous burden for him to give the customers their hot lunches and talk with them.

He successfully did his final exams in December 2006 to become a state-registered acupuncturist and shiatsu therapist. His last day in the supermarket was a Saturday before Christmas 2006. These two tasks that had been a tremendous burden to him were now over.

Three weeks later in January 2007, he had a myocardial infarction at a party. He fainted and woke up at the hospital. They kept him there for a week. He slept for almost the entire time. He took a three-week holiday to help him recover.

He started work as a therapist in February 2007. Harald has recommended that he take it easy and not to take on too much work and to work at a pace that he feels comfortable for him. He is following Harald's advice.

Preventing a fatal heart attack

When the knowledge of German New Medicine becomes universally available, its major impact will be in preventative medicine. Universal knowledge will enable us to take control of our health and our lives. People will still get biological shocks, but they will have the ability to deal with them effectively in order to prevent them becoming serious or fatal. The following story typifies an idyllic world, when the person concerned realises they have a severe territorial conflict, and takes the measures necessary to solve the conflict before it becomes fatal.

Heart attack case study 3: The businessman and his mild heart attack[302]

A successful Swiss businessman called Walter had been the managing director of a concrete manufacturer in the canton of Zurich for about thirty years. He had built the company up from one factory with 30 employees to its later size of several factories with more than 500 employees. The major shareholder was a man twenty years his senior with whom he had a very good relationship. This man owned the majority of the shares. The rest of the shares were owned by various individuals.

By 1999, Walter had every right to be happy with himself. He had a happy home life. His wife Margaret was a homeopath and they had two grown-up children who were doing well. He had been very successful professionally, and was proud of this company, which he regarded as his own, although he was not a shareholder. He was 55 years old and he was extremely healthy. Life couldn't be better.

The major shareholder, who was about 75 years old, wanted to hand it on to his sons. The sons weren't willing to take it over. In October 1999, the major shareholder called in a firm of management consultants, whose brief was to split up the company and sell. His sons were in favour of this strategy. Walter would have to give up the entire company that he had spent most of his working-life developing. Walter didn't want to start afresh. Walter was naturally opposed to any such decision. The sons wanted him fired so they could pursue their "asset-stripping" strategy.

Walter got a biological shock, a DHS that he was going to lose his company, his territory, his "baby" that he had built up over a large number of years. He decided to fight back to see if he could persuade the other shareholders to back him. But from the get-go his plan was already doomed.

Luckily Walter and his wife Margaret, a homeopath with a natural interest in "alternative medicine" or medicine outside the mainstream, had attended a seminar given by Harald about three months into Walter's conflict. They attended another seminar and then asked Harald for a consultation.

Walter is right-handed. Consequently his territorial-loss conflict affected his right brain hemisphere and therefore his coronary arteries.

He had already experienced severe chest-pain or angina pectoris and Walter knew from Harald's seminar that this was the symptom of a territorial-loss conflict in the conflict-active phase.

Walter and Margaret came to Harald with a brain CT scan (as recommended by Harald) for a consultation in early 2000. In one session, Harald was able to predict that Walter would have a severe but not fatal heart attack because he had already had an intense territorial conflict lasting for more than three months.

Walter was a decisive man. He retired immediately. He immediately solved his territorial conflict. He had negotiated a good pension and a lump-sum payment. This money was now his territory and was under his total control. The company that he had managed for thirty years was no longer part of his territory. It was in the distant past. He had definitively solved his territorial conflict. He had moved on for the good of his health. He could now fully devote his time to his wife, children, grandchildren and his new passion, German New Medicine.

Three weeks after solving his territorial conflict he had a massive heart attack. He was sitting down when it occurred. It was as if a thunderstorm was going on in his head and he felt massive pressure on his chest. Despite these terrible symptoms, he wasn't afraid. He feared going to hospital. He feared getting an infusion or drip because he knew that it would prolong the EC crisis and potentially cause a fatal heart attack. He was not afraid of the heart attack itself and neither was his wife, but he was afraid of going into a hospital. He stayed at home and weathered it. Slowly he recovered from his heart attack and he is now living a very active retirement today. Walter and his entire family are enthusiastic supporters of the German New Medicine.

Myocardial heart attacks and the five Biological Laws of Nature

First Biological Law: The DHS

The DHS for a heart attack is a feeling of being completely overwhelmed, of having way too much to do, and not enough time to do it, in most cases, or being cheated by somebody in other cases. This feeling has lasted for a long time.

Second, third and fourth Biological Laws

In the conflict-active phase of this conflict, the heart muscle weakens because it is overburdened. This is usually not noticed. In the first half of the reparation phase, the heart muscle strengthens itself. During the EC in the middle of the reparation phase, the heart muscle suddenly weakens again. This is what is called a myocardial infarction.

Fifth Biological Law: The quintessence

The biological purpose of a myocardial infarction or feeling of being completely overwhelmed and overburdened is in the reparation phase. It causes the heart muscle to be strengthened so that it can better withstand such intense and ongoing strain into the future.

Regular heart attacks and the five Biological Laws of Nature

First Biological Law: The DHS

The DHS for a heart attack is a territorial-loss conflict. It is an actual loss of territory as opposed to a "fear of loss of territory" which causes bronchial cancer.

Second, third and fourth Biological Laws

The arteries ulcerate during the conflict-active phase of a territorial conflict for a right-handed male. If the conflict is intense enough, angina pectoris is the result. The arteries refill themselves in the reparation phase. A heart attack occurs in the middle of the reparation phase during the EC if the conflict has built up enough mass.

Fifth Biological Law: The quintessence

The biological purpose of a territorial conflict is in the conflict-active phase. For example, the arteries of a right-handed man ulcerate in the conflict-active phase so that more blood flows into the heart and then through the body, which optimizes performance and gives the man the strength and energy required to win back his territory. A heart attack occurs in the middle of the reparation phase (EC).

You no longer fear a heart attack because you understand it. You can solve the conflict that caused it. You can take measures to prevent the reoccurrence of future heart attacks. Heart attacks are preventable: Nobody should die unnecessarily from a heart attack.

CHAPTER 34

Allergies

According to Modern Medicine, an allergy is an adverse reaction to an allergen—such as nuts or pollen—in our environment. These allergens are normally harmless to other individuals. The body reacts to allergens by releasing histamine from cells in our skin, lungs, nose or intestine, which causes inflammation. The symptoms might be itchy skin, tissue swelling or wheezing, and can lead to full-blown anaphylaxis and even death.[303]

Allergies provide further evidence about the craziness and inane stupidity of Modern Medicine. Why should a small group of people be allergic to certain substances like nuts or milk or eggs or to animals like dogs or cats? Are these people deficient in some way? Has God or Mother Nature failed these people in a cruel and heartless manner?

German New Medicine has an entirely different understanding of allergies. When a biological shock or DHS occurs, the human organism subconsciously picks up on certain things in the environment that were present when the DHS occurred. Clearly our body has a special ability to sense things like nuts, milk, eggs, cats, or dogs, and if any of these are present when a biological shock occurs, every time we encounter these items our body goes back onto the tracks of the original DHS. In the reparation phase of this track or if you will, a repeated biological shock or DHS to our subconscious, we get the symptoms known as an allergy such as a runny nose or rashes. These symptoms are to remind us that something bad occurred in a similar situation in the past and we should avoid these circumstances at all costs.

Allergy case study 1: The cow in the backyard[304]

A young five-year-old boy named Willy lived in the countryside in the canton of Appenzell in Switzerland. One summer's day in 1995 he was out playing in the back garden, in a sand-pit on his own. It was very windy, but he was very happily playing. A gust of wind caught him momentarily off-guard and when he looked around he saw an enormous cow in the back garden. His DHS was the biological shock at the sudden appearance of this huge cow. He screamed but was paralysed and couldn't move. Fortunately his older brother went outside, chased the cow away, and brought his brother into the house.

The shock must have been very strong because since then, he was allergic to cows, specifically cow-hair, and to certain pollen that were in the garden at the time.

He had it for about three years and received a mouth spray for acute situations. His parents had heard about Harald by word of mouth. They had a single 90-minute session with Harald around 1999.

Harald recommended a solution that would involve Willy playing with cows, going to a milking parlour and meeting with many cows, talking to them, saying moo-moo, touching one cow, stroking it and making friends with it. In this way the allergy could be solved. He would no longer associate cows with the biological shock he had and would no longer be allergic to cows.

The parents never came back to Harald. Harald does not know if they implemented his ideas, but the principles are the same for all allergies. Once you have no fear of the particular allergen and do not mentally associate it (even if subconsciously) with the event that caused your original biological shock, you can overcome your allergy.

Allergy case study 2: The nut allergy[305]

There is a compelling story on a GNM web-site about a German woman who overcame her allergy to nuts.

Ottilie did not even know that she was allergic to nuts, let alone that she had a general food allergy, until she went on a two-week vacation to China with her husband Leo in April 1994. While there she noticed that she didn't have mouth ulcers, this terrible allergy that had afflicted her all her life. When she came home she was convinced that her allergic reaction was in response to some kind of food. She then wrote down everything she ate. She examined the ingredients of what she was eating and came to the conclusion that the allergy got bad every time she ate nuts. She stopped eating nuts and told all her friends and relations that she had a nut allergy so that nobody would provide her with any food containing nuts. Ottilie had solved a problem that had afflicted her all her adult life. The symptoms of this nut allergy were severe mouth ulcers. These symptoms had adversely affected the quality of her life.

Ottilie came across the German New Medicine through a friend who lent her a few books written by Dr Hamer. She read them and understood GNM and, in particular, she understood that allergies are caused by the occurrence of a biological shock while the body picks up on all the surrounding circumstances. In her case, she was convinced that she must have had a biological shock while she was eating nuts. But Ottilie simply couldn't think of a shock that had occurred while she was eating nuts. Ottilie racked her brains, discussed it with her husband, but still couldn't think of any experience that would have caused a shock while in the presence of nuts.

Ottilie woke suddenly one night as if from a dream and remembered. When she was a young girl in the autumn of 1946 or 1947, their family were living with their grandparents. She and her sister were strictly forbidden to take the then ripe nuts from a nut-tree belonging to a neighbour because this neighbour was a difficult, fussy old woman.

Both Ottilie and her elder sister went out to the neighbour's backyard and took care to ensure that neither this fussy old woman nor their grandmother or mother could see them. They took the nuts and went back into their own garden and then threw them into the neighbour's garden to annoy her. The fussy old lady noticed this and opened her window and complained. Almost simultaneously her mother noticed what had occurred, and was furious, and called both daughters indoors. They were whacked by their mother and she threatened to kill them if they ever went near that nut-tree again.

It is interesting that Ottilie's sister, who was five years older, did not get a DHS in the exact same situation and had no subsequent allergy to nuts. This illustrates the wonder and the mystery of the human psyche. What causes a DHS for one person has no effect on another person. Ottilie told her then 90-year-old mother and her sister about the suspected cause of her allergy and both of them remembered the incident.

Every time Ottilie ate nuts after the incident, she came back on the tracks of the original biological shock. Her body warned her about this by responding with her allergic symptoms which occur in the reparation phase of this biological shock. Unfortunately she didn't know for many years that her body was responding to her eating nuts.

Ottilie had visited various MDs over the years. The first MD thought it was because of a vitamin B deficiency. An MD who was a professor at a skin clinic gave her a tincture and when that didn't work said it must be "genetic" even though there was no history of nut allergies in the family. The diagnosis of a "genetic" disease is the final admission that Modern Medicine can do no more for you. Over the years Ottilie tried everything all sorts of lotions and potions but nothing had worked.

Ottilie now knew the cause of her allergy beyond doubt. Two weeks after recalling the incident that had caused her allergy, she bought herself a bag of peanuts. She looked at them all day. That evening Ottilie told her husband Leo that she would eat the peanuts and nothing bad would happen because she wouldn't get whacked by her now 90-year-old mother or the long since deceased fussy old lady who owned the nut-tree.

With mixed feelings she opened the shell of the nut and ate both peanuts. She opened two or three more and ate the peanuts and repeated mentally to herself that nothing more should happen. She felt the inside of her mouth to be almost burning and noticed a dark red spot inside it. She got angry and looked at herself in the mirror and said this cannot happen again. The next day, the red spots were gone. She ate peanuts again, but no more spots appeared, and there were no more mouth ulcers.

Ottilie now eats all sorts of nuts with no allergic reaction. She had overcome the particular allergen, nuts, that were present when she had her biological shock. Ottilie had suffered these painful mouth ulcers for nearly fifty years but finally it was all over. She is very grateful to Dr Hamer that she is free from this terrible affliction.

Allergies and the Five Biological Laws of Nature

First Biological Law: The DHS

The person originally experienced a biological shock or DHS. The person subconsciously remembers the DHS and all the circumstances surrounding the DHS. Every time the person encounters any substance that was present during this biological shock, he gets a repeated DHS which is experienced subconsciously and which is immediately solved because there is no actual shock. In the reparation phase, the person gets the symptoms we call an allergy.

Second, third and fourth Biological Laws

Allergies are always linked to the original DHS that caused them. The repeated DHS occurs because of the recurrence of the allergen that was present when the original DHS occurred.

Fifth Biological Law: The quintessence

The biological purpose of an allergy is to remind us that we previously got a biological shock with the same allergens present. Our body is telling us to avoid doing whatever it is we're doing because we experienced a DHS in similar circumstances in the past.

Allergies are not a failure of Mother Nature, rather they can be regarded as an alarm bell which reminds us that something bad happened in the past when a particular substance or allergen or animal was present. Mother Nature is warning us to get away fast, or something similar might happen again. Animals do this instinctively, but civilized man has lost this ability.

Once we understand the DHS or the surrounding circumstances that caused the allergy, we can take steps to overcome our allergy. The allergen (what we are allergic to) did not cause the DHS. It was merely present when the DHS occurred. Your life does not have to be afflicted by your allergy. You can take measures to get rid of your allergy. Allergies can be overcome with patience and are reversible. Allergies are curable: Nobody should have their life blighted unnecessarily for years by them.

CHAPTER 35

Multiple Sclerosis (MS)

According to Modern Medicine, multiple sclerosis (MS) is a degenerative disease. According to the German New Medicine, MS occurs in the conflict-active phase and in the EC (middle of the reparation phase) of a particular type of biological shock. The brain relay controlling these muscle movements are in the cerebral cortex. In the conflict-active phase, instead of getting cancer you get what Dr Hamer calls a "cancer-equivalent" disease such as MS. By this all he means is that the disease works exactly like all cancers according to the five Biological Laws of Nature. In the case of MS during the conflict-active phase, you lose the ability to run, walk, or move your arms. In other words, you suffer a "functional-loss" instead of a cancer. In the terminology of GNM, MS is a cancer-equivalent disease. In the reparation phase, you regain your motor ability. MS does not have to be a one-track road to despair, decay and death. MS, like any other disease or cancer, is reversible and curable.

The causes of MS are biological shocks relating to events with themes such as: Not knowing what to do in a particular situation; not being able to keep up with someone; not being able to run away from or get away from someone or something; not being able to hold someone back; or feeling trapped by someone or something.

MS case study 1: I can't shoot the thieves[306]

In the following case study the biological shock leading to MS had a theme of: Not being able to execute a desired movement.

A Swiss man named Walter was at his home in a rural part of the canton of Aargau with his wife Sylvia and their ten-year-old son one weekday morning. Their seventeen-year-old daughter was away at college. Walter was a wealthy man with a printing business. He normally had a large sum of money in his current account.

Walter was a sharp-shooter in the Swiss Army. He went shooting regularly with Sylvia, it was a hobby that they both enjoyed. Walter could accurately hit a target at up to 1 km distance. Like all active and reserve Swiss Army members, he kept a rifle at home.

One weekday morning in 1999, there was a knock at the door. His ten-year-old answered it. Two armed men burst through and pointed a gun at Walter's son's head. They tied up his wife and their young son in the kitchen.[307] Walter was obliged to go to his bank with one of the thieves and withdraw around SF90,000 (€50,000) while the other guarded his wife and son. The security cameras in the bank were not working properly, a fact which must have been known to the thieves. They returned to the villa and Walter was shut in the cellar. Sylvia and son were still tied up in the kitchen. The thieves then set off, delighted with their success.

Hearing them leave the house, Walter slammed the cellar door open and quickly untied the ropes holding Sylvia and his son. Walter ran over to his rifle cabinet, unlocked it, took out his loaded rifle and ran outside onto the terrace.

He had a full view of the thieves running down a country lane. He raised the rifle and sighted it. He was just about to shoot the thieves when Sylvia pulled the rifle down preventing him from shooting them.

This was an enormous shock for him. He had the thieves in sight. All he had to do was press the trigger but he was prevented from doing so by his wife of twenty-two years. He probably would not have shot them in the back. He doesn't really know because he was never given the opportunity to shoot. He thinks he would have aimed above their heads and had some fun shooting at them, scaring them. This is what Walter believes to this day, but he doesn't really know.

Sylvia clearly acted in good faith. She knew her husband was an excellent shot and that if he had shot the thieves in the back he would have been jailed for murder. She did not want him to go to jail for killing these two thieves.

Walter and Sylvia had previously discussed many times what they would do if they were robbed. They had agreed that they would fight back. Walter felt an acute sense of betrayal by Sylvia in preventing him from shooting at the thieves. Sylvia wouldn't let him shoot at the thieves who had invaded their home, threatened their son in such a vicious manner and robbed them. And they had previously agreed that this is exactly what they would do.

Two or three days later Walter found that his motor movements were slightly impaired. They became progressively worse and worse. Within three months he was unable to move his arms at all and could not feed himself. He was dependent on his wife Sylvia to feed him.

Every time Walter saw his wife, he felt an acute sense of betrayal even though Sylvia had done the right thing. Walter was on the tracks of his original DHS every time he saw Sylvia.

This is clearly a vicious circle. Walter felt betrayed by his wife Sylvia, which caused his MS. Sylvia was now feeding him, and the constant presence of Sylvia, and the fact that he was now dependent on her to feed him, reinforced his DHS, which made his MS worse and worse.

Walter knew Arlette Büchel through some business dealings. Arlette must have spoken of Harald's work with the German New Medicine and Walter had remembered that conversation.

In February 2000, Walter came to see Harald for a single 90-minute session. Harald explained the types of biological shocks causing MS and Walter told Harald about the recent robbery. They discussed it and Walter understood immediately that this betrayal by his wife (as he saw it) had caused his MS.

In Walter's case, he couldn't shoot the thieves: he couldn't execute the movement of pressing the trigger and shooting the thieves, whether at them or above their heads is debatable, but he couldn't shoot at them, which is what he wanted to do. His body created the situation for him through MS where he could eventually not move his arms and was unable to feed himself.

Walter thought about it for a long time. The solution was that although he loved his wife, if he was going to live a healthy life again and recover his motor functions he couldn't see her again. They separated in September 2001 and divorced in 2003.

Their older daughter was fine with the divorce and she understood the reasons for it. Their young son was clearly not happy about his parents divorcing, but if this had not have happened his father would not have been able to eat, would have required 24-hour care, and would have probably died prematurely. His wife Sylvia understood the GNM and agreed that a divorce was the only practicable solution.

Walter's motor movement is much better. He has a slightly odd manner of walking and does not have full motor movement with his arms but otherwise he is fine. He can feed himself, drive his car and work normally. However he can no longer shoot.

MS and the five Biological Laws of Nature

First Biological Law: The DHS

The biological shock or DHS for MS is concerned with themes such as: Not knowing what to do in a particular situation; not being able to keep up with someone; not being able to run away from or get away from someone or something; not being able to hold someone back; not being able to execute a movement; or to feel trapped by someone or something.

Second, third and fourth Biological Laws

The brain relay controlling the innervation of the muscles is in the cerebral cortex. In the conflict-active phase of MS, one gets motor impairment or a functional loss in your motor movement. In the case of full resolution of the conflict, the functional loss is recovered in the reparation phase. In some cases it is fully recovered, in other cases it is almost fully recovered.

Fifth Biological Law: The quintessence

In the conflict-active phase of MS one creates the actual situation which caused the biological shock. If, for example, you cannot run as fast as your friend or child, or dance as well as you would like or jump as high as you would wish, and you get a DHS, then you will loose motor movement in your legs or they will be impaired and you will be physically unable to run fast, then walk. You create for yourself that which caused your biological shock, which you have imagined. For example, if you couldn't run as fast as your 9-year old son, and if this caused a shock for you, you will not be able to run, then walk because of MS: You create for yourself what was your biological shock. This seems heartless to me but so it is.

Nobody should fear MS once you understand it. You can solve the conflict that caused it. MS is not necessarily degenerative. MS is reversible just like all other cancers and diseases. MS is curable: Nobody should have their life blighted unnecessarily for years by it.

CHAPTER 36

Diabetes

The term diabetes is derived from a Greek word that literally means "passing through," or "siphon", referring to one of diabetes' major symptoms: excessive urine production.[308]

According to Modern Medicine there are two types of diabetes. In Type1 diabetes, symptoms tend to develop rapidly over a couple of weeks and are more severe. Type1 diabetes is said to affect young people particularly children but anybody under the age of forty. In Type 2 diabetes, the symptoms develop slowly and are usually milder. Type 2a diabetes is said to affect skinny people and Type 2b diabetes is said to affect fat people.[309]

Another definition of diabetes according to Modern Medicine is that patients with Type1 diabetes do not produce any insulin and people with Type2 diabetes do not produce sufficient insulin.

This apparent differentiation between Type1 and Type 2a diabetes appears to be scientific but is in fact meaningless. Older adults are in most cases more mature than children and have an increased ability to avoid the situation that gave rise to their original DHS. That's why the symptoms of diabetes take longer to appear with older people and are less severe.

Common symptoms of both types of diabetes (Type1 and Type2a) are:

1. Passing water frequently, especially at night;
2. Tiredness and fatigue;
3. Loss of weight;
4. Breath smells like nail polish.

Diagnosing diabetes

According to Modern Medicine, diabetes occurs when there is excess glucose present in the blood. This excess glucose is caused by too little or no insulin at all: insulin being necessary to regulate the blood sugar. Diabetes may be detected in a routine urine test. A blood test will confirm whether or not the underlying cause is diabetes.

Diabetes according to GNM

There are two sugar-centres in the brain. The under-sugar centre or the alpha islet cells is located in the left hemisphere of the cerebral cortex. The over-sugar centre or the beta islet cells is located in the right hemisphere of the cerebral cortex.

The theme of the biological shock is of "fear-disgust" or "repulsion" or "revulsion" or an "inner resistance to doing something that you don't want to do but that you still have to do or are forced to do". Depending on whether the person is male or female and their laterality, one side of the cerebral cortex is affected. The exact same biological shock (for example, fear-disgust or repulsion) can cause either the alpha islet cells in the left hemisphere or the beta islet cells in the right hemisphere to be affected causing completely different symptoms.

The disease diabetes is caused by a DHS with a fear-disgust or repulsion or revulsion theme affecting the beta islet cells in the right hemisphere of the cerebral cortex.

Laterality and cerebral cortex conflicts

For all biological shocks affecting the cerebral cortex, a right-handed man (with no other active biological conflicts), who experiences a DHS, his right brain-hemisphere will be first affected. A left-handed male will experience his first cerebral cortex DHS in the left-hemisphere. The situation is exactly reversed for women. A right-handed woman will experience her first cerebral cortex biological shock in the left-hemisphere; a left-handed woman in the right-hemisphere.

A qualifier to even more complicate matters, is that this all assumes that the woman is from a hormonal viewpoint a woman – she is not taking a contraceptive pill and has not been through menopause. Any woman who is post-menopausal or who is taking the contraceptive pill, will react to a biological shock like a male and not a female. It also assumes that the man is from a hormonal viewpoint a man. An older man will react to a similar shock like a woman and not like a pre-menopausal man, because of this change of post-menopausal hormonal balance.

A right-handed male with a fear-disgust or repulsion or revulsion conflict will always get diabetes, because the beta cells will be affected, if it is his first biological shock. If he already has an active conflict on his right cerebral cortex, the fear-disgust conflict will then skip the right cerebral cortex hemisphere and hit the left cerebral cortex hemisphere, affecting the alpha cells causing obesity. The same shock for a left-handed male will cause the alpha cells to be affected if it is his first biological shock.

This is all very complex but if it is the first active conflict on the cerebral cortex the brain hemisphere affected will follow the laws of laterality for the person concerned. If the person concerned already has an active conflict on their dominant brain hemisphere, the other brain hemisphere will be affected. This is an important caveat on the rule of laterality.

Fear-Disgust DHS: laterality and diabetes

If a right-handed male gets a "fear-disgust" or "revulsion" DHS, the right hemisphere will be affected. The HH controlling the beta islet cells will be "switched on" and in target configuration. This causes the classic diabetes, with a lowering of the insulin level and a consequent increase of the glucose level in the blood. This causes the urine to have a sweet taste, resulting in the name diabetes mellitus.[310]

Fear-disgust DHS: Laterality and obesity

A right-handed woman (who is sexually mature, not in menopause and is not taking the pill),[311] will react to the same fear-disgust DHS with the left hemisphere, and the HH controlling the alpha islet cells will be "switched on" and in target configuration. In this situation the woman will overeat particularly sugary foods in order to have sufficient glucose for her fear-disgust conflict. If this conflict is ongoing she will become obese. She has no personal choice in the matter.

Normally in the conflict-active mode of a cancer/disease one loses weight. However in the case of a fear-disgust conflict when the alpha islets are switched on, one gains weight and if the conflict is not solved or is ongoing one becomes obese.

According to the German New Medicine, too little sugar and consequently too high an insulin level is the major problem. In contrast too much sugar and too low an insulin level or the classic diabetes mellitus is considerably less dangerous.

Diabetes case study 1: Two old friends[312]

Two elderly ladies, one of whom was called Margaret, were in their 70s. They had been close school friends but had lost contact over the years, with getting married and raising a family. Both their husbands had recently died, and both were at a loose end, and had independently looked each other up in 1997.

They initially talked by telephone. They then decided to meet up for a meal in a restaurant. Finally they agreed to have a meal in each others apartment. They got on famously as old friends mostly do. The only thing that bothered Margaret about the other lady was that she had a slovenly manner in eating her meals, slurped aloud and sometimes drooled. This could perhaps be overlooked as a sign of old age.

Their first meal was in Margaret's apartment. Margaret cooked a nice meal and they had a great time. It was now time for a return visit to the other lady's apartment.

She cooked a nice meal and the dining table was nicely laid out and everything seemed to be fine. Margaret insisted on helping with the washing-up. Margaret went into the kitchen and got the dish-towel. Margaret was immediately disgusted and revolted by it. It was filthy. It was so bad, it should have been thrown out. Margaret was physically repulsed by the thought that she had eaten off dishes that had been cleaned with this disgusting towel. Once you notice something like this, you tend to notice more and more unhygienic habits, which Margaret did.

This was an intense fear-disgust biological shock for her. They continued to meet, and Margaret dreaded having to go to the school-friends apartment. She enjoyed her company, but was revolted by her personal hygiene.

She got the classic symptoms of diabetes mellitus. She had excess glucose in her blood and a low insulin level. Her MD gave her tablets to take to increase her insulin level and therefore reduce her blood-sugar level.

Margaret was a personal friend of Arlette Büchel. Arlette was friendly with Margaret's daughter whom she went to school with. They all met up at a birthday party. Margaret explained to Arlette that she had recently become a type 2a diabetic.

Arlette explained the GNM to her and tried to ascertain what the probable source of the fear-disgust/revulsion biological shock was.

Margaret was immediately able to identify her friend's disgusting personal hygiene as a probable cause.

Margaret was right-handed. She was in her 70s and clearly post-menopausal. She therefore reacted to all conflicts in a male manner. She had a fear-disgust conflict because of her friends disgusting personal hygiene. This conflict affected the right hemisphere of her cerebral cortex causing her beta cells or over-sugar centre to be affected. She had excess glucose in her blood and a low insulin level or diabetes mellitus.

Margaret thought about this for a while. She used a home-test kit to measure her blood-sugar level. After a visit to her friend, her blood-sugar level increased dramatically and then slowly decreased once the visit and the repeated DHS was over. She measured her blood-sugar obsessively and noticed it always increased when she visited her friend.

She went back to the MD for reassurance because she had stopped taking her diabetes pills. The MD took her normal blood-sugar level as proof that the pills were working.

However, Margaret now had normal blood-sugar level because she had solved her biological shock. The solution to her diabetes that she decided for herself was to avoid going to her friend's apartment for lunch, and over a period of a few months to avoid meeting her at all.

Diabetes case study 2: The mechanic and his son-in-law[313]

A self-employed 63-year-old mechanic with his own garage called Walter B was living a contented life in Switzerland. He had three adult children. His youngest daughter wanted to marry a man originally from Yugoslavia. The mechanic knew that his daughter was happy with this man. His only problem from Walter's viewpoint was that he was at that time unemployed and had difficulty speaking proper Swiss-German.[314]

The son-in-law set himself up as a mechanic in the neighbouring village. This clearly bothered the mechanic as he was now in competition with his son-in-law. The son-in-law came by every few days, and borrowed this and that, and never, not once, did he return any of the tools that he had borrowed.

During one of these occasions when the son-in-law came by to borrow the equipment, Walter must have gotten a "repulsion" biological shock. Because every time he saw this man driving up, he knew that this man, his son-in-law, would effectively steal more tools from him. He was equipping his garage in the neighbouring village with the tools that he had stolen.

Walter was right-handed. Although male, because of his age, he was post-menopausal and he reacted to this shock like a woman. Instead of his beta cells being affected, he reacted to his repulsion conflict with the alpha under-sugar centre in the left hemisphere of the cerebral cortex.

Every time Walter saw his son-in-law, he had a lowered glucose level in his blood, and a relatively increased insulin level. This lowered glucose level caused him to feel physically weak. His solution was to drink beer, eat some cake, or eat fructose every time after he saw his son-in-law.

Walter went to the MD and was diagnosed with type 2b diabetes. Diabetes can only be said to occur when you have a high blood sugar and a low insulin level. So why did Walter get such a diagnosis?

When Walter sees his son-in-law, he immediately gets a lowered blood sugar level and a higher level of insulin because his alpha cells are affected. When his son-in-law is away again, and his conflict is temporarily resolved, he gets a high blood sugar level in the reparation phase and a low level of insulin. The reason why he was diagnosed as being diabetic was because the MD saw him when he was in the reparation phase. If the MD saw him in the conflict-active phase, if his son-in-law had accompanied Walter on the visit, the MD would have not diagnosed diabetes because Walter would have had a high level of insulin and a low blood sugar.

The key issue is that the blood sugar level is not static in the body. It fluctuates and can fluctuate considerably. The analogy here would be with your heart-beat. Your heart beats slowly after a good nights rest. After running a few kilometres, your heart beats much faster; your heart beat obviously fluctuates depending on what you are doing. Similarly with blood sugar, or with cholesterol, their level varies depending on the various conflicts the person has.

Initially Walter accepted his prescription for diabetes and took some pills to increase his insulin level and to consequently reduce his blood sugar level. However Walter was interested in "alternative medicine". He was a distant relation of Arlette Büchel's father.

Walter had a single 90-minute session with Harald. He immediately understood the cause of his diabetes. He thought about his situation for a few months. His solution was to give his business to his son and retire. He would no longer have to endure the constant visits of his son-in-law which caused him a fear-disgust conflict. He also would avoid meeting his son-in-law as much as possible because every time he met him he ran onto the tracks of his revulsion biological shock, and went back into the conflict active phase, with a much lowered blood-sugar level.

He doesn't take any pills to increase his insulin level. He understands that this would be pointless. He still has to meet his son-in-law for family gatherings but he can manage the symptoms of his increased blood sugar level by eating some fructose. However he is obese because he cannot avoid meeting his son-in-law. Despite this, he is content with his life, and because of his age can live with his obesity.

Diabetes and the five Biological Laws of Nature

First Biological Law: The DHS

The biological shock or DHS for diabetes is a shock concerned with conflict of fear-disgust, resistance, repugnance, repulsion, revulsion and loathing. You are disgusted/repulsed by something (politics, relationships, smells, liquids, hair, snakes, or types of food) or you are being forced to do something that you simply don't want to do.

Second, third and fourth Biological Laws

The brain relay controlling the alpha and beta cells is in the cerebral cortex. Depending on whether the person is right-handed or left-handed, male or female, whether it is their first biological shock, and their hormonal status, the identical biological shock will cause either the alpha or beta sugar centre to be affected. The symptoms of diabetes are caused by the beta cells or over-sugar centre being affected by a Fear-Disgust biological shock. The exact same biological shock can cause the alpha cells or under-sugar centre to be affected causing obesity.

Fifth Biological Law: The quintessence

The biological purpose of diabetes mellitus lies in the conflict-active phase, to provide in a timely manner enough glucose (blood-sugar) because the act of struggling against, revolting, resisting or opposing something takes a lot of muscle exertion. Diabetes is curable: Nobody should have their life blighted unnecessarily by it.

CHAPTER 37

Obesity

I always thought that obesity was a personal choice. This misconception is widespread. It is also completely wrong. Obesity is not a personal choice: It happens for two major reasons. The first is cancer of the kidney-collecting tubules and the second is a fear-disgust/revulsion biological shock affecting the alpha cells.

Cancer of the kidney-collecting tubules

Dr Hamer calls the shock causing cancer of the kidney-collecting tubules a refugee conflict/existence conflict/feeling of being completely alone biological shock or conflict. The kidney-collecting tubules are made up of endodermal tissue. The brain relays controlling the right and left kidney-collecting tubules are in the brain-stem, which is part of the old brain. Consequently you get a multiplication of the cells in these tubules in the conflict-active phase. One can liken the working of these additional cells in a collecting tubule to that of a sponge: they can absorb much more fluid. The biological purpose of this multiplication of the cells in the collecting tubules is in the conflict-active phase that is, to create a much more powerful pump in order to enable the organism to retain more water so that the organism doesn't dry out. This fluid that is pumped out by the kidney collecting tubules is then stored in tissue distributed throughout the body causing obesity.

Life began in the oceans millions of years ago. If an organism was washed up onto a beach and then stranded on the beach when the tide receded, it had to survive by retaining as much seawater as possible so that it wouldn't dry out before the tide came in again so that it could return to its natural habitat the ocean.

These organisms developed the survival ability by increasing their capacity to retain the maximum amount of seawater from the puddle left on the beach after the tide had gone out. In this way the organism could best survive until the next tide came in to reclaim it back to the ocean.

These simple organisms got a biological shock of being out of their normal environment and grew extra cells in order to retain more liquid and not to dry out and survive till the next tide. Once the tide came in and the organism was safely back out to sea, into its normal environment, the biological shock would have been naturally solved, and the extra cells would have been discarded over time.

This million-year-old survival mechanism is now used by the kidney-collecting tubules, which causes them to enhance their capacity to retain fluid, when the organism, the human person, gets a biological shock, a shock that they are all on their own, which Dr Hamer calls an existence conflict/refugee conflict/ feeling of being completely alone conflict.

When a person gets this kind of biological shock, the cells in the kidney tubules multiply so that the organism retains as much water as possible. This results in the person not urinating as much as normal. An adult normally urinates about 1.5 litres per day. The kidney-collecting tubules are controlled by relays in the brain stem, which are endodermal in origin. There are two brain relays in the brain stem, one for the left kidney and the other for the right kidney. When one gets this biological shock that affects one brain relay, one set of kidney tubules is affected. If it is a very strong shock then both brain relays are affected and consequently the kidney-collecting tubules belonging to both the left and right kidneys are affected.

One existence conflict causes uraemia or the amount of urine produced each day to drop to 800 ml per day. A second such existence conflict, a double-sided existence conflict causes the production of urine to fall to 350 ml per day. It is such a double-sided and intense feeling of being all alone biological shock that causes both kidneys to be affected. One will not really notice much if only one kidney is affected but once the kidney-collecting tubules in both kidneys are affected, the result is immediately noticeable: obesity.

The result of cancer of the kidney-collecting tubules causes the person to become bloated. They put on weight because they are retaining as much water as possible and not eliminating the same quantity of urine as normal. Even if these people eat small quantities of food they continue to put on weight because they are not eliminating as much urine as possible.

Obesity case study 1: The gardener and cancer of the kidney-collecting tubules[315]

A young man called Hans came to Harald because his girlfriend had heard about the German New Medicine. She was concerned about her boyfriend's weight and felt that Harald might have a solution through the German New Medicine.

Hans was then working as a lorry driver and was very heavy. Hans had been twice to the South of France on vacation with his mother and girlfriend and each time he had to cut the holiday short after four or five days because he had a tremendous feeling of loneliness and homesickness and wanted to return home. In his work as a lorry driver, Hans noticed that each time he drove away from his home village he did not feel the need to urinate while away. When he came home he urinated a lot. Once while driving in the South of France he became completely disorientated and had to concentrate really hard so that he could make his way back home.

After a session with Harald, they discovered the original shock that had caused his DHS. It had all started when he went to primary school in his home village. He didn't like the teacher and would have preferred to have stayed at home with his mother. He felt completely out of his element. He got an intense feeling of loneliness of being all alone in a strange place away from his mother and his home. The situation worsened at secondary school because he had to cycle to the secondary school at the other end of the village and he did not like this at all. He had an existence shock because he felt all alone, like a fish out of water, at this school. He was heavy at secondary school but not particularly obese. The situation dramatically worsened when he did his military service with the Swiss Army. He was away from home for four months and put on 25 kg/56 lbs/4 stone in weight. He was conscious of this and was not overeating. In fact he was if anything under-eating because of his enormous weight gain. He was simply not urinating as much as normal and was retaining water, which meant he was becoming obese.

After coming home from military service, he lost a lot of weight but was still overweight but not obese. He got a job as a gardener and worked in his local village and enjoyed the work. However he had learned to drive a truck in the army and was now expected to drive the truck to other neighbouring villages and towns for gardening work. He did this work but somehow he didn't like it. He associated this dislike with the gardening work, but in reality it was because he got a feeling of being completely alone every time he left his home village, and had a strong feeling of wanting to return home as quickly as possible. He became a lorry driver and his weight problems got much worse and caused him to eventually look for a solution.

He could never fully get over this feeling of intense loneliness that had affected him all his life but the solution was to give up his job as a lorry driver and become a gardener again and work only in his local village. He is doing this and is now overweight but not obese.

Experiment to confirm cancer of the kidney-collecting tubules

There are enough morbidly obese people around to perform a simple experiment: Do they urinate very little? This simple experiment would prove that they retain as much water in their body as possible. A further anamnesis would confirm the biological shock causing them to retain water, which is some type of existence conflict.

If they are morbidly obese and overeat, the conflict causing them to overeat particularly sugary foods is a separate biological shock, a fear-disgust conflict that affects the alpha cells.

Further analysis would confirm cancer of the kidney-collecting tubules, that is, the additional cellular growth in the kidney-collecting tubules, which prevents them from expelling the normal amount of urine. Modern Medicine is completely oblivious to this.

Refugee/existence biological shock: Obesity and the five Biological Laws of Nature

First Biological Law: The DHS

The biological shock or DHS for some types of obesity is a shock concerned with a conflict of being a refugee, a stranger in a foreign place, a feeling of intense loneliness, a feeling of being out of one's element, a feeling of not belonging to the place where one is.

Second, third and fourth Biological Laws

The kidney-collecting tubules are made up of endodermal tissue. The brain relays controlling the right and left kidney-collecting tubules are in the brain-stem, which is part of the old brain. Consequently there is multiplication of the cells in the kidney-collecting tubules in the conflict-active phase. This causes the body to retain as much water as possible, thus causing obesity.

In the reparation phase, these additional cells in the kidney-collecting tubules are destroyed by the relevant microbes.

Fifth Biological Law: The quintessence

I personally prefer the term "existence-conflict" as opposed to refugee-conflict to describe cancer of kidney-collecting tubules. The biological purpose of such a conflict is to retain as much water in the body as possible. This biological purpose goes back millions of years to when simple life-forms that were washed up on a beach and had to survive till the next tide came in.

In the case of humans one must solve the "existence-conflict" that causes the person to retain fluid in their body. Once the conflict is solved, they will urinate excessively until they have finally rid their body of the excess water. They are no longer lost or refugees; they are now in their element and this feeling of intense loneliness is gone.

Fear-Disgust biological shock: Obesity and the five Biological Laws of Nature

First Biological Law: The DHS

The biological shock or DHS for obesity (caused by the alpha-cells) is a shock concerned with conflict of fear-disgust, resistance, repugnance, revulsion and loathing. You are disgusted at something or you are being forced to do something that you simply don't want to do. In the case of obesity this biological shock affects the alpha-cells or the under-sugar centre in the left brain hemisphere.

Second, third and fourth Biological Laws

The brain relay controlling the alpha and beta cells is in the cerebral cortex. Depending on whether the person is right-handed or left-handed, male or female, the identical biological shock will cause either the alpha or beta sugar centre to be affected. The symptoms of obesity are caused by the alpha cells or under-sugar centre being affected by a fear-disgust biological shock. The exact same biological shock can cause the beta cells or over-sugar centre to be affected, which causes the symptoms of diabetes.

Fifth Biological Law: the quintessence

The biological purpose of the fear-disgust conflict that affects the alpha cells and causes obesity in the conflict-active phase is to cause the person to eat additional food so that they have enough sugar in order to compensate for the low level of glucose in the body. They have no choice in this matter and if the conflict is ongoing, the person will become obese.

The biological purpose of obesity is that the person is compelled to eat, and thereby raise their blood-sugar level in order for the individual to survive until the biological shock affecting the alpha cells can be solved.

The syndrome

Cancer of the kidney-collecting tubules is a common "syndrome", or an additional biological shock which can make the symptoms of other ongoing biological shocks much worse. This syndrome can be explained with two simple examples. The syndrome is extremely important in the German New Medicine and is completely overlooked by Modern Medicine.

Syndrome: brain cancer

Let's take the example of a person in the reparation phase of a conflict and therefore with an expanding oedema around the respective HH. On its own, this can cause a severe headache, but if this is combined with an "existence" conflict the brain cannot expel the oedema, although it wants to because the refugee conflict demands that the water is retained. This makes the oedema last much longer, and therefore increases the probability of severe, ongoing headaches. If the person is unfortunate enough to go to an MD, or even worse an oncologist, they will probably be diagnosed with brain cancer and their life will be effectively destroyed.

Syndrome: morbid obesity

If a person is unlucky to have both a fear-disgust conflict affecting the alpha islets resulting in overeating particularly sugary food, plus an existence conflict resulting in water retention, and both these conflicts are ongoing, the person will become morbidly obese. The person overeats sugary foods becoming obese, and cannot expel enough waste products by urinating, thus becoming morbidly obese.

Obesity and personal choice

Obesity is not a personal choice. There must be a tremendous feeling of guilt by an obese person, when they eat the wrong foods, such as processed sugary foods and drinks. They know they are fat because they eat junk food and sugary drinks, but despite their guilt, they cannot stop consuming these processed foods and drinks, because they are compelled by their biological shock to get more sugar into them.

Diet programs, identifying the right types of food to eat and the correct quantities can be useful in helping a person get to their desired weight. But the reason why these programs fail for most obese people is because they haven't solved their DHS that caused them to overeat in the first place.

It must be a tremendous relief once you understand that you are not a bad person; that you are not a weak person; that you are not a glutton; that you are not a moral degenerate because of your eating habits and your obesity. Once you solve the conflict that caused your obesity, you will no longer feel compelled to overeat, and to eat the wrong types of foods, particularly processed sugary foods. Once this overriding eating compulsion is gone, because the biological shock has been solved, you will naturally lose weight with or without a diet programme.

Obesity is reversible, provided that the biological shocks that caused it are resolved. Obesity is curable: Nobody should have their lives blighted unnecessarily for years by it.

CHAPTER 38

Mental Disorders

Mental disorders such as suicide, schizophrenia, manic-depression, paranoia and psychoses of all types occur, because the person has two or more ongoing conflicts on both brain hemispheres, which bring the brain out of synchronisation. The MDs know that the brain is not operating properly, or is not in synchronisation, but they do not know why.

This is most apparent with territorial conflicts, which affect the cerebral cortex part of the brain.

The point about all so-called mental disorders, is that yes the person does crazy things but they do this because they have two or more active HHs/brain relays on both brain hemispheres. But they are not "crazy", they do crazy things, stupid things and occasionally criminal acts, but they are not mad. If any of us had the same active biological shocks as these people, we would also be mad. These people are not "mad"; they simply have two or more active territorial biological conflicts on both brain hemispheres. The "madness" can be permanently solved once the individual conflicts are solved.

This cannot be emphasised enough: The Cartesian division of Modern Medicine into mental and physical problems with the physicians attending to the physical problems and the psychiatrists attending to mental problems is absolute nonsense and is stupid. Worse, it is criminally wrong. The diagnosis of schizophrenia or a psychosis is another example of a life-long condition known as PFLS (Patient For Life Syndrome) where the patient is "maintained" on a drug therapy with occasional in-patient treatment. This is a lucrative business for the MDs, the hospitals and the pharmaceutical companies. It is debilitating for the patient at the very least.

Experimental proof for the origin of all mental disorders

The proof that mental disorders are caused by a "mad" person having two active biological conflicts on both hemispheres of the brain is to perform a brain CT scan on them. One will discover two or more active HHs, both in the active phase, with concentric rings around the HHs in both brain hemispheres. Most mental institutions have CT scanners at their disposal and this would be an almost cost-free experiment for them to perform.

This experiment would conclusively prove the real reason for "madness": ongoing biological shocks on both hemispheres. Once the individual biological shocks are solved, the "madness" will disappear.

Mental disorder case study 1: The Horse-buggy Museum[316]

A successful unmarried policeman called Georg was a local police officer in the canton of Bern in Switzerland. He was proud of himself and his social standing in the community. He had had a particular hobby for many years, which was restoring various types of horse-coaches or horse buggies. He read up about them, knew about their manufacturers and restored these horse-coaches to their original condition with painstaking care and devotion. He had restored many of these and he had them stored in his shed. He was now in his mid 50s, coming to the end of his career as a policeman and he wanted to have a legacy, something he could pass on to future generations.

He succeeded in building a museum for his horse buggies and had them displayed there. He was a very happy man. He had achieved all his goals in life. Life could not be any better. In 1999, there were extremely heavy rains and the museum was flooded with up to 2-metres or 6 feet of water. His life's work, all the horse buggies that he had painstakingly restored for decades were completely destroyed.

He had had a massive territorial conflict. It was a double-sided territorial conflict. It hit both sides of his cerebral cortex almost simultaneously. In such a situation the person can believe that they have almost no other choice but to commit suicide. He couldn't talk about this deep personal shock with anyone: The conditions for the DHS were met. As soon as he saw the damage done to his museum and to the coaches that he had spent his adult life restoring, he went down to the local river, took out his handgun and shot himself in the head.

The solution to intense suicidal feelings like Georg experienced is to break through the isolative aspect of the DHS. If Georg could have talked with a good friend, he might have been able to reduce the conflict mass and reduce the isolative aspect of the DHS.

The best preventative measure for suicides is for people to be aware of German New Medicine and of the isolative aspect of the DHS.

In Ireland, I have noticed a huge increase in suicides among young men in recent years. This frequently happens after they have been "dumped" by their first serious girlfriend. These young men can suffer such an intense territorial-loss that they get a DHS on both brain hemispheres. In situations like this one must have a number of good friends in order to break through the isolative aspect of the DHS and prevent the conflict mass increasing.

Mental disorder case study 2: Our marriage is over[317]

A 35-year-old Swiss man called HO was living in Bogota, Colombia with his wife Christine and their two children. He worked as a teacher and was very content with his life in Colombia. Shortly after the birth of their third child, his wife Christine told him that she didn't want to be in a relationship with him any more.

This was a double territorial conflict for him. The shock hit both sides of his cerebral cortex simultaneously. He had lost his wife and children. This is what Dr Hamer calls a "schizophrenic constellation". He was now officially "crazy". He had a nervous breakdown; he had total hopelessness; he was depressed and apathetic. He also had black-outs and absences when he couldn't remember what he had been doing.

In 1984, one month after his wife threw him out of their home, he was committed to an asylum in Bogota, Colombia. His parents flew over a few days later, rescued him, and he was committed to an asylum back home in Switzerland.

He was there on and off for a few years. He was most fortunate to be cared for by, among others, a nurse called B. They fell in love. His madness was over when she told him that she was pregnant and wanted to marry him. He had regained his territory; he had a new wife and a new child. It was a great relief for him, his madness was over; he could now resume his life as a teacher in Switzerland. This he has done most successfully.

Bone cancer case study 1: Our marriage is over[318]

As an interesting aside I would like to tell the story of another Swiss, Tony who suffered almost the exact same fate as HO except he didn't become "mad" and become a schizophrenic. Instead, he got bone cancer.

Tony was not a patient of Harald. He was an acquaintance who had served in the Swiss Army with him. Harald met him again in 1994 after an absence of a few years. Harald was shocked. His friend Tony had shrunk by about 12 cm. Tony was right-handed. At this stage Harald knew about the GNM and knew that he must have suffered a severe devaluation conflict affecting people he considered to be his partner, which affected the right-side of his vertebrae, and either his mother or his children, which affected the left-side of his vertebrae. Both left and right sides of the vertebrae of his back would have simply collapsed. It must have been an enormous self-devaluation conflict.

Tony was happily married, or so he thought. His wife had just given birth to their third child at a hospital in the canton of Bern. He called by for a visit with a bunch of flowers and some chocolates for his wife. She brutally told him that she now had all the children she wanted, that he was merely the donor and she had never loved him.

In a situation very similar to this, HO experienced a double-side territory loss and went into a schizophrenic constellation and was declared by the MDs to be a schizophrenic and to be permanently mad.

In this situation, Tony took this loss of his wife and children not as a territory loss, but as a major self-devaluation conflict. He was worthless as a father. His wife regarded him as merely a sperm-donor for their children and not as a father. He was also worthless as a husband, because she had never loved him. Over a period of six months both left and right sides of his vertebrae collapsed and he shrank by about 12 cm or 5 inches in total.

I tell this story to illustrate the point that, in an almost identical situation, two different people can interpret the exact same shock from a circumstantial viewpoint, with a very different theme, and with a consequent different biological shock.

HO interpreted the loss of his wife and children with a double sided territorial-loss conflict causing schizophrenia whereas Tony interpreted the exact same loss of his wife and children with a major self-devaluation conflict that caused him to shrink considerably. This story illustrates the mystery of the human psyche which is unique to every individual.

Mental Disorders and the five Biological Laws of Nature

First Biological Law: The DHS

The biological purpose of being "mad" is that these intensely felt territorial conflicts do not build up enough conflict-mass. For example, if a right-handed male has an intense territorial conflict lasting many months and resolves it, he will probably get a fatal heart attack in the middle of the reparation phase during the EC (Epileptoid Crisis). The right-handed male has to solve his conflict in a certain amount of time or else he will die in the reparation phase. However if he has had such a severe territorial conflict that it hits both sides of his cerebral cortex almost simultaneously, he is in a "schizophrenic constellation" according to the German New Medicine. God or Mother Nature has granted him more time to solve his territorial conflicts, and when he solves them, he will not get a fatal heart attack, because each of the individual conflicts will not have built up the conflict mass necessary to cause a heart attack, even though these individual conflicts might have lasted for many decades.

Second, third and fourth Biological Laws

We deal with each individual territorial conflict that makes up the schizophrenic constellation. Each of these individual conflicts work as a normal territorial conflict but in tandem they make the affected patient mad or schizophrenic. Each of the separate conflicts affecting the patient can be dealt with and resolved.

Fifth Biological Law: The quintessence

Mental disorders illustrate the absolute wonder of Nature. Neither God nor Mother Nature has run amok. There is a logic or rationale behind the person going "mad" so that the individual conflicts do not build up enough conflict mass, to be able to survive longer and to give him enough time to solve each of his individual territorial conflicts. Mental disorders are curable: Nobody should die from them or have their life blighted for years by them.

CHAPTER 39

Outcome

Modern Medicine is a world religion based on the sacred scriptures that make up the Biomedical Paradigm. Modern Medicine cannot change itself because of its irrational and unscientific belief in these medical dogmas. Modern Medicine cannot be reformed or transformed from within.

The key dogma of the Biomedical Paradigm is the Germ Theory of Disease, which is based on the medical myth that germs cause disease. Germs do not cause disease but are present and active in the reparation phase of all cancers/diseases. The Germ Theory of Disease states that many diseases are caused by viruses. The problem with the concept of pathogenic viruses is that they simply do not exist! This is the Achilles' heel[319] of Modern Medicine and is the only way the Biomedical Paradigm can be overcome.

The MDs and other white-coats repeatedly state that viruses exist. In science, if an assertion is made that something is true, the scientist is duty bound to prove it. This assertion must be reproducible in all circumstances by other scientists. Only then can one state with scientific certainty that the assertion is true.

As a young student Dr Lanka discovered a virus in sea algae. He proved its existence by isolating, photographing and biochemically characterising the virus. He then discovered that there was no proof for the existence of any pathogenic viruses that are said to exist such as HIV, mumps, measles, rubella and bird flu. He tried to persuade other scientists and MDs but this was impossible because they were all devoted followers of the Biomedical Paradigm.

Dr Lanka and Karl Krafeld established Klein-Klein-Aktion with the objective that ordinary people would ask the authorities for proof of the existence of these alleged viruses. The authorities can provide no such proof because viruses do not exist. They currently get away with this because few people have asked them for proof of the existence of these allegedly pathogenic viruses. The Germ Theory of Disease medical myth can be revealed to be the key dogma of Modern Medicine if many hundreds of thousands of ordinary people ask the relevant authorities for proof of the existence of these viruses. Our respective governments will only respond when enough of us demand that these authorities are brought to account.

The outcome will be a true, open international scientific debate about the proof for the existence of any virus. This great debate will enable us to understand that the Germ Theory of Disease is an enormous criminal and scientific fraud with horrendous consequences. This great international debate will mark the beginning of the Turning Point, the point at which the scientific elites finally agree that the infamous Germ Theory of Disease medical myth is clearly false.

Once the Germ Theory of Disease is accepted to be scientifically and medically wrong, and that pathogenic viruses do not exist, the whole edifice of Modern Medicine will crash down. It will be replaced by a true scientific and medical understanding of the origin and nature of all cancers and other diseases: German New Medicine.

You now have a good understanding of the origin and mechanism of a number of major cancers and some cancer-equivalent diseases. They are all MBPs (Meaningful Biological Programs of Nature) and are effectively explained using the five Biological Laws of Nature.

More importantly, you understand how one can become cured from these cancers and various diseases. We have no reason to fear them: We simply have to understand them and solve the conflict that caused them. We are in charge of our own return to health. We are no longer "treated" but we effectively treat ourselves. There is much more to learn about GNM, but you now have a good understanding of the essential points. You now know more valuable information about medicine than any MD and hopefully you now know this to be true.

The most important aspect of GNM is in preventive medicine. If we are aware that we have suffered a biological shock, we can take steps to solve it immediately so that it has no organic manifestations. If we do not solve the conflict in time and the organic manifestation of the biological shock occurs, we have been given notice by God to quickly solve our conflict or else...

German New Medicine has been tested many times before. That it could not be accepted by the MDs is absolute proof of the Semmelweis Reflex: the automatic dismissal of new empirical and incontrovertible medical evidence by the medical profession without due consideration.

There are various testing protocols one could use. Dr Hamer could be given a number of patients with specifically determined medical conditions and be asked to determine the nature of the shocks that had caused these conditions. In other words, Dr Hamer could determine the nature of the shock as experienced by the patient in his psyche from a determination of the cancers/diseases affecting the organs of the patient.

Alternatively, Dr Hamer could be given a brain CT scan and be asked to determine the cancers/diseases affecting the various organs of the body and the nature and theme of the shock that had caused these cancers/diseases. German New Medicine is a natural science. Therefore it is reproducible and other people can be trained to understand the CT scans and determine the organic symptoms of a cancer/disease from the brain level of the human trinity.

German New Medicine is an over-determined system: Once you know what is happening on one level of the human trinity, you can predict exactly what is occurring on the other two levels. Give Dr Hamer or Harald Baumann or another GNM therapist one level such as the organ level or the brain level or the psyche level, and they will describe in precise detail what is happening on the other two levels.

I personally believe that the best way to prove and openly demonstrate the German New Medicine is to appropriately treat a small group of willing patients with one specific disease or cancer and who understand the five Biological Laws of Nature. Another small group of patients with a similar cancer/disease would be treated according to Modern Medicine. A third group with the same cancer/disease would not be treated at all.

These treatment regimes would be done with the active consent of the patients concerned. It is self-evident that no patient can be "treated" using GNM if they do not understand the five Biological Laws of Nature and the specific DHS or biological shock that caused their cancer/disease. Those patients opting for Modern Medicine or German New Medicine would be giving their active consent as would those patients who choose to do nothing at all.

The progress of the three groups of patients would be followed in a reality TV format. One would observe how patients with a specific cancer/disease are treated by Modern Medicine and see the actual outcome. In contrast, one would then observe how patients with a full understanding of the five Biological Laws of Nature of German New Medicine effectively resolve the conflict that caused their cancer/disease, treat themselves and become cured. One would compare both sets of treatment protocols with the benchmark group, the third group who choose to do nothing.

This could be done with a number of different cancers or other diseases. It would be simpler for the viewers if the patients only had one specific cancer/disease, as it would be much easier to follow. It would be compulsive viewing. It would also be the impetus behind getting German New Medicine accepted as the true scientific medicine.

This will only happen when enough people demand change from our respective governments. This can happen in the free world because our governments do eventually respond to public opinion.

But how do we get German New Medicine officially tested? It will depend upon individuals making their voices heard and persuading others. It will depend on us all spreading the good news of the German New Medicine. It will only happen because enough of us write to the authorities and ask them for the scientific proof for the existence of these viruses. It will only happen when we demand from our governments that these white-coats respond to our legitimate queries. It will only happen when enough of us sign a petition and demand that the German New Medicine is openly tested and verified.

It will only happen when we realise the true evil nature of the Biomedical Paradigm and the absolute truth that God is perfect and that we do not get cancers randomly or because of perceived failures of Mother Nature but because of specific shocks that have occurred in our lives.

It will only happen because we have made the most wonderful voyage of discovery possible and now see with new eyes.

5

Correspondence

Government is never more dangerous than when our desire to have it help us blinds us to its power to harm us.
Ronald Reagan (40th US President, 1911–2004)

Our lives begin to end, the day when we become silent about things that matter.
Martin Luther King (American civil rights leader, 1929–1968)

All that is necessary for the triumph of evil is that good men do nothing.
Edmund Burke (Irish/British philosopher and statesman, 1729–1797)

First they came for the Jews
and I did not speak out
because I was not a Jew.
Then they came for the Communists
and I did not speak out
because I was not a Communist.
Then they came for the trade unionists
and I did not speak out
because I was not a trade unionist.
Then they came for me
and there was no one left
to speak out for me.
Pastor Martin Niemöller (German Christian minister, 1892–1984)

... the hottest places in hell are reserved for those who in a period of moral crisis maintain their neutrality.

Ask not what your country can do for you – Ask what you can do for your country.
John F Kennedy (35th US President, 1917–1963)

Be the change you want to see in the world.
Mahatma Gandhi (Indian Prime Minister and philosopher, 1869–1948)

The journey of a thousand miles begins with one step.
Lao-Tse (*Chinese philosopher, 604–531 BC*)

CHAPTER 40

Virus Correspondence with the Irish Experts

Dr Darina O'Flanagan Director HPSC

By March 2006, I had read many books and countless articles on the Internet. I had studied German and had read with some difficulty a number of books in German published by the Klein-Klein publishing press and some books by Dr Hamer himself. I had lots more to read and to understand. However it was time for me to become involved and do something as well.

Klein-Klein-Aktion encourages people to take action themselves. Dr Stefan Lanka, Karl Krafeld (co-founders of Klein-Klein-Aktion) and the Klein-Klein web-site don't ask people to believe them or to trust them. This is not a new religion. They ask people to question the authorities themselves; to ask them for the direct evidence for the existence of any so-called disease-inducing or pathogenic viruses.

There was an article in early 2006 in the *Sunday Business Post*[320] about Dr Darina O'Flanagan, Director of the Health Protection Surveillance Centre (HPSC) in Dublin. She was a strong advocate for vaccinations. I subsequently discovered that she favoured the reduction of child benefits from the Irish Government for those parents that rejected vaccinations for their children.[321] One day at work I decided to look up this government agency, HPSC, on the Internet. At this stage of my life, every day, I thought about and read about and talked about the German New Medicine and the fact that the Germ Theory of Disease is an absolute moral and scientific fraud and is the major dogma of the Biomedical Paradigm. It was, and is, constantly on my mind.

According to its web-site, HPSC is Ireland's specialist agency for the surveillance of communicable diseases. They were responsible for monitoring all these so-called infectious diseases and were the responsible authority in Ireland for vaccines. I wrote an e-mail on

Thursday 30th March 2006 at lunch-time to the Director of the HPSC, Dr Darina O'Flanagan.

Dr O'Flanagan. My name is James McCumiskey. I unfortunately had my children vaccinated in the Republic of Ireland because I believed the medical profession to be correct about the existence of so-called infectious diseases. I understand that your organisation the Health Protection Surveillance Centre is responsible for the provision of information about infectious diseases in Ireland.

I have studied the work of a number of leading medical dissidents (particularly Dr RG Hamer about the true cause of cancer and other diseases) and also Dr Stefan Lanka. Dr Lanka got a doctorate after discovering a real virus in seawater: So he knows how to isolate a real virus according to established scientific criteria. After discovering this real virus he set about reading about the HIV virus and he read all the published literature. He made a truly incredible discovery: Not only did the HIV virus not exist but neither did any of the so-called disease inducing viruses like measles, mumps, rubella etc.

These following questions have already been placed to the WHO (World Health Organization) and the German Health ministry. I would like the definitive response of your organisation to these questions.

1) What publication (no secondary literature please) contains the proof that the viruses that supposedly cause disease, do actually exist (polio, hepatitis A and B, influenza, measles, mumps, rubella etc)?
2) What publication shows that a virus (if it actually exists) or a bacteria can actually cause a certain disease that is that a person infected with the virus gets the disease?
3) What publication proves that vaccines actually protect people from certain diseases and does not harm them?
4) In Ireland, do you check the patient's vaccinal condition after the diagnosis of a viral or bacterial disease, and if so, does it show up in the statistics?

Best Regards
James McCumiskey[322]

As I review this e-mail, I should have been more polite. There was no "Dear Dr O'Flanagan". I had obtained the above four questions from the Klein-Klein-Aktion web-site; the questions were all right. However I should not have mentioned that my children had been vaccinated. I was bringing emotion into it. It would have been better to stick to the scientific facts. But one does get emotional when babies are being poisoned for no other reason than the fact that the medical profession believes in the Germ Theory of Disease. Nonetheless, it was an awful e-mail for many reasons. However it was sent and there was no point in worrying about it.

Dr Darina O'Flanagan responded promptly later that day at 17.30.

Dear James McCumiskey,

1 and 2. I recommend Mandell Bennett and Dolin on Principles and Practices of infectious diseases. You will find plenty of primary references in there.

3. I recommend Plotkin and Orenstein on Vaccines 4th edition. The evidence on benefits and adverse effects is outlined in this publication.

4. Unfortunately we cannot routinely link vaccine status with infectious disease diagnosis. This would require a unique personal identifier to be used in all contacts with the health system as is done in Scandinavian countries.

Yours sincerely
Darina O'Flanagan

Dr Darina O'Flanagan had responded with secondary sources: text books. I had asked for primary sources: the original paper in which these viruses were isolated, photographed and biochemically characterised.

I sent Dr O'Flanagan's reply to the Klein-Klein-Aktion web-site and asked for help in dealing with it. Susanne Brix contacted me and told me to ask again for primary references; quoting text books was simply not good enough. She gave me three examples of primary references concerning the virus Dr Lanka had discovered in seawater. This was the first of many e-mails with Susanne. She was surprised that somebody far away in Ireland had heard about the "missing viruses". Apparently I was the first non-German to question the existence of these viruses. I explained to her how I came across Klein-Klein-Aktion and the work of Dr Lanka through Harald Baumann.

Armed with information from Susanne, I e-mailed Dr Darina O'Flanagan on Monday the 3rd April 2006.

Dear Dr Darina O'Flanagan

I got a lot of help and information from Susanne Brix of the Klein-Klein-Aktion group in Germany. I am copying this e-mail to her and the Klein-Klein-Aktion organisation in Germany.

I asked you for PRIMARY literature proving the existence of disease-inducing viruses. You gave me SECONDARY literature that apparently contains primary references. This is the secondary literature you quoted to me:

1) Principles and Practices of infectious diseases by Gerard Mandell, John Bennett and Raphael Dolin.
2) Vaccines, Fourth edition by Plotkin and Orenstein.

I do not want to look for the primary references in these above books. I want you to give me (and then through me the Klein-Klein-Aktion organization) the primary references that your organisation uses to justify say the MMR vaccine in the Republic of Ireland. I want the primary references that prove the existence of the measles, mumps and rubella viruses and therefore the alleged necessity for the MMR vaccine. Surely as the organisation responsible for promoting the benefits of the MMR vaccine you can do that?

I can give you an example of a primary reference. It's the publication of the virus Dr Lanka discovered:

1) Title: A Virus Infection in the Marine Brown Alga Ectocarpus siliculosus (Phaeophyceae) Autoren: D.G. Müller, H. Kawai, B. Stache, and S. Lanka, Fundstelle/Zeitschrift: Botanica Acta 103 (1990) 72-82
2) Title: Genome Structure of a Virus Infecting the Marine Brown Alga Ectocarpus siliculosus Autoren: Stefan T.J. LANKA, Michael KLEIN, Uwe RAMSPERGER, Dieter G. MÜLLER, and Rolf KNIPPERS, Fundstelle/Zeitschrift: Virology 193, 802-811 (1993)
3) Title: Coat Protein of the Ectocarpus siliculosus Virus, Autoren: Michael KLEIN, Stefan T.J. LANKA, Rolf KNIPPERS, and Dieter G. MÜLLER, Fundstelle/Zeitschrift: Virology 206, 520-526 (1995). This can be viewed at the address below
Coat Protein of the Ectocarpus siliculosus Virus

I want the primary references for the existence of the measles, mumps, and rubella vaccines such as those above which show how a real virus but not a pathogenic virus was isolated from seawater.

I should point out that although I currently live in the North of Ireland I am a citizen of the Republic of Ireland and my two sons (now aged 5 and 8) received their vaccines in the Republic of Ireland including of course the MMR vaccines.

Best Regards
James McCumiskey[323]

I sent a number of e-mails in April to Dr Darina O'Flanagan requesting the primary sources for the existence of these viruses. First thing on the morning of Wednesday 19th April 2006, I e-mailed her again. I was annoyed with the complete lack of response to my e-mails. At lunch-time that day I decided to phone Dr Darina O'Flanagan. Apparently she was at a meeting. Within a few hours I got the following reply:

Dear Mr McCumiskey

Dr O'Flanagan has received your emails. We regret we can assist you no further in this regard. HPSC has supplied you with references and if you do not choose to follow these up there is nothing further we can do to assist you in this matter.

Yours sincerely,
xxxxx
PA to Director

Well, that seemed to be it. Dr Darina O'Flanagan did not appreciate being challenged. However, Dr Darina O'Flanagan wasn't going to have the last word. I e-mailed her again on Thursday 20th April 2006.

Dear Dr Darina O'Flanagan,

You provided me with the titles of two text-books which allegedly contain primary references for the existence of the measles, mumps and rubella viruses. I did not ask you for any such secondary sources. Instead I asked you for primary sources for the existence of these viruses, which you have refused to provide me and the Klein-Klein-Aktion organisation.

There are two arguments against vaccinations: One is on the grounds of safety and the second is on the grounds of effectiveness. Dr Gerhard Buchwald in his book "Vaccinations - A business based on fear" has clearly demonstrated the dangers of vaccinations in terms of new diseases like sudden infant death syndrome, shaken baby syndrome, autism, attention deficit disorders etc. On safety grounds alone vaccines should be banned.

Dr Buchwald and Thomas McKeown (medical historian) have also successfully proven that vaccinations had no effect on the incidence of so-called infectious disease. They have conclusively proven that so-called infectious diseases had declined in incidence for at least a hundred years prior to the introduction of vaccines and continued this long-term decline after the introduction of vaccines. The vaccine industry including your organisation has of course taken the credit for this actual decline. The only explanation of the real reason for the actual decline in so-called infectious diseases is that offered by Thomas Mc Keown in his book "The Role of Medicine". This explanation was that it was hunger, a constant actual hunger that made children susceptible to these diseases and caused their deaths, that is the children were already weakened through hunger by the time they got the so-called infectious diseases. So it was hunger, malnutrition that really killed the child and not the so-called infectious disease.

Dr Lanka has conclusively shown that the Germ theory of Disease as promulgated by Pasteur and Koch is an absolute moral and scientific fraud. This is because these so-called disease inducing viruses do not actually exist! These viruses have never been isolated and photographed and biochemically characterised according to established scientific criteria. Dr Lanka has clearly shown how this was done in the three primary references I have previously given you regarding a virus he identified in seawater.

There is no basis for vaccinations because these disease-inducing viruses simply do not exist. There is no virus to vaccinate against!

In post-war Germany most of the adult population excused themselves by stating that "they did not know" about the genocidal campaign of the Nazis. You have no such excuse in the silent holocaust of children through vaccinations, particularly in the third world where the children are already suffering from malnutrition. You know (or certainly have the ability to ascertain the truth) but you have chosen to do nothing.

Shame on you.[324]

Yours Sincerely
James McCumiskey

The "Shame on you" might seem strong but it is true. If you call yourself a scientist, you should be willing to test all your preconceived ideas and to continually query your own assumptions and hypotheses. She couldn't do that because she is an MD and a devoted follower of the Biomedical Paradigm. Dr O'Flanagan cannot use the "I did not know "argument to justify her position.

A few days later on Tuesday 25th April 2006, I decided to call her bluff and e-mailed her. I pretended that I personally and also the Klein-Klein-Aktion team had read her text-books even though I was positive from their web-site that these text-books contained no such primary references.

Dear Dr Darina O'Flanagan:

After careful examination of the two text-books listed below, which you have given me as secondary sources, the Klein-Klein-Aktion Organisation have not been able to find any primary sources for the existence of the measles, mumps and rubella viruses.

1) Principles and Practices of Infectious diseases
2) Vaccines

Can you please tell me on which page, and which primary references you are referring to for the alleged existence of the measles, mumps and rubella viruses.

Best regards
James McCumiskey[325]

This e-mail stated exactly what I wanted: primary sources for the existence of these viruses. I did not expect an immediate reply. Hell would freeze over before she would reply to me. It was time to park the measles, mumps and rubella correspondence with Dr Darina O'Flanagan and move on.

Flu vaccine

On Tuesday, October 17th 2006, there was a three-quarter page article entitled" Building defences against cold war" in the *Irish Times* medical supplement. It enraged me. Elderly people will prematurely die because of this article. I felt obliged to write again six months later after my MMR correspondence to Dr Darina O'Flanagan.

Dear Dr Darina O'Flanagan,

I read with tremendous interest and absolute horror the propaganda about the flu vaccine in the medical supplement of the Irish Times on Tuesday 17th October 2006.

I have a few questions. How do the all-knowing Seers in the WHO know in advance which flu virus is going to affect us in Ireland this winter? Will a different flu virus occur in China or the US? Do they have different flu vaccines for these countries? Are there some countries with a mixture of flu viruses that are deemed likely by the WHO to occur, maybe Russia for example because it is between China and Europe?

If these viruses exist, your organization should be able to produce a scientific publication which demonstrates how the "Influenza-A Flu virus" - H3N2 or H1N1 or even the bird flu virus - the H5N1 virus were isolated, biochemically characterised and photographed.

If your organisation manages to isolate the HIV virus please tell Luc Montagnier who as you know allegedly discovered the HIV virus and now admits there is no scientific proof that it exists.

In the hopefully not too distant future, when you are successfully prosecuted for criminal negligence, you will not be able to claim the "I did not know" defense in relation to the non-existence of any virus: flu, bird flu, measles, mumps and rubella etc. You do know: You have been repeatedly told about it by me but have chosen to do nothing.

I will not give up my pursuit of the truth that there is no scientific evidence for the existence of any virus.

Yours Sincerely
James McCumiskey[326]

Needless to mention, Dr Darina O'Flanagan did not respond to this e-mail.

The Irish Medicines Board (IMB)

Trawling through the internet one night, I came across an organisation called the Irish Medicines Board (IMB). They seem to be responsible for licensing medicines in Ireland. I wasn't entirely sure, but it seemed that the HPSC were responsible for determining what diseases had to be vaccinated against and the IMB were responsible for licensing the vaccines. On the 30th November 2006, I sent an e-mail to the IMB:

To whom it may concern,

I understand you are responsible for licensing medicines in Ireland?

My question is in relation to the MMR vaccine. I have asked Dr Darina O'Flanagan Director of the HPSC the same question but she has refused to answer my question.

Presumably the MMR vaccine is necessary because the measles, mumps and rubella viruses exist? Can you please give me primary evidence from a scientific journal for proof of the existence of the measles, mumps and rubella viruses?

This putative article would have to show how the measles, mumps and rubella viruses were 1 isolated, 2 photographed and 3 biochemically characterised.

I am not interested in a medical text-book which would be a secondary source of evidence. I want the primary source that proves the existence of these viruses.

Yours Sincerely
James McCumiskey

I received a reply a few days later on Tuesday morning, 5th December 2006, from the Information Officer at the IMB.

Dear James,

Your query does not fall within the remit of the Irish Medicines Board.

The IMB is responsible for the authorisation of vaccines (assessing quality, safety and efficacy).

The Department of Health and Children (www.dohc.ie) decide which of the licensed vaccines are part of the national immunisation schedule based on epidemiology data.

Regards
Jackie Cottell
Information Officer

I responded a few hours later:

Dear Jackie,

Having examined your response to my e-mail, I believe that my query does also fall within the remit of the IMB. How can you measure the efficacy of a vaccine against viruses such as measles, mumps and rubella when there is no scientific proof for the existence of these viruses?

I think your organisation should be equally concerned about the non-existence of any scientific proof for the existence of these viruses.

Yours Sincerely
James McCumiskey

Jackie Cottell replied back on Friday afternoon, 8th December 2006, and asked me to send any further queries to the British MHRA. I was really going around in circles. I had already been onto the MHRA and the Department of Health in the UK. Now almost 100 years after Irish independence from Britain, the IMB is relying on their British counterpart for advice. Apparently they cannot provide this information themselves! That annoyed me. I sent her the following e-mail a half-hour later on Friday 8th December and phoned her and left her a voice-mail message.

Hi Jackie,

I am an Irish citizen and as such I want the IMB to provide the scientific publications which prove the existence of the measles, mumps and rubella viruses. If you cannot prove the existence of these viruses then how can you measure the efficacy of these vaccines? This query of mine, which is apparently stupid, is not so simple is it, because these viruses do not exist?

Because I currently live in Northern Ireland , I felt duty-bound to question the UK authorities about the proof for the existence of the measles, mumps and rubella viruses. I dealt with the MHRA, who couldn't answer my queries. They referred me to the Immunization Policy branch of the Department of Health; there I dealt with a Kalpana Chauhan.

Kalpana Chauhan provided me with scientific papers, which allegedly contained photographs of the measles, mumps and rubella viruses. However I challenged these so-called photographs from these scientific publications, because nowhere in these publications does it state that these viruses have been isolated and biochemically characterised. Some of this correspondence is published on www.klein-klein-aktion.de.

I do not think it is good enough for the IMB to rely on foreign regulatory agencies, namely the British MHRA. Please give me the scientific publication which proves the existence of the measles, mumps and rubella viruses. If you cannot prove the existence of these viruses, there is not much point in having a vaccine against them? The efficacy of such a vaccine is clearly in doubt?

This scientific publication proving the existence of the measles, mumps and rubella viruses must show how these viruses were 1) isolated, 2) photographed and 3) biochemically characterised.

Yours Sincerely
James McCumiskey[327]

Late on Thursday 13th December 2006, I decided to up the ante.

Hi Jackie,

Should you be able to provide a scientific publication proving the existence of the measles, mumps and rubella viruses, I know enough myself about real viruses to be able to give an informed opinion on it, but Susanne Brix and Dr Lanka are on standby in Germany to give an expert opinion.

We are keen to have an open public scientific debate about this. Are the relevant experts in the IMB happy that there is direct proof for the existence of the measles, mumps and rubella viruses? If so please provide me with the evidence. If there is no direct proof and I am positive that there is no direct proof, because these viruses do not exist in humans, animals or plants, then I am anxious to discover what the basis is for the belief in the existence of these viruses. Is it a belief in "dominant medical opinion", or is it the "indirect evidence argument" on the basis of so-called antibodies? The dominant medical opinion argument or the indirect evidence argument is not sufficient proof for the existence of these viruses, at least not in a court of law.

This is an extremely serious matter as I'm sure you will appreciate. The ramifications of the missing evidence for the existence of these "viruses" will be enormous.

Yours Sincerely
James McCumiskey[328]

I was happy enough with the content of these e-mails. It was very simple. Please give me the direct evidence for the existence of these viruses. This time I will not reveal my hand by stating that the Germ Theory of Disease is a major criminal fraud. I simply want the proof for the existence of these viruses. Period.

I e-mailed Jackie again on St Stephen's day, 26th December, 2006:

Hi Jackie,

I hope you had a peaceful and happy Christmas, I have so far and I feel very much refreshed. I will be having an extremely busy year in 2007, not least concerning the "virus question".

I am establishing a paper-trail for legal action against the IMB and HPSC concerning the absence of evidence for the existence of any virus, in particular the measles, mumps and rubella viruses. My recourse to the courts will be because I have not been provided with any primary evidence by neither the IMB nor the HPSC proving the existence of these viruses.

In a court of law the IMB and HPSC, will be asked for the primary evidence which is the direct evidence establishing the proof of the existence of these viruses.

I am asking you once again; please provide me with the scientific publication proving the existence of these putative viruses. In the event that your organization realizes that there is no direct primary evidence please publicly admit it.

It is possible to prove the existence of a virus by means of biochemical characterisation techniques available since the early 1970s and to photograph such a virus by means of an electron microscope which was invented in the early 1930s. The technology is available to directly prove the existence of viruses by 1) isolating them, 2) photographing them and 3) biochemically characterising them.

The key issue I believe for a court of law is; if it is technologically possible to directly prove the existence of these alleged viruses, why have these techniques never been employed before?

And then we are at the kernel of the question: Why does the medical profession and the associated "white-coats" in the scientific community believe in the existence of these viruses, and that so-called indirect evidence such as antibodies etc. proves the existence of these alleged viruses when there is absolutely no direct scientific evidence and this is technologically possible?

Happy New Year
James McCumiskey[329]

I put in the business about the courts of law because I had served on a three-day jury trial in December 2006 and had an insight into the way the legal system operates. The burden of proof always rests with the prosecution who assert that the defendant is guilty. In the case of legal action concerning the "virus issue", the burden of proof would rest with the people who claim that these viruses exist.

Jackie wrote back on the 9th January 2007 with the following brush-off e-mail.

Dear James

Thank you for your e-mail dated 26 December 2006. Unfortunately there is nothing further I can add to my previous e-mails other than to refer you to the published data on these viruses.

Yours sincerely,
Jackie Cottell
Information Officer

The correspondence was now over for a while. So much for freedom of information. The Information Officer is more like the Minister for Information in a communist/totalitarian state, who should really be called the Minister for Disinformation, the Minister for keeping the truth from the masses. In the case of the IMB, there is no information at all, just rhetoric. The whole point of my correspondence with Jackie Cottell of the IMB is that there is no scientific publication in existence proving the existence of any pathogenic virus, and she still refers me to non-existent published data on the existence of these viruses.

Never wanting anybody to have the last word, particularly a Prevention of Information Officer, I wrote back the next day, 10th January 2007:

Dear Jackie,

The published data on these so-called viruses does not claim to have proven them to exist. The Immunisation Policy Branch of the Department of Health in England provided me with almost 20 such publications but none of them claimed to have proven these viruses to exist.

Jackie, Your job-title is Freedom of Information Officer for the IMB. What scientific publication proves the existence of these putative viruses? Please cite it? If you can't, then at least publicly admit there is no direct evidence for the existence of these viruses but only indirect evidence using antibodies etc.

It is technologically possible to directly prove the existence of these viruses. Viruses do not exist in humans, animals or plants. I repeat this; viruses do not exist in humans, animals or plants. One cannot vaccinate against viruses that don't exist!

The fact that your organisation licences the MMR vaccine for these three viruses that don't exist and your organisation is unconcerned about the fact that these viruses don't exist is a savage indictment of your organisation. The MMR vaccine licensed by your organisation is unnecessary and is both toxic and iatrogenic, causing diseases such as autism, SIDS, SBS, attention deficit disorders etc.

I intend to be in a position to issue you with a subpoena in the next few months compelling the IMB to provide an Irish court with the scientific publications proving the existence of these viruses.

The game will get interesting then.

Yours Sincerely
James McCumiskey[330]

Jackie did not reply. At this stage, I had no way of pursuing this matter in a law court, but having served on a jury, I was convinced this was the only effective means of determining the complete lack of evidence for the existence of these putative viruses. But I was bluffing and my bluff was called.

CHAPTER 41

Virus Correspondence with Irish Politicians

The Taoiseach[331]

With no effective response from the Irish pseudo-virologist, MD and white-coat Dr Darina O'Flanagan, I decided to exert some political pressure on her. A friend lived in Dromcondra, Dublin near Mr Bertie Ahern the Taoiseach (Irish Prime Minister). He e-mailed the Taoiseach on the 12th April 2006 and requested that he get Darina O'Flanagan to respond to my request for the proof of the existence of the measles, mumps and rubella viruses.

After reading his e-mail, I responded directly to An Taoiseach Bertie Ahern on Wednesday 26th April 2006:

An Taoiseach,

A friend of mine xxxxx, who is also a constituent of yours, asked you if you could persuade Dr Darina O'Flanagan to respond to my information request. I am now again pleading with you to use the power of your office to enforce this information request.

I am certain that Dr Darina O'Flanagan cannot give any primary sources for the existence of the measles, mumps and rubella viruses, because as unbelievable as it sounds, they do not exist. These viruses have never been isolated, photographed in an electron microscope and biochemically characterised because they simply do not exist.

If there is no primary evidence for the existence of these viruses, there is no need to vaccinate against them.

I appreciate any help you can give in getting Dr Darina O'Flanagan to respond to my very fundamental questions concerning the primary sources for the existence of these viruses.

I have a copy of an e-mail I sent her attached below.

Yours Sincerely
James McCumiskey[332]

On Friday 28th April 2006 (less than 2 days later), I received an e-mail from an Assistant Private Secretary to the Taoiseach. I was impressed by the efficiency of his private office. Mr Bertie Ahern is probably the best constituency politician in the world. He is always out meeting the people and is known to respond to all queries from his constituents and also from the wider Irish public. He is extremely likeable but is impossible to pin down on any issue: a true politician, one of the best.

Dear Mr McCumiskey,

The Taoiseach, Mr Bertie Ahern T.D., has asked me to refer to your recent e-mail, the contents of which have been noted.

The Taoiseach has asked me to say that he has forwarded your letter to his colleague Ms Mary Harney T.D., Tánaiste and Minister for Health and

Children for her attention and consideration. The Taoiseach has asked the Tánaiste to respond to you directly on this matter.

The Taoiseach has asked me to pass on his best wishes to you.

Yours sincerely,
xxxxx
Assistant Private Secretary to the Taoiseach

The Irish word Tánaiste[333] means Deputy Prime Minister. At this time the Minster for Health Ms Mary Harney was also the Tánaiste. The abbreviation T.D. means Teachta Dála or Member of Parliament (MP) in English.

I loved the line, "The Taoiseach has asked me to pass on his best wishes to you". This is a real Bertie-stroke; he makes people believe that he is really interested in what they have to say. As I said, he is a masterful politician.

Although Mr Bertie Ahern passed on his best wishes to me, he nonetheless attended an AIDS conference a few weeks later, and gave €70m of Irish tax-payers money to an AIDS charity fronted by former US President Bill Clinton.

In early May, my friend received a letter from Dr Darina O'Flanagan. An Taoiseach, Bertie Ahern was making sure that a government employee responded directly to a query from his constituent. I was angry with Dr Darina's response to my friend as is evident from my e-mail On Wednesday, 5th May 2006.

Dear Taoiseach,

My friend, xxxxx, who is your constituent, recently received a letter from Dr Darina O'Flanagan (Director of HPSC) with regard to the proof of the existence of the measles, mumps and rubella viruses. In this letter she stated that I didn't like her references. It is not a question of me liking or disliking her references.

I am asking for primary references for the existence of the measles, mumps and rubella viruses. She gave me two text-books which allegedly contain these references. We (Klein-Klein-Aktion) checked out these text-books. They contain no such primary references.

As an analogy, if I were to allege that little green men from Mars cause the measles virus, there is no point in giving me a novel or text-book which states this to be a fact. You would have to give me primary evidence, a photograph etc, to prove the existence of these little green men.

What I want is the primary references which state how the measles, mumps and rubella viruses were isolated, photographed and biochemically characterised. There are no such primary references.

Taoiseach, we have learned to our horror that just because a man is a priest that he can still be guilty of horrendous crimes against children. The prevailing wisdom a few decades ago would have been that a Man of God, a priest would have been incapable of such acts.

Lord Denning in his infamous "appalling vista" judgment found the Birmingham Six to be still guilty because if they were innocent this would mean the English police would have been guilty of torture, perjury, falsifying evidence, etc. This was too horrible for him to contemplate.

Likewise the prevailing wisdom in medicine is that these pathogenic viruses exist. Is it such an appalling vista to consider that the medical profession and Dr Darina O'Flanagan are wrong about these so-called viruses?

Taoiseach, the proof is simple, please ask Dr Darina O'Flanagan for the primary evidence demonstrating how these viruses were isolated, photographed and biochemically characterised.

Yours Sincerely
James McCumiskey[334]

On Wednesday, 10th May 2006, I received a stock-response e-mail from an Assistant Private Secretary to the Taoiseach to the effect that my e-mail had been referred to the Tánaiste and Minister for Health and Children, Ms Mary Harney.

Appalling vista

The "appalling vista" reference is an expression used by Lord Denning when rejecting an appeal by the Birmingham Six against their conviction. The IRA (Irish Republican Army) bombed two pubs in Birmingham in 1974 killing twenty one people. Naturally the English public were righteously outraged and the English police were under intense pressure to arrest the Irish terrorists who committed this horrific act. Unfortunately they arrested and subsequently convicted six wholly innocent Irishmen.

In rejecting one of the Birmingham Six's appeals against their unjust conviction, as one of his grounds, Lord Denning said that the six men must be guilty because if they were innocent, this would mean that the English police had tortured them, fabricated evidence and forced them to sign a confession. Such a course of events would be such an "appalling vista", that it could not be possibly contemplated: Therefore the Birmingham Six were guilty.

I followed the Birmingham Six case at the time as they were going through the appeals process. It was obvious to anyone who took the slightest interest in this case that these men were entirely innocent.

It was indeed an appalling vista that the Birmingham Six, along with other innocent Irish people, were wrongly imprisoned during what is called the "Troubles".[335] However this appalling vista only directly affected the wrongly convicted Irish people and their immediate families.

The appalling vista that one cannot verify Dr Lanka's discovery that these alleged viruses do not exist because it would mean that Modern Medicine was completely wrong, and that its central dogma, the Germ Theory of Disease is a huge moral and scientific fraud, is such an appalling and horrifying vista that it cannot be possibly contemplated.

An Tánaiste Mary Harney Minister for Health[336]

On the 1st June 2006, I finally decided to e-mail the Tánaiste Mary Harney who was also the Minister for Health directly. I was reluctant to e-mail her because I had no confidence in her ability to do anything meaningful. My impression of her was that she was completely bought into the Biomedical Paradigm. However she was Minister for Health, and I was duty bound to inform her of my concerns regarding the complete absence of any evidence supporting the existence of these viruses.

Dear Tánaiste,

I have in several e-mails dated March 2006 and April 2006 requested the primary references that Dr Darina O'Flanagan (Director HPSC) relies upon for the existence of the measles, mumps and rubella viruses.

I have also requested the Taoiseach for assistance in this matter and I understand that he has forwarded my previous e-mails to you for your attention. With respect to this matter, I am working with the Klein-Klein-Aktion organisation (www.klein-klein-aktion.de) in Germany.

I asked Dr Darina O' Flanagan in my first e-mail dated 30th March 2006 for the primary literature proving the existence of disease-inducing viruses. Instead she replied on the 31st March 2006 with two secondary sources that apparently contain primary references. This is the secondary literature she quoted to me:

1) Principles and Practices of Infectious diseases
2) Vaccines

The klein-klein-aktion organisation have examined these text books and can find no primary references for the existence of the measles, mumps and rubella viruses. Can Dr Darina O'Flanagan tell me the page number on these text books and the specific primary reference that confirm the proof of the existence of these viruses?

As an example, if I were to allege to you that little green men from Mars caused the mumps virus, you would ask me for proof, a photograph etc. In a likewise manner I am asking for primary references concerning the existence of these three viruses. The fact that they are stated to exist in a text-book does not provide sufficient proof.

In order to clearly illustrate the type of documentation that I require, I am providing you with three examples of primary references concerning the virus Dr Lanka (co-founder of the Klein-Klein-Aktion organisation) discovered in seawater:

1) Title: A Virus Infection in the Marine Brown Alga Ectocarpus siliculosus (Phaeophyceae) Authors: D.G. Müller, H. Kawai, B. Stache, and S. Lanka, Botanica Acta 103 (1990) 72-82
2) Title: Genome Structure of a Virus Infecting the Marine Brown Alga Ectocarpus siliculosus Authors: Stefan T.J. LANKA, Michael KLEIN, Uwe RAMSPERGER, Dieter G. MÜLLER, and Rolf KNIPPERS, Virology 193, 802-811 (1993)
3) Title: Coat Protein of the Ectocarpus siliculosus Virus, Authors: Michael KLEIN, Stefan T.J. LANKA, Rolf KNIPPERS, and Dieter G. MÜLLER; Virology 206, 520-526 (1995). This can be viewed at the address below
Coat Protein of the Ectocarpus siliculosus Virus

Is it possible to get similar primary references for the existence of the measles, mumps and rubella viruses?

The primary references must show how the measles, mumps and rubella viruses were isolated, photographed and biochemically characterised. This is the burden of proof currently required by science.

I appreciate any help you can give me in directing Dr Darina O'Flanagan to provide these primary references for the existence of these viruses. The implications of what I am requesting are immense: If these viruses cannot be proven to exist, then why do we vaccinate against them? This then opens up the question of the damage caused by these unnecessary vaccines that are administered to our children.

This e-mail is also being copied to the Klein-Klein-Aktion organisation.

Yours Sincerely
James McCumiskey[337]

I received a letter dated 23rd June 2006 from a Private Secretary to the Minister for Health. He stated that the matter was closed because I had received the relevant references from Dr Darina O'Flanagan. I was absolutely livid. On Sunday evening/early Monday morning, 2nd July 2006, I e-mailed the office of the Minister for Health who at that time was also the Tánaiste or Deputy Prime Minister.

Dear Tánaiste,

Thank you for the letter I received from xxxxx, Private Secretary, dated 23rd June 2006. In this letter xxxxx stated that I had received the "relevant references" from Dr Darina O'Flanagan concerning the existence of the measles, mumps and rubella viruses.

I received references to two text-books from Dr Darina O'Flanagan called:

1) Principles and Practices of Infectious diseases
2) Vaccines

These text-books are secondary sources and do not provide any proof for the existence of the measles, mumps and rubella viruses. I asked Dr Darina O'Flanagan to inform me of the page number on these text books and the specific primary reference that confirm the proof of the existence of these viruses? She has refused to answer my question.

As an example, if I were to allege to you that little green men from Mars caused the mumps virus, you would ask me for proof, a photograph etc. In a likewise manner I am asking for primary references concerning the existence of these three viruses. The fact that they are stated to exist in a text-book does not provide sufficient proof.

In order to clearly illustrate the type of documentation that I require, I am providing you with three examples of primary references concerning the virus Dr Lanka (co-founder of the Klein-Klein-Aktion organisation) discovered in seawater:

1) Title: A Virus Infection in the Marine Brown Alga Ectocarpus siliculosus (Phaeophyceae) Authors: D.G. Müller, H. Kawai, B. Stache, and S. Lanka, Botanica Acta 103 (1990) 72-82

2) Title: Genome Structure of a Virus Infecting the Marine Brown Alga Ectocarpus siliculosus Authors: Stefan T.J. LANKA, Michael KLEIN, Uwe RAMSPERGER, Dieter G. MÜLLER, and Rolf KNIPPERS, Virology 193, 802-811 (1993)
3) Title: Coat Protein of the Ectocarpus siliculosus Virus, Authors: Michael KLEIN, Stefan T.J. LANKA, Rolf KNIPPERS, and Dieter G. MÜLLER; Virology 206, 520-526 (1995). This can be viewed at the address below
Coat Protein of the Ectocarpus siliculosus Virus

I want Dr Darina O'Flanagan to give similar primary references for the existence of the measles, mumps and rubella viruses. The primary references must show how the measles, mumps and rubella viruses were isolated, photographed and biochemically characterised. This is the burden of proof currently required by science.

I know it sound unbelievable but there exists no such primary evidence for the existence of these viruses. If "viruses" existed the way Dr Darina O'Flanagan states they exist, then it would be possible for Dr Darina O'Flanagan's microbiologists and virologists, to get a blood sample from a child in Ireland suffering from measles, mumps or rubella, isolate the respective "virus", biochemically characterise it and photograph it.

They will not be able to do this apparently simple experiment because these viruses do not exist! If the HPSC personnel were real doctors and scientists, they would accept my challenge and try and isolate these viruses themselves. Unfortunately they are highly-paid charlatans masquerading as scientists, paid for by the tax-payer and apparently unaccountable to a simple enquiry from an Irish citizen.

Tánaiste, accepting the word of Dr Darina O'Flanagan of the Health Protection Surveillance Centre (HPSC) that she has provided me with "relevant references" will not absolve you of political responsibility and more importantly criminal negligence in not ensuring that Dr Darina O'Flanagan is challenged either:

1) To provide the relevant primary references or
2) Get the HPSC to isolate, photograph and biochemically characterise these viruses themselves.

I have helped translate some key articles explaining this and have published my correspondence with Dr Darina O'Flanagan on the klein-klein-aktion web-site - www.klein-klein-aktion.de

As a citizen of the Republic of Ireland, I absolutely insist that my request for the provision of the primary references for the existence of these viruses is complied with. Tánaiste, as Dr Darina O'Flanagan's employer, you have the duty to force her to comply with my request. However as Minister of Health you have a much more important duty to the children of our country to ensure that they are not poisoned by vaccines against these phantom viruses. Diseases caused by for example the MMR vaccine include autism, sudden infant death syndrome, attention deficit disorders etc.

Dr Darina O'Flanagan will not be able to provide any primary references for the existence of these viruses.

This e-mail is also being copied to the Klein-Klein-Aktion organisation and will be published on their web-site.

Yours Sincerely
James McCumiskey[338]

This letter was strong in tone. I was hoping that the strength of my argument would convince her to force Dr Darina O'Flanagan to provide the relevant primary references. But if I were to bet on it, I would bet that the Minister is relying on expert opinion and is dismissing my e-mail as that of a psychotic crank. I was certainly obsessed by all this but certainly not psychotic: Not yet, anyway!

CHAPTER 42

Virus Correspondence with the UK Experts

MHRA (Medicines and Healthcare Products Regulatory Agency)

As I currently live in the North of Ireland and as Northern Ireland is an integral part of the United Kingdom (UK), I decided to contact the relevant UK authorities. I read a few anti-vaccine articles on the internet written by UK-based authors. I e-mailed a few of them and one of them gave me an e-mail address for the Department of Health in England who referred me to the MHRA (Medicines and Healthcare Products Regulatory Agency). They said that they were the responsible authority for vaccines. I e-mailed them on the 18th May 2006.

To whom it may concern,

I understand that the MHRA is the authority responsible for vaccines in the UK.

In the last five months I have studied the work of Dr Stefan Lanka and the Klein-Klein-Aktion organisation (www.klein-klein-aktion.de). Dr Lanka states emphatically that no viruses exist in plants, animals or humans. He has asked people not to believe him directly but to question the authorities directly themselves.

I would like the primary references, (please no text books or secondary sources) which conclusively prove the existence of the measles, mumps and rubella viruses.

I can give you examples of the type of primary references I am looking for. Please find below three primary references concerning the virus Dr Lanka discovered in seawater:

1) Title: A Virus Infection in the Marine Brown Alga Ectocarpus siliculosus (Phaeophyceae) Authors: D.G. Müller, H. Kawai, B. Stache, and S. Lanka, Fundstelle/Zeitschrift: Botanica Acta 103 (1990) 72-82
2) Title: Genome Structure of a Virus Infecting the Marine Brown Alga Ectocarpus siliculosus Authors: Stefan T.J. LANKA, Michael KLEIN, Uwe RAM-

SPERGER, Dieter G. MÜLLER, and Rolf KNIPPERS, Fundstelle/Zeitschrift: Virology 193, 802-811 (1993)
3) Title: Coat Protein of the Ectocarpus siliculosus Virus, Authors: Michael KLEIN, Stefan T.J. LANKA, Rolf KNIPPERS, and Dieter G. MÜLLER, Fundstelle/Zeitschrift: Virology 206, 520-526 (1995). This can be viewed at the address below
Coat Protein of the Ectocarpus siliculosus Virus

The primary references must show how the measles, mumps and rubella viruses were isolated, photographed and biochemically characterised.
I am copying this email to the Klein-Klein-Aktion organisation.

Best Regards
James McCumiskey[339]

I was happy with this e-mail. There was no emotion involved. It was very simple; please give me the primary references for the existence of these three viruses. There are three examples of primary references attached. Please give me similar references. I received a reply a week later on the 26th May 2006.

Dear James McCumiskey

Thank you for your recent enquiry to the MHRA, for which we have liaised with the Immunisation Branch within the Department of Health.
There are numerous resources we could provide you with, one of these is 'Vaccine', edited by Plotkin and Orenstein and the last edition was published in 2004. This book describes the identification processes of measles, mumps and rubella viruses.
If you do not feel this publication addresses the concerns you have, we suggest you ask a library to conduct a literary search on your behalf.

Kind Regards,
Central Enquiry Point
Information Centre
Medicines and Healthcare products Regulatory Agency

This was clearly a stock response. They were quoting the same text-book that Dr Darina O'Flanagan referred to. The last sentence in the e-mail was a bit cheeky. The e-mail bothered me and it had to be responded to, but with some reflection. I responded a few days later on Tuesday, 30th May 2006.

To whom it may concern;

Please find attached a link to the text-book (Vaccines: Plotkin and Orenstein) you recommended to me for proof of the existence of the measles, mumps and rubella viruses.

1) Vaccines by Plotkin and Orenstein

The Klein-Klein-Aktion organisation have examined this publication and can find no primary references for the existence of the measles, mumps and rubella viruses. Can you tell me which page number on this book and which primary reference confirms the proof of the existence of these viruses?

As an example, if I were to allege to you that little green men from Mars caused the mumps virus, you would ask me for proof, a photograph etc. In a likewise manner I am asking for primary references concerning the existence of these three viruses. The fact that they are stated to exist in a text-book does not provide sufficient proof.

Once again, I will give you examples of the type of primary references I am looking for. Please find below three Primary references concerning the virus Dr Lanka discovered in seawater:

1) Title: A Virus Infection in the Marine Brown Alga Ectocarpus siliculosus (Phaeophyceae) Authors: D.G. Müller, H. Kawai, B. Stache, and S. Lanka, Fundstelle/Zeitschrift: Botanica Acta 103 (1990) 72-82
2) Title: Genome Structure of a Virus Infecting the Marine Brown Alga Ectocarpus siliculosus Authors: Stefan T.J. LANKA, Michael KLEIN, Uwe RAMSPERGER, Dieter G. MÜLLER, and Rolf KNIPPERS, Fundstelle/Zeitschrift: Virology 193, 802-811 (1993)
3) Title: Coat Protein of the Ectocarpus siliculosus Virus, Authors: Michael KLEIN, Stefan T.J. LANKA, Rolf KNIPPERS, and Dieter G. MÜLLER, Fundstelle/Zeitschrift: Virology 206, 520-526 (1995). This can be viewed at the address below

Coat Protein of the Ectocarpus siliculosus Virus

There are in fact thousands of viruses in a litre of seawater, but we do not get an infectious disease when we go for a swim in the sea?

Is it possible to get similar primary references for the existence of the measles, mumps and rubella viruses?

The primary references must show how the measles, mumps and rubella viruses were isolated, photographed and biochemically characterised.This is the burden of proof required by science. The Klein-Klein-Aktion organisation are positive that there are no such primary references for the existence of these viruses, that is these "viruses" do not actually in fact exist.

Best Regards
James McCumiskey[340]

I was being a bit flippant about the thousands of viruses in a litre of seawater. Although this is true this sentence was perhaps a little derogatory. Dr Lanka wrote that it was just as well that the health authorities did not know about the millions of viruses we encounter every time we go for a swim in the sea: Otherwise we'd all have to wear an all-body condom to protect us from these deadly allegedly infectious viruses!

I got the "Little Green Men from Mars" analogy from Karl Krafeld.[341] At this stage I was a real admirer of Karl. He teaches us how to think and his analogies are excellent.

This reply came a day later on the 31st May 2006.

Dear James McCumiskey

Thank you for your recent enquiry to the MHRA.

We responded to your original request with a reference, as requested. If you do not feel this is conclusive enough you should re-direct your enquiry to the Immunisation Policy branch of the Department of Health as this issue falls within their remit, not that of the MHRA: DHmail@dh.gsi.gov.uk

Kind Regards,
Central Enquiry Point
Information Centre
Medicines and Healthcare products Regulatory Agency

The official in the MHRA was still polite but clearly this correspondence was getting a tad tedious. In true civil-service fashion it was time to pass the buck back to the Immunization Policy Branch of the Department of Health.

Immunization Policy Branch of the Department of Health

Well I certainly wasn't going to give up. I e-mailed a similar query to the Immunization Policy branch as I did to the MRHA giving them three examples of primary references describing the virus that Dr Lanka had isolated and requesting them to provide similar references for the proof of the existence of the measles, mumps and rubella viruses.

A reply came less than two weeks later on the 13th June 2006. It certainly wasn't a stock reply and the author had clearly engaged.

Dear Mr McCumiskey,

Thank you for your email of 31 May to the Department of Health about MMR viruses. Your email has been passed to me for reply. It would appear from the contents of the web-site www.klein-klein-aktion.de that there is little or no knowledge of either vaccination or immunisation. The web-site professes not to have had a response from any of the august organisations they have approached. This can only be presumed to be because there doesn't appear to be any properly defined question being asked. More importantly, there are no references to any authors in the site, other than those you mention in your email. They are certainly not recognisable names in the field of vaccination and immunisation, and further searches have not revealed any useful information on their credentials.

However, to respond, as you have requested on your "little Green Men from Mars" analogy, I would refer you to The Big Picture Book of Viruses: Paramyxoviridae which has referenced information on every virus, including measles, mumps and rubella.

The text-book Vaccines you refer to is regarded as the definitive document on the subjects of vaccination and immunisation. There are separate chapters covering each of the vaccine preventable diseases, all of which are fully referenced, and give clear accounts of the history of each disease, and the scientific achievements in the identification of the causative organisms (either bacteria, viruses or toxins) and development of safe and effective vaccines.

Thank you again for writing.
Yours sincerely,
Kalpana Chauhan
Customer Service Centre
Department of Health[342]

Kalpana (I didn't know the gender or origin of this name at the time) had certainly engaged. The first paragraph was the formalities. He/she got stuck into Klein-Klein in the second paragraph. I figured a male. It had to be a he. The third paragraph gave me a web-site address where there were loads of photographs of alleged viruses. The fourth paragraph clearly justified the text-book *Vaccines*.

I had already helped translate some articles Dr Lanka had written, explaining to non-virologists/microbiologists, explaining to the layman how to identify a real isolated virus.

I looked at a few of the pictures. I wasn't over-awed by them. I knew they were false. I did a first draft that night. In my first draft, I used phrases like "virology for dummies". I toned it down and sent the following e-mail one night later on the 14th June 2006.

Dear Kalpana Chauhan,

Thank you for responding to my e-mail. I am an accountant and not a virologist. But I have helped translate a number of Dr Lanka's articles, which should be published on the Klein-Klein web-site in the near future. In the process of translation I worked with Susanne Brix from Klein-Klein and from our countless e-mails I believe I can answer your points directly myself and pose questions of my own.

I am surprised that you state that "there doesn't appear to be any properly defined question being asked". On the contrary!

Dr Lanka discovered a virus in seawater. There are three publicly available scientific publications where he clearly demonstrates how this virus was isolated, biochemically characterised and photographed. The relevant scientific publications once again are:

1) Title: A Virus Infection in the Marine Brown Alga Ectocarpus siliculosus (Phaeophyceae) Authors: D.G. Müller, H. Kawai, B. Stache, and S. Lanka, Fundstelle/Zeitschrift: Botanica Acta 103 (1990) 72-82
2) Title: Genome Structure of a Virus Infecting the Marine Brown Alga Ectocarpus siliculosus Authors: Stefan T.J. LANKA, Michael KLEIN, Uwe RAMSPERGER, Dieter G. MÜLLER, and Rolf KNIPPERS, Fundstelle/Zeitschrift: Virology 193, 802-811 (1993)
3) Title: Coat Protein of the Ectocarpus siliculosus Virus, Authors: Michael KLEIN, Stefan T.J. LANKA, Rolf KNIPPERS, and Dieter G. MÜLLER, Fundstelle/Zeitschrift: Virology 206, 520-526 (1995). This can be viewed at the address below
Coat Protein of the Ectocarpus siliculosus Virus

Have you read Dr Lanka's publications so that you are familiar with the type of evidence I want? All I am looking for is similar type publications that prove the existence of the measles, mumps and rubella viruses.

You provided me with a link (The Big Picture Book of Viruses: Paramyxoviridae) which allegedly gives photographs of these apparently pathogenic viruses. Will you please tell me the names of the scientific publications which describe how these three viruses (measles, mumps and rubella) were isolated, biochemically characterised and then photographed. I hope you understand this to be a "properly defined question".

In the course of translating Dr Lanka's article, I learned that photographs from an electron microscope are always in back and white. Can you confirm this? The relevance of this question is that we are looking for the primary evidence, the original photograph from an electron microscope and not a doctored image.

I also learned that all viruses of a particular type, all have the same shape and consistency. The one thing all these photographs have in common is that they all show viruses with different shapes. Dr Lanka states emphatically that these so-called pictures of viruses, do not show a virus that is isolated from its host cell.

I am only concerned with a true scientific understanding of what is being shown in these photographs of these so-called disease-inducing viruses. I have accepted Dr Lanka's challenge for ordinary people to request the authorities for information so that Dr Lanka's incredible allegations can be rebutted. Please help me! If you can show me a photograph of a virus and the scientific publication which demonstrates how this virus was isolated and biochemically characterised I would be most grateful. I require this information for the measles, mumps and rubella viruses.

This e-mail is of course being copied to the Klein-Klein-Aktion organisation (www.klein-klein-aktion.de) for their attention.

Yours Sincerely
James McCumiskey[343]

Kalpana responded on Thursday 13th July, almost a month after my original e-mail. Clearly this correspondence was becoming more serious. Kalpana had attempted to provide me with scientific journals that allegedly prove the existence of these viruses.

Dear Mr McCumiskey,

Thank you for your further email of 14 June to the Department of Health about publications proving the existence of measles, mumps and rubella viruses.

There are numerous publications that describe the investigation and visualisation of measles, mumps and rubella viruses (see links below) and a description of their identification and isolation are described in virology text books (such as Vaccines, fourth edition by Plotkin and Orenstein 2003). In addition, these viruses have been sequenced and their molecular structure determined.

For information on genomic sequences and three dimensional structures, you may like to visit the National Centre for Biotechnology Information website at: Entrez, The Life Sciences Search Engine

Further links to electron microscopy publications are listed below:

Immuno-Electron Microscopy of the Morphogenesis of Mumps Virus

Hemadsorption of Mumps Virus Examined by Light and Electron Microscopy Electron Microscopy of Monkey Kidney Cell Cultures Infected with Rubella Virus

Antibody-induced capping of measles virus antigens on plasma membrane studied by electron microscopy

Electron microscopy of the development of rubella virus in BHK-21 cells

Electron Microscopic Study on the Development of Measles Virus in Cultured Cells

Fine Structure of Cellular Inclusions in Measles Virus Infections

Observations of Measles Virus Infection of Cultured Human Cells: I. A Study of Development and Spread of Virus Antigen by Means of Immunofluorescence

Immuno-Electron Microscopy of the Morphogenesis of Mumps Virus

Electron Microscopy of Monkey Kidney Cell Cultures Infected with the Rubella virus

Electron microscopy of the development of rubella virus in BHK-21 ...

I hope this reply is helpful.

Yours sincerely,

Kalpana Chauhan
Customer Service Centre
Department of Health[344]

I initially looked at these pictures and knew straight away that they did not show isolated viruses because they were not all of equal size and disposition. However I asked Susanne Brix to have a look at them and to respond back. At this stage of our correspondence I wrote my e-mails to her in English and she wrote back in German. Susanne responded back and really all she did was look at the captions on the photographs and on the tile of the journal. There was no need to read all the material contained in the journal. And anyway it was all mumbo jumbo to me; I'd have to take a few courses in virology to appreciate what they were writing. Two weeks later, very late on Tuesday evening, 25th July, I responded to Kalpana Chauhan. My response to Kalpana in English was more or less what Susanne had written to me in German.

Dear Kalpana Chauhan,

Thank you for responding with the scientific publications. I will respond individually to each of the publications you have given me in my quest for proof of the existence of the measles, mumps and rubella viruses. I stated that the isolation, biochemical characterisation and a photograph of the measles, mumps and rubella viruses would be sufficient to prove their existence.

1) Entrez, The Life Sciences Search Engine

This is a Life Science web-site and not a scientific publication. It is not possible to produce a genomic sequence and three-dimensional structure of something that has never been proven to exist.

Therefore this reference did not interest me at all. I was however interested in the scientific publications you gave me.

2) Immuno-Electron Microscopy of the Morphogenesis of Mumps Virus

There is no photograph of an isolated virus contained. Isolated viruses are of equal size and disposition. These are not shown here. The authors don't even claim that the photographs are of isolated viruses. For example Pictures 19-24 show "virus particles" but do not claim to show isolated viruses.

3) Hemadsorption of Mumps Virus Examined by Light and Electron Microscopy

Again just by looking at the picture titles in this publication, it is immediately clear that the author is not claiming to have isolated the mumps virus. In fact what these pictures show are solely components of cells which by definition one cannot isolate.

4) Electron microscopy of the development of rubella virus in BHK-21 cells

Again just by looking at the picture titles in this publication, it is immediately clear that the authors are not claiming to have isolated the rubella virus.

5) Electron Microscopy of Monkey Kidney Cell Cultures Infected with Rubella Virus

This publication looked interesting because of the title of the article. "Electron Microscopy of Monkey Kidney Cell Cultures Infected with the Rubella Virus". Maybe I would finally see the Rubella virus? Unfortunately not. The Picture tiles state "infected cells" but nowhere does it state that the Rubella virus has been isolated.

6) Antibody-induced capping of measles virus antigens on plasma membrane studied by electron microscopy

Again just by looking at the picture titles in this publication, it is immediately clear that the authors are not claiming to have isolated the measles virus. Nowhere in this publication is there any acknowledgement that the measles virus has been isolated.

7) Electron microscopy of the development of rubella virus in BHK-21 cells

Again just by looking at the picture titles in this publication, it is immediately clear that the authors are not claiming to have isolated the measles virus.

8) Electron Microscopic Study on the Development of Measles Virus in Cultured Cells

This publication looked interesting: "Development of Measles Virus in Cultured Cells". However the problem is it doesn't evince any evidence of how the alleged measles virus was isolated, biochemically characterised and photographed.

9) Fine Structure of Cellular Inclusions in Measles Virus Infections

Again just by looking at the picture titles in this publication, it is immediately clear that the authors are not claiming to have isolated the measles virus.

10) Observations of Measles Virus Infection of Cultured Human Cells: I. A Study of Development and Spread of Virus Antigen by Means of Immunofluorescence

Again just by looking at the picture titles in this publication, it is immediately clear that the authors are not claiming to have isolated the measles virus.

11) Immuno-Electron Microscopy of the Morphogenesis of Mumps Virus

Again just by looking at the picture titles in this publication, it is immediately clear that the authors are not claiming to have isolated the mumps virus.

12) Electron Microscopy of Monkey Kidney Cell Cultures Infected with the Rubella virus

This publication looked interesting because of the title of the article. "Electron Microscopy of Monkey Kidney Cell Cultures Infected with the Rubella Virus". Maybe I would finally see the Rubella virus? Unfortunately not. The picture tiles state "infected cells" but nowhere does it state that the rubella virus has been isolated.

13) Electron microscopy of the development of rubella virus in BHK-21 ...

Again just by looking at the picture titles in this publication, it is immediately clear that the authors are not claiming to have isolated the rubella virus.

I wonder did you do a search for publications with the words "measles", "mumps", or "rubella" contained therein? Because although all of these publications allegedly show pictures of these viruses none of them claim to have isolated these viruses. Even if you ask the authors none of them will claim to have isolated these viruses. Please do!

I should point out that the research on these publications was done by Susanne Brix from Klein-Klein-Aktion who is by profession a tax accountant and not a virologist.

I suggest that you ask the best virologist or microbiologist in the Department of Health for help! Either find the relevant publication or even better do the experiments and try and isolate these viruses yourselves.

When you cannot find any proof of the existence of these viruses and that their existence is purely because of a medical dogma - the Germ Theory of Disease -, please publicly admit it.

Yours Sincerely
James McCumiskey[345]

Almost a month later, on the 23rd of August 2006, I received the following brush-off e-mail.

Dear Mr McCumiskey,

Thank you for your further email of 25 July about MMR.

As your opinions appear to be in direct opposition to scientific evidence, the Department of Health is unable to help you further.

Yours sincerely,

Kalpana Chauhan
Customer Service Centre
Department of Health

My last paragraph about the Germ Theory of Disease medical myth did not go down too well. I thought about this e-mail for a while and came up with the following response on the 5th September 2006.

Dear Kalpana Chauhan

I am responding to your e-mail dated 23rd August, where you have cut off communication on the basis that you have no interest in discussing my opinion on the Germ Theory of Disease. I too have no interest in discussing my opinions with you either. In my discussions with you, I am only interested in scientific facts.

What I am specifically interested in is this: Proof that allegedly disease-inducing viruses such as measles, mumps and rubella exist. Your organisation promotes vaccinations against these putative viruses. Surely it is not unreasonable to request the evidence for the existence of these viruses?

As stated many times in previous correspondence, any proof of the existence of a pathogenic virus would have to show how the virus was 1) isolated, 2) photographed and 3) biochemically characterised.

I have in previous correspondence provided you with three scientific references for the existence of a virus that Dr Lanka discovered in seawater. In accordance with the strict scientific standards of reproducibility Dr Lanka has clearly demonstrated how this virus was isolated, photographed and biochemically characterised.

Dr Lanka further states that there are millions of viruses in a litre of seawater. Yet these viruses are clearly harmless, otherwise we would have to wear a total-body condom before going for a swim in the sea!

In a previous e-mail you provided me with scientific papers which allegedly contained photographs of the measles, mumps and rubella viruses, which you claimed proved the existence of these three viruses. I responded to your e-mail and demonstrated that they clearly did not show pictures of an isolated measles, mumps or rubella virus. I challenged you to even ask the authors of these papers whether they had claimed to have isolated these respective viruses.

I am still awaiting a scientific paper which proves the existence of these alleged viruses.

If you provide me with proof for the existence of the measles, mumps and rubella viruses then I will admit I am wrong and will then have to revise my opinion concerning the Germ Theory of Disease.

Yours Sincerely

James McCumiskey[346]

The point of this e-mail was to draw back from any opinion I have on the Germ Theory of Disease and to make it clear that all I am interested in is scientific papers proving the existence of the measles, mumps and rubella viruses.

I did not get any response.

CHAPTER 43

New Medicine Correspondence with the Irish Health Minister

On Thursday 13th April 2006, I decided to inform the Tánaiste (Irish Deputy Prime Minister) who is also the Minister for Health about the German New Medicine. I did not want her or her officials in the Department for Health in the future saying, "I did not know". I do not know whether her officials actually got her to read this e-mail.

Dear Tánaiste,

My name is James McCumiskey. I am an Irish citizen currently living in Belfast. I have no medical training. However I have been studying German New Medicine (GNM) for the last few years. GNM is the result of the life's work of a Dr Ryke Geerd Hamer.

Briefly Dr Hamer was a successful 43 year old Internist in 1978 when his son Dirk died in very tragic circumstances. Dr Hamer developed several months later testicular cancer. He had his right testicle removed but he declined any further radiation treatment and nearly died himself.

He wondered was there a connection between him getting testicular cancer and the shock he experienced at the unexpected death of his son Dirk. He investigated this connection and came up with what is now called German New Medicine.

While GNM explains the mechanism of every disease it is easier to understand (for the layman) in relation to cancer. With the application of GNM, 95% of cancer patients could survive at a cost at least 75% less than what we currently pay. GNM has been tested on numerous occasions but has not found favour with the medical profession for reasons that will become apparent to you as you learn more about GNM.

There are a few web-sites explaining GNM in English. I have also written a book explaining the five Biological Laws of GNM. I would be happy to forward it to you if you are interested.

GNM will be the medicine of the future and should be the medicine of today.

Best Regards
James McCumiskey[347]

On reflection, the e-mail was weak. It looks like I'm trying to push my book, which I was. The claims about the cure rates and the cost of GNM might seem to be too good to be true. 99% of the time anything that is too good to be true is usually not. In the case though of the GNM, this is not true. But neither the Minister for Health nor her officials will know that.

I did not receive a reply to my e-mail. I'm not sure if this is an example of the sheer incompetence of Ms Mary Harney personally or of the officials in her Department. Six months after my first e-mail concerning German New Medicine on the 19th September 2006, I decided to e-mail her office again. At this time she had resigned the office of Tánaiste (deputy Prime Minister) but was still the Minister for Health.

Dear Minister of Health, Mary Harney TD,

Minister, I note that the Taoiseach has launched an "active citizenship" program recently about trying to get citizens to engage fully in our Republic. I believe I am being a good and active citizen in bringing to your attention as Minister for Health the work of Dr Ryke Geerd Hamer and his body of work known as German New Medicine.

Briefly,

German New Medicine (GNM) has five Biological Laws. It explains the mechanism of every cancer and disease except diseases caused by malnutrition, poisoning, trauma etc.

1 The first Biological Law is known as the Iron Rule of Cancer or IRC.

It is called the Iron Rule of Cancer because when Dr Hamer discovered it he thought it only applied to cancers. He subsequently proved that the IRC applies to all diseases. Every disease is caused by a biological shock or Dirk Hamer Syndrome (DHS). The DHS is a difficult, highly acute, dramatic and isolating shock occurring simultaneously on the three levels of the human trinity:

1 Psyche

2 Brain

3 Organ

2 The second Biological Law is known as the Law of Two-phases

The first phase is the "conflict-active phase", which occurs after a DHS or biological shock has occurred. There is a [348] *"healing-phase" after you have resolved the conflict in your psyche.*

The conflict-active phase is also called the "cold phase". When the body is under stress the blood vessels are constricted resulting in cold hands and cold feet, a cold skin, chills, shivers, or cold sweats. In the conflict-active phase one is thinking compulsively about the event that caused the biological shock.

The healing phase is also called the "hot phase" because the blood vessels are widened resulting in warm hands, warm skin, and possible fever. There is a feeling in the mind or psyche of great relief that the conflict is finally over.

3 The third Biological Law is called The Ontogenetic System of Tumours and Cancer-equivalent diseases.

This third Biological Law states that the symptoms of a cancer or other disease in the conflict-active phase and the reparation phase are dependent upon the germ layer that the respective organ is made up from.

There are three germ layers; the endoderm or inner germ layer, the mesoderm or middle germ layer and the ectoderm or outer germ layer. These germ layers are built up in the first 15 days of the life of a newly created Baby or Embryo.

4 The fourth Biological Law is called the Ontogenetic System of Microbes

The fourth Biological Law states that the types of microbes operating in the reparation phase are dependent upon the germ layer that the diseased organ is made up from.

The microbes only operate in the reparation phase and do not operate in the conflict-active phase. The microbes fungi operate on Endodermal tissue, bacteria on Mesodermal tissue and smaller microbes on Ectodermal tissue.

5 The fifth Biological Law: Meaningful Biological Program of Nature – the quintessence

The quintessence of Hamer's German New Medicine is that every so-called cancer (or disease) has to be understood as a Meaningful Biological Program of Nature (MBP) created to solve a biological shock.

By applying these five Biological Laws to common cancers one can avoid costly and ineffective medical treatments and more importantly save annually thousands of patients' lives that would otherwise be prematurely dead because of conventional medical treatments.

A brain relay is "switched on" in the conflict-active phase and in the reparation phase, which can be observed on a CT scan of the brain. In fact merely by examining a CT scan of a patient, Dr Hamer or any other GNM doctor/therapist would be able to ascertain what diseases the patient had.

Disease example Glandular Breast Cancer

Let us take as an example a woman who is walking with her toddler on the pavement. The toddler breaks free from her mother's hand and runs out onto the road. The toddler gets knocked down by a car and is seriously though not mortally injured.

The mother gets a biological shock or Dirk Hamer Syndrome - DHS (first Biological Law). Her beautiful daughter has been knocked down and she is blaming herself. She is compulsively thinking about the accident. She is in the conflict-active phase of Glandular Breast Cancer. This tissue in this part of the breast is mesodermal in origin, which means that a tumor grows in the conflict-active phase and is degraded in the reparation phase (third Biological Law). The specific type of microbe involved is mycobacteria (fourth Biological Law).

The reason why a tumour would grow in the conflict active phase is because in biological terms, an injured offspring recovers faster when it receives more milk. Extra milk production is immediately stimulated by increasing the number of breast gland cells. This tumor is not a meaningless cancer but a Meaningful Biological Program of Nature (fifth Biological Law) designed to produce extra milk for the injured child. Even if the woman is not breast feeding, the biological shock still triggers the onset of this response as it has been doing over millions of years. As long as a woman is in the conflict-active phase (because her child is still in hospital), the breast cells will keep dividing and multiplying, forming what is commonly called a glandular breast tumour.

Breast cancer vividly demonstrates the principle of laterality – whether the woman is right-handed or left-handed. If the woman is right handed, the tumour will be in her left "child"-breast; if she is left handed her right breast will be affected.

As soon as the conflict is resolved in a meaningful way for the mother (when her child is well again and released from the hospital), the tumour immediately stops growing (second and third Biological Laws). Since the child is out of danger, there is no longer a need to produce extra breast gland cells. During the reparation phase the now superfluous cells are broken down with the help of mycobacteria. The tumour will be completely removed by these microbes with the completion of the healing process (fourth Biological Law).

Having examined hundreds of patients with "glandular breast cancer" Hamer established that this type of cancer concerned worries or arguments within what a woman terms to be her "nest", For example her home, her children, her partner, her workplace.

This is one example of a cancer. Dr Hamer has a disease chart that explains the mechanism of all cancers and other diseases.

Conclusion

There is no point in me or you as Minister for Health notifying the Irish medical profession because they will automatically dismiss the work of Dr Hamer without seriously considering it – a known medical condition called the Semmelweis Reflex.[349]

What I want is to have Dr Hamer's five Biological Laws tested in Ireland. The testing protocols could be agreed within a matter of weeks. I can understand a reluctance to test the German New Medicine on the basis of one e-mail from an ordinary citizen – but this I understand to be the basic principle of active citizenship. There is also an enormous amount of published literature explaining GNM which I can put at your disposal.

In Italy and Switzerland, 50,000 signatures are required to force the government to act on a particular petition. Petitions concerning the testing of German New Medicine are currently underway in these countries. Is there a similar law in Ireland that can force you as Minister of Health to test the five Biological Laws that Dr Hamer has discovered? If there is I will personally organise a similar petition.

However I implore you to voluntarily agree to openly test these five Biological Laws of Dr Hamer. If you agree to do so, Ireland will be the first country in the world to verify this wonderful New Medicine. History will judge you very kindly for such a brave decision.

Yours Sincerely
James McCumiskey[350]

This e-mail was reasonably all right, except in the original e-mail I had left in the title of the third Biological Law in the title of the fourth Biological Law. The fourth Biological Law was, of course, the Ontogenetic System of Microbes. This was a major error! I had learned to curb my anger and hopefully appeal to her common humanity. I sent the e-mail without expectation of a response just so that she could not later deny that "she did not know". Even if she was never given the letter, some senior officials in her department could not deny subsequently any lack of knowledge.

I am sure that they will use the excuse that they relied on expert opinion. However I was not an expert when I first came across German New Medicine, but I was able to form an opinion and then able to read and inform myself further. Surely the officials in the Department of Health can also do that? I doubt it.

I received no response.

CHAPTER 44

Other New Medicine Correspondence

The Catholic Church

As a Catholic specifically, and more importantly as a Christian, I felt it important to inform the Pope about the German New Medicine. I looked up the Vatican web-site and found an e-mail address. I didn't know if it was the direct e-mail address for the Pope, but I'm sure that with a few prayers on my part and the help of Vatican officials the e-mail might receive the attention of the Pope himself.

His Holiness Pope Benedict XV1 is German. I wrote the e-mail in English. Susanne Brix from Klein-Klein-Aktion translated it into German. I agreed her translation with some minor changes. I sent the German version of the e-mail to the Pope. I felt that as a German he could better read it in his mother tongue. I also felt that he might be surprised to get a letter written in German by an Irishman. The novelty factor alone might encourage him to read it.

Would he get it? Would he read it? Would he act upon it? Only time would tell.

Holy Father,

I am a 41-year-old Catholic living in Belfast, Ireland. I am married with two young boys, 5- and 8-years old. I work as an accountant and have a degree in engineering. However my letter to you is as a lay-member of the Catholic Church, from one Christian to another.

My father died from primary liver cancer in October 2002, shortly before his 65th birthday. Since that time I have become extremely interested in medical matters.

I came across what is now called German New Medicine. This is the life-work of a Dr Ryke Geerd Hamer. In it he describes the mechanism of every cancer and most other diseases (except those caused by malnutrition, poisoning etc).

Dr Hamer has conclusively proven that every cancer/disease is caused by a "biological shock". He was a 43-year-old doctor in 1978 when his son Dirk died in tragic circumstances. Dr Hamer subsequently got testicular cancer. He had been healthy all his life and resolved that when he recovered from cancer that he would investigate the link between the shock he experienced at the tragic loss of his son and him getting testicular cancer.

He has proven the connection between a shock and a particular disease. For example, liver cancer is a starvation conflict. This is why liver cancer rates are the most commonly occurring cancer in countries where there is a real danger of starvation. Another example: testicular and ovarian cancer occur because of the shock associated with the loss or disappearance of a loved one etc.

Depending on the nature or theme of the "shock-experience" one gets different forms of cancers or other diseases. Holy Father, Dr Hamer has scientifically proven the mind-body connection. There is a clear connection between a shock with a particular conflict-theme in the pyche, the affected brain relay (which is observable on a CT scan) and the organ that is affected. The connection is clear: Psyche -> Brain -> Organ.

In the last year I have come across the work of a Dr Stefan Lanka and his organisation Klein-Klein-Aktion. Dr Lanka has scientifically proven that the Germ Theory of Disease is an absolute moral and scientific fraud. No virus such as measles, mumps or rubella have ever been scientifically isolated, photographed and biochemically characterised. His organisation are requesting the health authorities in a number of European countries for scientific evidence of the existence of these viruses. No such evidence has been produced nor can it be produced.

The Germ Theory of Disease is to orthodox medicine what the Resurrection is to Christianity. If Jesus did not rise from the dead on the third day, then he is not the Son of God and Christianity is meaningless. Similarly with orthodox medicine, its most important dogma or belief is that of the Germ Theory of Disease. We have experienced the destructive secular religions of communism and fascism. However the most destructive secular religion of all-time is that of orthodox medicine. It has managed to convince most of humanity that the diseases that afflict us come from the outside and not from within.

If we can reorient ourselves to the fact that diseases come from within, we can collectively reconnect our bodies to our psyche and then to our soul, to the Holy Spirit that is in each of us. In this way the world will become much better, more spiritual and truly Christian.

Once the mechanism of disease according to Dr Hamer is generally accepted, namely that of Psyche -> Brain -> Organ, this equation can be modified to account for the Holy Spirit, the third person of the Blessed Trinity: Spirit -> Psyche ->Brain -> Organ.

The rediscovery of the absolute scientific truth of the mind–body connection will allow the Christian Church to overcome the present-day dominant secular religions of orthodox medicine and pseudo-science.

Holy Father, Jesus says in John 8:32 "And you will know the truth, and the truth will set you free". The truth of the German New Medicine, and the absent evidence of any disease-inducing viruses will set us free from the secular religion of orthodox medicine and allow mankind to once again discover the truth of the risen Christ.

Holy Father, in the words of your dear friend John Paul 2: "Be not afraid".

Yours Sincerely
James McCumiskey[351]

This letter summed up my beliefs. I am a Christian. I believe that Jesus Christ is the son of God, that he was crucified and died on the Cross and rose from the dead on the third day. But I realise this is a belief, a faith; there is no scientific evidence for it. But I do know that without this belief in Jesus and without the help of the Holy Spirit, I would have long ago given up on this endeavour. This faith sustains me now as it always has. This is all I believe in. I do not believe in anything else.

Fascism is a secular religion based upon the false premise that some races are inherently superior to others. Communism is a secular religion based on the false premise of enforced equality of income and wealth by an all-knowing state. Modern Medicine is a secular religion built around the Biomedical Paradigm, which in time will be universally accepted to have killed and injured many times more people than both fascism and communism combined.

Dr Hamer and Dr Lanka are not my personal gurus. I read what they have to say, very slowly, and repeatedly (my German isn't very good) and I try to understand it. Dr Lanka's discovery that there is no such thing as a virus ties in with Dr Hamer's fourth Biological Law: that microbes (fungi, bacteria and smaller microbes that are "virus-like") are only present in the reparation phase of a disease, in the "hot-phase", usually accompanied by a fever.

Dr Lanka and Karl Krafeld fully accepted Dr Hamer's wonderful discovery of the German New Medicine and Dr Hamer likewise accepted that there was no such thing as viruses and so-called infectious diseases. It all fitted together beautifully.

It is remarkable that all these discoveries are by Germans: They are going to save us all from the Horror of Modern Medicine.

The President of the Bavarian Cancer Society

The President of the Bavarian Cancer Society issued the following statement which was published in Passauer Woche on 8th March

2006. The translation is by Caroline Markolin, who published the letter on her web-site[352] in mid-June 2006.

"German New Medicine" (GNM) is the obtuse and pseudo-scientific doctrine of an outsider, which has been developed and propagated by the former medical doctor Dr Ryke Geerd Hamer, and is apparently the result of the dramatic death of his son Dirk that caused Hamer's testicular cancer a few months after his son's passing.

Recent epidemiological studies clearly show that there is no increased risk of developing cancer with people who suffer from depressions or from severe psychological stress (Source: Dalton et al. 2002 and 2004).

There is also no evidence that people with a so-called "cancer personality", that show certain characteristics and attitudes would be at greater risk of developing cancer (Source: Schwarz et al 2001).

Hamer claims that the cause of every disease, including cancer, is always a "biological conflict", a serious dramatic shock, which he calls a "Dirk Hamer Syndrome", and which typically shows as a "Hamer Focus" (German: Hamerscher Herd) on a computer tomogram of the brain. Hence, the resolution of the underlying conflict ("conflictolysis") is said to be the prerequisite for the natural healing process in every phase of an illness such as cancer. Cancer is, according to Hamer, a "Meaningful Special Biological Program" and already part of the healing process itself. Chemotherapy is viewed as a pseudo-treatment that stimulates the cancer growth and is seen as equal to exorcism.

Regretfully, there have been some cases where patients, who blindly turned to his absurd teachings (Hamer promises a 95% success rate with cancer), died despite of a curable disease, like testicular cancer, by depriving themselves from the conventional, allegedly "Jewish", treatment. Several deaths that could have been avoided are documented in Germany as well as in France.

Hamer's doctrine is irrational and is lacking in scientific or empirical evidence; based on the aforementioned fatalities, it has to be considered as extremely dangerous.

The potential legal consequences for medical doctors, who on the basis of this method discontinue or stop conventional treatments, is to be charged with negligence in providing medical assistance or to possibly lose their medical license.

In 1986, Hamer himself was stripped of his medical license. But, he continued to practice illegally. In December 2004, he had been imprisoned in France for a three-year term for the illegal practice of medicine. He is facing other jail sentences in Austria as well as in Germany. The Bavarian Cancer Society expressively warns patients not to trust into this kind of treatment.

All available judicial means must be generated to stop any further dissemination of this doctrine.

Professor Dr Reiner Hartenstein,
President of the Bavarian Cancer Society[353]

This statement was revealing for a number of reasons. The principal reason was that the statement was issued in the first place. Clearly people are becoming aware of the German New Medicine and are asking the oncologists (cancer MDs) about it. This bothers them. Good! Let's hope that millions more people begin to hear about it and query their respective oncologists and MDs.

Professor Hartenstein confuses the Dirk Hamer Syndrome with a cancer personality/depression/severe psychological stress. It is none of these things. It is a shock that has caught the patient off-guard, on the wrong foot and completely unawares. There is no "mumbo-jumbo" involved in a DHS. The patient will have a clear recollection of the DHS, the sleepless nights and the constant obsessing about the circumstances of the DHS. The DHS has nothing to do with any pseudo-scientific theory of a cancer personality.

He calls German New Medicine obtuse and pseudo-scientific. Nothing could be further from the truth. In fact, these adjectives are absolutely accurate about Modern Medicine.

In challenge, Dr Hamer told Professor Hartenstein that he was willing to demonstrate the Biological Laws of the GNM on any number of patients in front of a video camera. Naturally, the Professor won't accept the challenge. However, I feel that this open verification, preferably in a reality TV format, is the only way for the general public to be able to clearly view the German New Medicine for what it is. Let the public and the afflicted patients make up their minds.

He states that all judicial means must be used to stop the spread of German New Medicine. In fact that has already happened. Hamer has twice been jailed for the crime of "agitation against orthodox medicine" or stating very clearly that orthodox medicine is wrong. This is truly incredible that an MD cannot act outside the "thought-police" of his own profession without being indicted.

Most worryingly, the professor made a remark about the conventional, allegedly "Jewish" treatment for cancer. The professor has identified Dr Hamer's great weakness, his Achilles' heel.

Dr Hamer cannot understand why the German New Medicine has not been already implemented worldwide. Unfortunately Dr Hamer believes that there is a conspiracy to apply the German New Medicine exclusively for the Jews and not for the benefit of the rest of humanity.

I have applied my common sense and my own personal experience of life in my study of the German New Medicine. GNM makes sense, I understand it and in particular I understand the five Biological Laws of Nature. Dr Hamer's claims are simple: let us openly test the German New Medicine on patients with specific diseases. Let it be openly proven or disproven. This is surely not too much to ask for?

However I cannot accept the assertion that Jews as a religious group are deliberately suppressing the implementation worldwide of German New Medicine. The suppression of the German New Medicine is because of the irrational and unscientific belief of the MDs and other white-coats in the Biomedical Paradigm. The white-coats cannot accept any new medical and scientific evidence that proves the Biomedical Paradigm to be a scientific and criminal fraud, which is the Ultimate Conspiracy.

I signed Caroline Markolin's petition to Professor Dr Reiner Hartenstein. I was disappointed by the number of signatories, hundreds in the English-language petition and only a few thousand in the German-language petition. GNM was not reaching a wide enough audience.

I knew that this oncologist, this white-coat would not dare openly test German New Medicine. But with enough pressure, some day soon, some government in the free world will eventually test this wonderful New Medicine. This has to be the goal.

CHAPTER 45

Active citizenship

Active Citizenship

I thought deeply about my correspondence with Dr Darina O'Flanagan, Director of the HPSC (Health Protection Surveillance Centre) in Ireland. I had made a complete mess, but I still wanted an answer to a simple question. Could she provide me with a scientific publication that proved the existence of the measles, mumps and rubella viruses? I e-mailed her on Wednesday night, 21st September 2006, and copied it to the Minister for Health, the Taoiseach (Prime Minister), and Susanne Brix of Klein-Klein-Aktion. I included in the e-mail the response I sent to Kalpana Chauhan regarding the pictures of the alleged measles, mumps and rubella viruses.

Dear Dr Darina O'Flanagan

Please find attached a copy of an email I sent to the Immunisation Policy branch of the Department of Health in England. At least they have engaged and are attempting to provide a scientific publication which proves the existence of the measles, mumps and rubella viruses.

You and your organisation strongly recommend vaccinations against the measles, mumps and rubella viruses. I am asking for the scientific publications which prove the existence of these viruses, which demonstrates how these viruses were 1 isolated, 2 photographed and 3 biochemically characterised.

I believe that what I am doing constitutes what the Taoiseach calls "active citizenship". In the spirit of citizenship and true republicanism, if no such scientific publication exists would you please inform the Minister for Health and the Irish public?

Yours Sincerely
James McCumiskey

I was absolutely certain at this stage that the approach initially advanced by Karl Krafeld of Klein-Klein-Aktion was absolutely correct: Ordinary citizens must ask the relevant authorities for proof of the existence of these alleged viruses. It is the only way to get to the truth of the non-existence of any virus.

The paragraph about "active citizenship" was in reference to an initiative recently launched by the Taoiseach (Prime Minister) about getting people to actively participate in our Republic. I didn't expect a reply from Dr Darina O'Flanagan. I do wonder though if she or anybody else in her organization or in the Department of Health are taking any of this seriously. Probably not. They could dismiss me as a crackpot or a fanatic, but the allegations I make are extremely serious. I believe that in a true republic these government officials would be duty-bound to investigate these claims.

On Friday 22nd September 2006, two days later, I received an acknowledgement of my copy e-mail to An Taoiseach. My query had been referred to the Minister for Health and Children for her attention.

The Taoiseach was again delegating this e-mail for the attention of the Minister for Health. It is a health matter, but this health matter should be of concern to everybody and not just the Minister for Health. This e-mail was clearly a stock reply e-mail that was almost exactly the same as previous responses, only the date had changed. I responded that night to the reply from the Taoiseach's Office:

Dear xxxxx,

Please thank the Taoiseach sincerely on my behalf and please send him my best wishes.

Given past correspondence from the Minister for Health, I do not expect her to act on this e-mail. In my last round of correspondence with the Minister for Health she stated that I had been provided with the "relevant references" by Dr Darina O'Flanagan Director of the HPSC.

Dr Darina O'Flanagan has given me the names of two text-books which allegedly contain primary references for the existence of the measles, mumps and rubella viruses. The Klein-Klein-Aktion organisation has examined these text-books and can find no such primary references.

What I am asking for is primary references (which are published in a scientific journal) for the existence of the measles, mumps and rubella viruses. These primary references must show how the respective virus was 1 isolated, 2 photographed and 3 biochemically characterised - in accordance with current scientific standards.

Believe it or not but this simple and apparently stupid request cannot be complied with by Dr Darina O'Flanagan because no such primary references exist because these viruses do not exist!

Please compel Dr Darina O'Flanagan to provide the relevant primary references; one reference per virus would be sufficient.

I believe that what I am doing constitutes "active citizenship". If you as Taoiseach act on my request and compel Dr Darina O'Flanagan to answer my request you will be proving that Ireland is a truly great republic.

I am also copying this e-mail to Dr Darina O'Flanagan and the Klein-Klein-Aktion organisation.

Yours Sincerely,
James McCumiskey

I addressed the e-mail to a Private Secretary as if I were writing to the Taoiseach. Anyway the message was clear. I had copied Dr Darina O'Flanagan in the hope but certainly not the expectation that she would try and ascertain the truth of what Dr Lanka was saying: that these viruses simply do not exist.

President Thabo Mbeki and the HIV-AIDS medical myth

The South African President, Thabo Mbeki, is the only worldwide leader to have questioned the HIV-AIDS medical myth. His misfortune has been to have the wrong medical dissidents advising him and telling him that the HIV virus exists but does not cause AIDS.[354] But President Thabo Mbeki is clearly an intelligent man and has indeed woken up. He is a unique man and if he acts and questions the existence of these viruses he will become a truly great world leader. We need to reach him and other politicians like him to effect a change, to make the general public realise that these viruses do not exist.

On Tuesday evening, 26th September 2006, I wrote an e-mail to President Mbeki or at least to an official in his Presidential Office.

Dear President Mbeki,

I have just read a number of articles by you questioning the HIV-AIDS link. I admire your strength of character in attempting to get real answers to the HIV-AIDS question. In pursuing this course of action you have incurred personal ridicule from the scientific and media establishments in the Western world. I respectfully suggest that the reason why you have not succeeded publicly in getting to the heart of the HIV-AIDS question is because you have not asked the key question.

The key question is this:

Can the scientists/virologists/MDs prove that the HIV virus exists in the first place? For a virus to be proven to exist it must be 1 isolated, 2 photographed and 3 biochemically characterised. Even Luc Montagnier who discovered the alleged HIV virus does not claim that the HIV virus has been isolated. Believe it or not there are no scientific publications worldwide that proves the existence of this HIV virus.

AIDS is a man-made creation. It is simply a collection of different diseases. In Africa this collection of diseases are as you have correctly stated "diseases of poverty" not diseases caused by the phantom HIV virus.

You are also correct in your questioning why AIDS affects homosexual men and drugs users in the Western world and somehow affects heterosexuals in Africa. This doesn't make any kind of common sense but somehow is accepted by the vast majority of people.

Once you accept the proposition that the phantom HIV virus does not exist, then you have to question the existence of the viruses that cause so-called infectious diseases like measles, mumps, rubella, etc.

Again, these viruses have not been 1 isolated, 2 photographed and 3 biochemically characterised. I am working with a German group (www.klein-klein-aktion.de) who are campaigning against vaccinations because there is nothing to vaccinate against - these viruses simply don't exist.

There is a huge body of literature proving that vaccinations had nothing to do with the decline in the incidence of so-called infectious diseases - most of the decline preceded vaccinations and this decline merely continued on post vaccinations. There is overwhelming evidence to prove that vaccines cause new diseases like sudden infant death syndrome (SIDS), autism, shaken baby syndrome, attention deficit disorders etc. However much harm these vaccinations cause in well-nourished children in the Western world, their effect is absolutely catastrophic for poor, badly-nourished children in Africa.

Dr Stefan Lanka co-founder of Klein-Klein-Aktion in the early 90s discovered a real virus in sea algae. He isolated it, photographed it and biochemically characterised it. Around this time the AIDS hysteria had started. He searched all the scientific publications available and could find no single publication proving the existence of the HIV virus.The same is also true for all the so-called infectious diseases that we vaccinate against. The measles virus does not exist, neither does the mumps virus etc.

There is an English-language page on the Klein-Klein-Aktion web-site where I have been asking the relevant authorities in Ireland and England for proof of the existence of these viruses.

I believe that the best way to expose this massive scientific and moral fraud is for your Government to offer a substantial bounty of €10m or even €100m to any scientist who can say prove the existence of HIV or indeed any other virus said to affect humans. When nobody can claim the bounty (because these viruses simply don't exist), then perhaps the rest of mankind will "wake up" and question the prevailing dogma as you have already done.

Please contact Dr Lanka directly for more information at www.klein-klein-aktion.de

Best Regards
James McCumiskey[355]

The bounty idea was my own or so I thought. Apparently bounties have already been offered, but they are not yet widely known. I really believe that this bounty idea would appeal to the imagination of the wider public and make them realise that there is something to these extremely serious allegations and question themselves the existence of these alleged viruses.

I said that the AIDS hysteria had started in the early 90s, but it was the early 80s. This is a major error and the whole content of the e-mail could be rejected because of this error, because maybe there were other errors, and maybe the whole e-mail was wrong?

I read an article on the Internet where the subject (a former insider in the pharmaceutical industry) had claimed that President Mbeki was also suspicious about vaccinations but was reluctant to say anything because of all the personal vitriol he had experienced over the AIDS issue.[356] The point of my e-mail to President Mbeki was to link in his known doubts about the HIV-AIDS medical myth to his allegedly private suspicions about the dangers of vaccinations. The connection is of course the fact that all these viruses simply do not exist.

If his government would offer a substantial bounty, the Ultimate Conspiracy would finally start to unravel. It would mark the beginning of the end of the Biomedical Paradigm.

CHAPTER 46

Virus Correspondence with the Media

RTE[357] – The Irish TV and Radio broadcasting organisation

On the 11th July 2006, I e-mailed Pat Kenny, an Irish broadcaster. He has a live TV chat show every Friday night and a morning radio show on RTE, the Irish national broadcasting organisation. He is also a graduate chemical engineer and prides himself on his intelligence and general scientific knowledge.

Hi Pat,

I know that you have a special interest in matters scientific. In recent years I have become particularly interested in the "Germ Theory of Disease" medical dogma and also other medical related matters.

The Germ Theory of Disease is to Modern Medicine what the Resurrection is to Christianity. If the Resurrection did not occur, then Jesus would not be the son of God and the Christian religion would have no meaning. The Germ theory of Disease is exactly analogous for Modern Medicine. Most of Modern Medicine becomes redundant if the Germ Theory of Disease is shown to be wrong.

As an example of a so-called infectious disease I have repeatedly asked Dr Darina O'Flanagan, Head of the HPSC (Health Protection Surveillance Centre) for primary evidence for the existence of the measles, mumps and rubella viruses. She has refused my request to provide me with the primary sources for the existence of the measles, mumps and rubella viruses?

As an analogy, if someone were to allege that little green men from Mars caused the measles virus, you would ask that person for proof, for a photograph etc. What I want is the primary references which demonstrate how the measles virus was isolated, biochemically characterised and photographed. This is the burden of proof required in science in order to determine the existence of a virus.

Please find below a copy of one of my e-mails to Dr Darina O'Flanagan and her inadequate response. I am requesting Dr Darina O'Flanagan for the primary sources. As incredible as it sounds this primary evidence does not exist and can never exist. There is no such thing as a pathogenic virus!

I have also requested the Taoiseach for his assistance in demanding that Dr Darina O'Flanagan provided these primary references. He referred the matter to the Tánaiste, the Minister for Health. She had a Private Secretary write to me stating that Dr Darina O'Flanagan had provided me with the "relevant references". All I received from Dr Darina O'Flanagan was references to two text books neither of which contain any relevant primary references.

Please check out the German web-site www.klein-klein-aktion.de for further information. There is an English language page on this web-site, where I have helped translate a number of key articles. You can also see my correspondence there with the relevant Irish and UK authorities requesting the relevant primary references.

Best Regards
James McCumiskey[358]

I wondered if Pat Kenny even got to read this e-mail. It probably didn't even get past a junior researcher because I received no reply and no acknowledgement even that the e-mail had been received.

Given the trials and tribulations of Dr Hamer and Dr Lanka and my own limited experience of the media, I have no confidence in the media having any ability to break this story. There was no point in trying to convince them.

Horizon science show on BBC television: Pandemic, November 7th 2006

However, I felt obliged to continue my correspondence with the media about the allegedly probable future bird flu pandemic which could kill tens of millions of people because of a masterful piece of TV propaganda for the Biomedical Paradigm called Pandemic.

The Horizon show is a long-running and respected science show on BBC[359] television. On Tuesday 7th November 2006, they had a show that lasted 90 minutes called Pandemic. It was about the prospective bird flu pandemic. It was prime-time television starting at 9pm. The BBC have no commercials, so it was 90 minutes of pure propaganda designed to instil fear about this would-be bird flu virus and encourage people to take Tamiflu and other anti-viral drugs in the hope that they would be protected.

In summary, the bird flu virus starts in a small village in South-East Asia and rapidly spreads all over the world.

Evidence of the existence of this deadly bird flu virus was given by the fact that thousands of migratory birds allegedly died from H5N1 on a lake somewhere in China. At the time, I missed the name of the lake and specific details of the incident from the TV show. However, I subsequently read an article about an incident which almost certainly provides the inspiration for the pandemic show. Apparently there was an alleged mass outbreak of H5N1 among geese in Qinghai Lake, Northern China. The white-coats constructed a theory that the H5N1 virus was then carried westwards by migratory birds to Kazakhstan, Russia and even Turkey.[360]

But bird conservationists and notably the organisation, BirdLife International, pointed out that Qinghai Lake has many surrounding poultry operations. They also noted that there is a fish farm in the area that the FAO (Food and Agricultural Organisation) helped construct, and that chicken faeces are commonly used as food and fertiliser in fish farms in China. This confirmed my original assumption that these geese must have died from poisoning. They certainly didn't die from any phantom bird flu virus.[361]

However, the Chinese white-coats somehow discovered that they had died from the alleged bird flu virus H5N1, which was rapidly confirmed by the WHO white-coats. This sets the scene for the Pandemic show: Bird flu does exist and has killed thousands of migratory birds. What would happened if these migratory birds spread it to poultry and then onto humans?

The vaccine experts tell us that there can be no effective vaccine until they know the particular strain of bird flu about 5 months or 6 months after the pandemic has started. The only hope apparently is to use anti-viral drugs like Tamiflu, which apparently must be used quickly to be effective.

The Pandemic show speculates that somewhere between 1% and 10% of the population will die from bird flu. We will all know somebody that died. 40% of the workforce will not or cannot go to work because of fear of getting bird flu. Professor of virology, Professor John Oxford tells us with imperial certainty, that not only will millions of people die from bird flu, but millions of apparent survivors will get "encephalitis lethargica" or sleeping sickness and die horribly from this disease a few years later.

Encephalitis lethargica attacks the brain, leaving some victims like human statues, speechless and motionless. The victims seem to go to sleep and do not wake up. Between 1917 and 1928 over 5 million people died from this epidemic of encephalitis lethargica.[362]

Professor John Oxford clearly associated this terrible disease with the Spanish flu of 1918 and as proof cites the example of some South Seas island that had no Spanish flu and no encephalitis lethargica.

There is of course an alternative explanation. The Spanish flu was caused mostly by vaccines. Encephalitis lethargica or "sleeping sickness" has all the hall-marks of vaccine-damage, which appears a few years after having been vaccinated.

This documentary will be seen in time as pure nasty propaganda about a would-be virus causing a deadly flu, which can only be actually caused if we take the putative vaccines for bird flu or the anti-viral drugs.

It is this fear of a non-existent bird flu virus engendered by alleged science shows like Horizon that will cause the next pandemic because of fearful people taking repeated doses of future bird flu vaccines and anti-viral drugs.

I was extremely angry that night. I couldn't believe what I had seen. I knew that 99% of people watching this show would have accepted everything on it as being scientific and true. It was a surreal experience to watch a show like this and know that although the program-makers and the experts all believe it to be true, they are absolutely wrong and their error has deadly and horrendous consequences. I looked at the web-site and found that one could e-mail questions to the so-called experts on the show. I chose Professor Oxford because he is a professor of virology and specifically an expert on the bird flu virus.

I debated with myself about what to write. Should I keep it simple and just ask him for proof of the existence of the virus and not mention anything about Klein-Klein-Aktion. I finally decided to ask him for proof for the existence of this virus and also to state my position as a member of Klein-Klein-Aktion and that more generally Klein-Klein-Aktion states that there is no evidence for the existence of any virus.

Dear Professor Oxford,

With regard to the Horizon program on BBC 2 television at 9pm on Tuesday 7th November 2006 concerning the bird flu pandemic, I have a simple question.

Can you please give me the scientific publication which demonstrates how the H5N1 virus was:

1 Isolated

2 Photographed

3 Biochemically characterised

I completely disagree with your bird flu pandemic hypothesis. My central point is that the H5N1 virus does not exist! My source for this is Dr Stefan Lanka from Klein-Klein-Aktion, a German action group that is questioning the authorities for proof for the existence of any virus. Their web-site is www. klein-klein-aktion.de.

Klein-Klein-Aktion's arguments are not based on some new-age religious dogma. They are purely scientific. All we require is the scientific publication which shows how the H5N1 virus was 1 isolated, 2 photographed and 3 biochemically characterised.

Yours Sincerely
James McCumiskey[363]

A few weeks later the BBC displayed eleven FAQs (Frequently Asked Questions) about the bird flu virus. All these questions assumed that the basic premise of the program was correct, that the H5N1 virus does actually exist. The BBC did not acknowledge my question and did not explain why it was not presented to Professor Oxford. Obviously my question was unfortunately unique and hadn't been asked frequently. As far as the BBC was concerned I was an idiot, a crank and a moron.

Letters to newspapers about the English bird flu scare of February 2007

In early February 2007 there was a bird flu scare at a turkey farm in England. Almost 160,000 turkeys were slaughtered "to prevent the virus from spreading". This was front-page news for a few days. As the bird flu virus was now topical, I felt obliged to have one final go at correspondence with the media. I wrote the following e-mail to a number of newspapers in Ireland and England.[364]

Dear Sir,

With regard to the bird flu/H5N1 virus, I have an apparently ridiculous but very simple question for the relevant scientists and government agencies: What proof is there for the existence of the H5N1 virus?

The current proof offered by scientists for the existence of the H5N1 virus is through indirect methods which are so convoluted as to be completely meaningless. By means of an analogy, a flattened corn-circle could provide indirect evidence for the existence of a UFO (Unidentified Flying Object); it could support the hypothesis that a UFO had landed. However a thousand such corn-circles do not prove the existence of a UFO. One would still need direct evidence such as a photograph to directly prove the existence of the

UFO. Similarly one needs direct evidence for the existence of the H5N1 virus in order to prove its existence: Indirect evidence is simply not sufficient, particularly when it is technically possible to directly prove the existence of any virus.

To prove that a virus exists according to modern scientific standards, it would have to be 1 isolated, 2 photographed and 3 biochemically characterised. One could photograph the putative H5N1 virus with an electron microscope which was originally invented in the early 1930s. Biochemical characterisation techniques were originally invented in the early 1970s. Thus it is currently technically possible to directly prove the existence of the alleged H5N1 virus.

In summary, I am looking for the direct evidence; the primary reference which is the original scientific publication that proves the existence of the so-called bird flu /H5N1 virus.

Yours Sincerely
James McCumiskey[365]

I was happy with this e-mail. I had examined it repeatedly for a few days. I was just asking for proof for the existence of the H5N1 virus. There was nothing about the fact that I question the existence of all pathogenic viruses. There was nothing about the fact that I question the Germ Theory of Disease. I was only looking for proof concerning the existence of the H5N1 virus.

I had no great expectations that the media would publish this letter. They didn't surprise me. But I felt that it was a good letter with a straightforward question: What is the direct evidence for the existence of the H5N1 virus? The burden of proof is on the white-coats to prove the existence of any pathogenic virus. If enough people question the authorities, they will be forced to respond by our Governments and then we will get a real scientific debate.

The scientific debate will signal the end of the Germ Theory of Disease medical myth, which is the central dogma of Modern Medicine. Once this occurs, the era of Modern Medicine will be over. The German New Medicine will then be belatedly allowed to be publicly tested and verified.

Future historians will state that this great debate marks the beginning of the Turning Point.[366]

6

The Turning Point

There is nothing more powerful than an idea whose time has come.
Victor Hugo (French writer, 1802–1885)

All great truths start out as blasphemies.
George Bernard Shaw (Irish writer, 1856–1950)

All truth passes though three stages: firstly it is ridiculed, secondly it is violently opposed, and thirdly, it is accepted as self-evident.
Arthur Schopenhauer (German philosopher, 1788–1860)

A truth can only become a reality when the recipient is ready for it.
Christian Morgenstern (German writer and poet, 1871–1914)

"You will know the truth, and the truth will set you free".
John 8:32

Fear not the path of truth for the lack of people walking on it.

Few will have the greatness to bend history; but each of us can work to change a small portion of events, and in the total of all those acts will be written the history of this generation.
Robert F Kennedy (US Attorney General, 1925–1968)

"You didn't have enough faith," Jesus told them. "I assure you, even if you had faith as small as a mustard seed you could say to this mountain, `Move from here to there,' and it would move. Nothing would be impossible."
Mathew 17:20

One night I had a dream:
We shall overcome – one day.
Deep, deep in my heart, I do believe.
We shall overcome. One day.
Martin Luther King (Christian pastor, US civil-rights leader 1929–1968)

Go into all the world and preach the Good News to everyone.
Mark 16:15

Be not afraid.
Joshua 1:9

CHAPTER 47

The Key Players and the Blame Game

The key players in the Biomedical Paradigm are the pharmaceutical industry, the cancer and AIDS charities, MDs, other white-coats, major worldwide organisations like WHO (World Health Organization), the media, government agencies such as the FDA (Federal Drugs Administration), CDC (Centre for Disease Control), EIS (Epidemiological Information Service) in the US, the European Agency for the Evaluation of Medicinal Products (EMEA), our politicians and finally us the general public.

The Turning Point will be the recognition by the scientific elites that the Germ Theory of Disease is wrong, that pathogenic viruses do not exist and that the five Biological Laws of Nature are 100% correct.

When the Turning Point has been reached by the scientific elites, the general public will finally understand the fact that the greatest and most infamous medical dogma of all—The Germ Theory of Disease medical myth—is a moral, scientific and criminal fraud. They will finally understand the truth of the five Biological Laws of Nature of the German New Medicine. There will be an enormous public anger and a demand that the key players are brought to account.

The pharmaceutical companies

Pharmaceutical companies do not attempt to look for the cause of any disease. They do not attempt to find a cause for any disease and then cure it. There is not a single prescription drug that cures any disease. Their business model is based on managing the symptoms or in the jargon, "sustainability".[367]

Patients are sustained rather than cured. Why? Because the pharmaceutical industry can only make money from sick people who can afford to pay for their expensive medicines: sick people with health insurance or sick people in wealthy countries who have their drugs paid for by their government.

The basis of creating a new pharmaceutical drug is to identify the symptoms of a disease and synthesize a drug to offset those symptoms. These drugs are typically derived from plants or other natural sources. They simply mimic Mother Nature. Unfortunately they carry large amounts of risk due to fast absorption into the bloodstream. They are also very toxic because the body does not recognize them as being natural.[368]

All pharmaceutical companies attempt to deal with the symptoms of a disease through their drug therapies. They do not attempt to cure the disease because fundamentally they have no understanding of the origin of disease: They have no idea as to the "why" or the origin of a particular disease.

All cancer and AIDS charities can be included under the umbrella of the pharmaceutical industry. The only research they support is the drug therapies favoured by the pharmaceutical companies. The work done by these charities is an enormous boost to the pharmaceutical industry. The cancer charities are an integral part of the Biomedical Paradigm. Although most people working for these charities believe they are doing good work, Hell is nonetheless paved with good intentions.[369]

Although the pharmaceutical companies cannot, by their absolute adherence to the Biomedical Paradigm, understand the mechanism of disease let alone be interested in the cause of disease, they are wholly culpable for the horror that has been created.

Their guilt is most apparent in relation to vaccines and the clear and unequivocal evidence of the harm done by them.

Government agencies

Government agencies are meant to protect the general public. The FDA (Federal Drug Administration), the CDC (Centre for Disease Control and Prevention) and the EIS (Epidemic Intelligence Services) in the United States are wholly culpable in disseminating and promoting the Germ Theory of Disease medical myth and all the other associated medical myths such as the HIV-AIDS myth and the bird flu myth. Their equivalents in Germany, the PEI (Paul Ehrlich institute and the RKI (Robert Koch Institute) are equally culpable. Every country has a number of government agencies that promote the central

Germ Theory of Disease medical myth. They are all culpable in this criminal fraud.

The key players at the top of these government agencies worldwide do know the truth about the missing viruses, but are covering it up because of their irrational and insane belief in the Biomedical Paradigm.

The MDs

I did not bother to e-mail Irish MDs about the German New Medicine. I knew it would be a complete waste of time and energy. Why? The University of Tübingen medical school has refused and continues to refuse to test the five Biological Laws of Nature in the first place. In September 1998, the University of Trnva (in Slovakia) tested the five Biological Laws of Nature on a number of patients, verified them and then ignored them. Both these medical schools could not break free from the straitjacket of thinking that is the Biomedical Paradigm.

There was also no point in informing the medical profession in Ireland about the missing evidence for the existence of these viruses. They probably would refer me back to the relevant experts, and I had already dealt with them.

Although I did not write to them, I believe the MDs are absolutely culpable in what they are doing, and in refusing to verify the German New Medicine. Modern Medicine is meant to operate according to the latest scientific advances. I am positive that the Irish medical profession will be no different from the German, the Slovakian and all the other medical professions. The fact they are unwilling to consider Dr Hamer's and Dr Lanka's discoveries means they are criminally negligent.

Dr Buchwald testified that he too believed everything he had been told about vaccinations at medical school without question. Until his son was brain damaged as a result of vaccination he continued to believe that vaccinations were beneficial. It was only as a result of huge personal trauma that he too began to question the prevailing dogmas of Modern Medicine concerning vaccinations.[370]

I too only began to question the Biomedical Paradigm because of the death of my father from liver cancer. It was a slow process because I had no medical training and I was doing this in my spare time, but I was able to ask questions and to find compelling answers.

If I can do it, I see no reason why the MDs, (whose whole vocation is meant to be health care) cannot also think for themselves and question the Biomedical Paradigm. For this reason I believe they are all wholly culpable and guilty of criminal negligence. They administer the vaccinations; they provide the chemotherapy and other toxic treatments for cancer; they are responsible for what they are doing and must be held to account. One brave MD to publicly renounce Modern Medicine is Patrick Quanten. He issued a public statement on November 1, 2001.

Personal Statement by Patrick Quanten MD

Today is a sad day for me.

I became a doctor with the firm intention of wanting to help people, wanting them to "heal". My initial disappointment when I experienced that this was not happening, turned into great excitement when I learned that there were other things one could do, outside the medical text-books. I even ignored the opposition I encountered. Soon my new found enthusiasm started to wane too, because although everything seemed to have its uses, nothing was definitive.

Looking for the answers to health and illness, using my knowledge and the science available, slowly became a crusade. Mathematics, physics, chemistry, astrology, as well as ancient medical systems, it was all explored in search of more complete answers.

More and more compelling evidence appeared, and eventually the camel's back broke. Being confronted with the fact - no more excuses available - that my way of helping people, that my medicine - the truth beyond a shadow of a doubt - was not only preventing people from recovering from illness, but was actually introducing illness, more illness and suffering than ever before in the whole history of humanity. That shocked me to the core. The realisation of all the damage I personally have caused in the name of "making people better" is sickening me.

Today is a sad day for me.

I worked hard because I was convinced that Western Medicine could change. Now I know it can't. The change involved is a complete U-turn; the truth lies in the direction totally opposite to the one in which Western Medicine is going. As a direct result of that realisation I have to get off this wagon here and now. I can no longer justify being a member of this sect and I hereby resign my post as a medical doctor.[371]

No further comment by me is necessary.

My Swiss GNM teacher, Harald Baumann told me two contrasting stories about two MDs. One MD, a surgeon, who having studied the German New Medicine, found he could no longer continue to practice Modern Medicine, and gave up his lucrative profession as a surgeon and became a gardener. At least he was doing something useful so he could live at peace with his soul.[372]

The other story concerned a psychiatrist. Having discovered the New Medicine, he was initially very enthusiastic and began to practice it and to spread the good news. He later came back to Harald and privately told him that he had been pressured by his wife and children to practice psychiatry according to Modern Medicine. They did not want him to probably become disbarred from the extremely lucrative psychiatric profession. [373]

You begin to die the day you know something is wrong but do nothing about it.[374] This psychiatrist is a weak individual; he will have a moneyed but unhappy existence.

The pseudo-virologists and pseudo-scientists

My own personal absolute contempt is for the white-coats, the pseudo-virologists and the pseudo-scientists who pontificate on the existence of phantom viruses like bird flu (H5N1), HIV, measles, mumps and rubella but do not tell the general public that they have no direct evidence for the existence of these viruses. These viruses are only deemed to exist because of allegedly indirect evidence based on an irrational, unscientific, superstitious and criminal belief in the Germ Theory of Disease medical myth. They discuss photographs of these viruses as though they were true photographic representations as we would normally understand what a true photograph is.

They do not publicly admit that no scientific publication exists in which these phantom viruses are proven to exist, where these viruses have been 1) isolated, 2) photographed and 3) biochemically characterised.

In relation to the HIV-AIDS myth, millions of people have died and sub-Saharan Africa has been damned to Hell on the strength of their determination about the existence of the HIV virus.

Politicians

The Taoiseach (Irish Prime Minister) correctly devolves all responsibility for health matters to the Minister for Health. The Minister for Health (who usually is not an MD) relies on her relevant experts such as Dr Darina O'Flanagan in relation to viruses.

A review of the German correspondence on the Klein-Klein-Aktion web-site confirms this delegation of responsibility. Ultimately the Minister for Health in any country devolves responsibility for answering queries about viruses to the relevant government agencies.

I have discussed this issue with many friends and acquaintances. I would say that at least 95% of people accept the Germ Theory of Disease to be an absolute truth. So much so, that they consider it almost a personal affront if you actually dare to question them about this central dogma of the Biomedical Paradigm. So as an ordinary citizen, I cannot blame the Irish Minster for Health personally for being negligent in not following through on this issue, because the vast majority of Irish people wouldn't. But she is not an ordinary citizen; she is the Minister for Health. Ditto for the Taoiseach (Irish Prime Minister). I have given the Minister for Health and the Taoiseach enough information and despite typographical errors in my original e-mails, I have presented the information in a reasonable enough fashion for it to be acted upon, if we were living in a properly functioning democracy where the queries and concerns of an individual citizen would be given due care and attention.

However, their defence will be that they relied on the opinion of the relevant experts, the dominant medical opinion. Unfortunately they couldn't use their own common sense.

The Minister for Health in Ireland clearly has direct responsibility for health-related matters. She can tinker with this system; she can substantially increase the amount of tax-payer money being wasted on it, she can subsidise more pharmaceuticals for more people but she cannot make the system work because Modern Medicine is based on a secular religion called the Biomedical Paradigm, which is inherently wrong.

If the Minister for Health in Ireland ever actually responds to my enquiries, she will almost certainly delegate any response to them to her MDs. They will automatically reject the truth of what Dr Hamer is saying, which proves yet again the endemic condition in Modern Medicine called the Semmelweis Reflex.

The media

The media will not investigate anything like this. They have a complete inability to use their own individual common sense. They will accept the word of the relevant experts and not pursue these serious allegations. I think a huge part of the problem with the media is that the vast majority of them are trained only in the humanities or law. Most of them never studied science at an advanced level at school and they naturally enough consider science and medicine to be too complicated and best left to the relevant experts, which is proof of the tyranny of the experts.

The Western media are overwhelmingly secular. They are secular fundamentalists and reject any notion of God; they have a secular fundamentalist belief in the so-called Age of Enlightenment and have bought into the Biomedical Paradigm hook, line and sinker. This is evident from reading the daily newspapers and watching the nightly TV news. They will not break any story that destroys their ideas about the world. They will only follow their audience, their viewer, their reader, when their audience awakens and becomes strong enough and vocal enough and demands change, only then will the media follow.

The general public

However, the fundamental problem is not with the pharmaceutical companies, nor with the cancer charities, nor with the government agencies, nor with the MDs, nor with the other white-coats - the pseudo-virologists and pseudo-scientists, nor with the politicians, nor with the media but with all of us: the general public. We are all so busy in our daily lives, working very hard, working too hard in most cases, running around here, there and everywhere, that in all our busyness we have forgotten how to think for ourselves.

We read all this rubbish about migratory birds spreading the bird flu, the H5N1 virus, and we believe it all. Despite the fact that only poultry that are factory-farmed die from H5N1, and that the so-called diseased migratory birds fly non-stop for weeks spreading the bird flu virus but do not get diseased nor die themselves. Of course they are probably "carriers". A medical dogma to explain another medical dogma to explain it all away within the straitjacket of thinking that is the Biomedical Paradigm. And we continue to believe all this?

What needs to happen is that we need to wake up, emerge from this self-inflicted nightmare and start to think for ourselves. Before we point the finger of blame at anyone we have to examine our own conscience, are we also to blame, are we also partly responsible? Nobody puts it better than Jesus Christ:[375] "Let him who is without sin cast the first stone".

Actions not blame

Before we throw stones at the key players and excoriate them, we must be sure that each of us has a clear conscience in relation to the

Ultimate Conspiracy; that we have played our part in revealing the truth of GNM and the absolute horror that is Modern Medicine.

In post-World War 2 Germany, children asked their parents what they did to help defeat fascism. Most parents had done nothing. They mostly pleaded the "I did not know" defence in relation to the evil perpetrated by the Nazis. The vast majority of these parents were good people that simply ignored what the Nazis were doing. Just like the children that grew up in post World War 2 Germany, our children and grandchildren will ask us what we did to overcome the Biomedical Paradigm. The vast majority of us will have done nothing; we will tell our children and grandchildren that we believed the relevant experts. Most of us will have ignored what Modern Medicine is doing on our behalf in the name of science and progress, but some of us will become part of the "resistance" that will eventually overcome the Biomedical Paradigm one day.

The Germ Theory of Disease is the most infamous medical dogma of all. It is also the weakest link in the chain that is the Biomedical Paradigm. Viruses are deemed to exist because of an irrational, unscientific and criminal belief in this medical dogma. I believe the fact that viruses simply don't exist in humans, animals or plants; that there is no direct evidence for their existence even though this is technologically possible; that the only evidence for the existence of viruses is indirect evidence that seems to support this fraudulent dogma; to be the Achilles' heel of the Biomedical Paradigm. If the general public can be persuaded that viruses simply don't exist; this would mark the beginning of the end of the Biomedical Paradigm.

Klein-Klein-Aktion believe that the only way to force the authorities to admit that there is no such thing as a disease-inducing/pathogenic virus is to get ordinary citizens to write directly to the relevant authorities asking for direct proof for the existence of these viruses.

I am certain they are correct in this approach. But the experts can continue to sit back in their comfortable armchairs in their permanent, pensionable positions and rubbish Lanka and all those stupid morons like me who ask ridiculous questions.

But the only hope is that enough people ask these questions and make their opinions known to the politicians in order to force them to demand a reason from these experts as to why they cannot produce a scientific publication which demonstrates how a virus (any virus) was isolated, photographed and biochemically characterised.

If enough pressure is put on the politicians they will eventually demand an answer from these white-coats; MDs, pseudo-scientists, pseudo-experts and pseudo-virologists. This matter must be dealt with on a global scale. I believe that the best way to achieve this objective would be to have a bounty of say €10,000,000 or even €100,000,000 provided by some wealthy individual or a government for any pseudo-virologist worldwide to prove the existence of any common virus such as measles, mumps, rubella, HIV, or bird flu.

Once this huge bounty is put on the table, it would force the ordinary citizen to wake up and question why, and maybe read a bit and explore the web, and ignore the propaganda promulgated by the MDs, other white-coats and their accomplices in the mass media.

A thousand pieces of indirect evidence does not provide scientific proof for the existence of any virus.[376] If all these MDs, scientists and virologists, white-coats all, can give no direct evidence for the existence of these putative viruses, then maybe we will all realise that the reason why they can give no direct evidence is because these viruses do not exist and are only stated to exist on the basis of indirect evidence which apparently supports the key dogma of Modern Medicine: The Germ Theory of Disease.

Once most people are convinced that viruses do not exist, that the Germ Theory of Disease is a gigantic fraud, I believe that they will be more than willing to have the German New Medicine openly verified.

I think the only way to get the German New Medicine openly tested is to get a petition signed by as many people as possible. The magic number of signatories required will vary depending on the country. But if enough people sign a petition, the Minister for Health in any country, being primarily a politician (and in the free world, very much interested in getting re-elected) will eventually have to concede these reasonable demands and have the German New Medicine openly verified.

Dr Hamer has been through the verification process successfully many times before, most infamously with the medical school in Trnva, Slovakia. This time we need to do this in a completely open and transparent manner.

As well as the MDs and other white-coats working on behalf of Modern Medicine, we need engineers, physicists, mathematicians and statisticians to verify the five Biological Laws of Nature. It needs to be made public and the best way of doing this is in a reality-TV format.

This is a put-up or shut-up proposition. German New Medicine makes many claims. Let them be openly verified. Let the MDs and other white-coats try and explain away the scientific certainty of the five Biological Laws of Nature. Let the people decide, if they can manage to wake up.

The key question we have to ask ourselves is this: What will we tell our children and grandchildren when they ask us what we did to overcome the Biomedical Paradigm?

CHAPTER 48

The Paradigms of German New Medicine

Medical Therapy of the German New Medicine

The approach of the MDs practicing Modern Medicine concerns procedures, tests, more tests and operations. They measure and quantify the symptoms and try to cure them. They do not have to; in fact they are not expected to listen to the patient's story. The MD knows best. The MD doesn't have to keep quiet and listen carefully to the patient. The MD tells the patient what will be done to him.

This approach of Modern Medicine called "symptomatic medicine" goes all the way back to the founder of Medicine: Hippocrates. The MDs measure and quantify the symptoms, and try to treat them by various methods such as bloodletting for over a thousand years and in modern times by chemotherapy, radiation therapy or radical surgery.

The approach of the GNM therapist is to keep quiet and listen intently to the patient's story. The patient tells his story and the GNM therapist must understand that story from the patient's viewpoint. To understand the patient's story the GNM therapist must understand the psyche of the patient. This takes time. The GNM therapist can get a CT scan and other diagnostics to confirm the nature of the shock on the three levels of the human trinity – the psyche, the brain and the organ. These will be explained to the patient and the patient will fully understand his particular biological shock and the organic symptoms emanating from it. The patient is in charge of his own return to health.

The paradigms of German New Medicine will underpin this new therapeutic approach and must be fully understood by the general public.

The paradigms of German New Medicine

The Greek myths of Hygieia and Asclepius[377] symbolise the two views of health that have been with us for thousands of years. The followers of Hygieia believe that health is the natural order of things, that health is something that we are all entitled to if we live our lives well. The followers of Hygieia believe that the most important function of medicine is to teach the natural laws. These natural laws will ensure a healthy mind in a healthy body. This is what Dr Hamer has given humanity with his German New Medicine and his five Biological Laws of Nature: the ability to allow all of us re-establish control over the most important part of our lives – our health.[378]

The followers of Asclepius believe that the key role of the physician is to treat disease, to restore health by correcting any alleged imperfections of Nature. Modern Medicine has followed the approach of Asclepius. The MDs try to cure the disease, or more accurately try to deal with the symptoms of the disease, whereas the practitioners of German New Medicine (the followers of Hygieia) try to get the patient to understand why they got their disease, not to be afraid and then to allow the patient cure himself.[379]

The Turning Point will have occurred when the paradigms of German New Medicine have finally been accepted by most of the population. The Turning Point will have occurred when most people regard the Germ Theory of Disease and the thousands of dogmas that make up the Biomedical Paradigm of Modern Medicine with absolute contempt, in the same manner as we currently regard anybody who believes that the Earth is flat.

Health comes from within. Listen to your soul, your psyche, and to your dreams. Once you give away the control and power over your health, you are in deep trouble. When we know something is wrong, we need to stop and think and get out of the busyness of life, turn off the TV and radio and in silence listen to our own body, our psyche and to our soul.

When we accept the truth of GNM and the non-existence of any virus, we are set free from fear: To live well all we need to do is to be in tune with our psyche and our soul and God.

GNM has four key paradigms or patterns of thinking underlying its philosophy.

The first paradigm is that God and Mother Nature are perfect. Cancers or diseases are not meaningless failures by God or Mother Nature but rather are Meaningful Biological Programs (MBPs) designed to help the individual overcome a particular biological shock. Nature doesn't harbour any malignant germs or cancer cells: we do not self-destruct through cancer in a horrible manner. Nature always works in a goal-oriented manner and the ultimate purpose of Nature is to secure its own survival.

The second paradigm is that disease is caused from within and not from without.

The third paradigm is the absolute scientific truth of the mind–body connection. There is a clear and provable connection between a specific conflict or biological shock in the psyche and the concerned brain relay and the affected organ.

The fourth paradigm is that we as individuals must accept full responsibility for our personal health. When we get ill as we all do, we must understand what caused our cancer or other disease and must be the boss of our own treatment. We will use GNM therapists for advice and comfort but we will effectively treat ourselves. We will have sole responsibility for our own health.

The patient is the key "change agent" in the treatment of his disease. He assumes responsibility for resolving the biological conflict which caused his cancer/disease. Even with the active support of a GNM therapist the patient must resolve the conflict on his own. The solution should in ideal circumstances be as real as possible in order for it to work. Sometimes it is not possible to get a real solution. It might be impossible to avoid seeing your son-in-law, or mother-in-law so that an intellectual/spiritual/religious solution might be a second-best solution. The patient is the "boss" of his therapy, assisted if required by a GNM therapist.

The Turning Point will have occurred when these paradigms of German New Medicine are deemed to be obvious by the scientific elite and most of the population. It will probably take generations for the scientific truth of the German New Medicine to be accepted by over 99% of the population. But once most of the population have made the mental leap and can now see with new eyes the Turning Point will be complete, the Horror of the Biomedical Paradigm will be finally over and we will have entered into a new era of medicine and of life on this planet.

CHAPTER 49

2020 Vision[380]

I woke up feeling good. It was a Tuesday in mid-October 2020. I was in the shower humming a song made famous by Louis Armstrong called "What a wonderful world".[381] I can't sing at all, but I sang quietly my favourite part of the song and the only part I know off by heart:

I hear babies cryin'....I watch them grow
They'll learn much more.....than I'll ever know
And I think to myself.....what a wonderful world
Yes, I think to myself.....what a wonderful world

An image of my father came into my mind. I stopped singing. I was about to visit his grave in Galway. It was coming up to the 18th anniversary of his death. If he had survived the liver cancer he would be now 83 years old. If the cancer had been diagnosed earlier so that we could have met the GNM therapist earlier, more importantly if the knowledge of GNM had been commonplace he could have survived. If only...

If only the knowledge of German New Medicine had been universally available at that time, he would still have had a severe cancer, liver cancer, but he would have had at least a 95% chance of successfully solving his conflict. The choice in this case is stark, certain painful death if you do not solve the conflict or its painful resolution and life.

His dying and awful death got me interested in German New Medicine. Every year up to now, I measured myself by what I had achieved by the anniversary of his death, what I had learned about GNM and how I had spread the word. Had I done enough in the previous year? I never had, of course.

I suddenly remembered what I had to do. I'd read the *Irish Times* that Tuesday and make a note of all the medical stories for that day.

This would guide me to setting my goals for the next year. I quickly got dressed and went to the front door. The *Irish Times* had been delivered. I took it, didn't look at it, nervously walked into the kitchen and put it face down on the kitchen table.

I made myself a nice cup of tea, Barry's Tea; my favourite way to start the day. I'd work my way through the *Irish Times* from the back-page. It was like opening up an examination paper all over again: That's the way I used to read them all, from back to front.

The first thing I noticed was there was no medical supplement. Great! No more fairy-tales and no more brainwashing of the masses about the Biomedical Paradigm. I religiously read that medical supplement every Tuesday for way too many years. How I never got diabetes[382] from it, I will never know, but I read it compulsively and was always appalled and disgusted by what I read. It reinforced my determination to keep on with my task of revealing the truth behind Modern Medicine.

In the business section there was an article about health costs in the developed countries continuing to fall as the German New Medicine was being rolled out worldwide. This was great news. It had really happened.

There was another article about a pharmaceutical company called Generic New Medicines (sic) which manufactured the few key drugs that were still useful according to the German New Medicine. There was an oblique reference to the collapse of the pharmaceutical industry. It was all happening the way I had dreamed about for years.

I moved impatiently on. I wanted to get to the front page. In the middle of the paper there was a four-page life-style section. I looked at it and smiled with pure joy.

An article about how to avoid a myocardial heart attack for top athletes…

Another article on allergies and how someone overcame their allergy to peanuts…

An article on meditation, and how one can calm the psyche and have a shortened conflict-active phase after a DHS. God, the article even mentioned people who believed they didn't get cancers or other diseases at all in the first place because of their practice of meditation…

An article on prayer and forgiveness and its importance in preventing biological shocks…

An article on prostate cancer. It explained the nature of the conflict. The article quoted from a recently published book about men who had all overcome prostate cancer by solving their individual conflicts. Some of the DHSs that had caused the prostate cancer were amazing. You couldn't have made them up!

An article for kids explaining measles according to the German New Medicine. The article was based on a booklet about measles produced in 2003 by Harald Baumann and Daniela Amstutz called "The Strong Family and their Medical Adventures".

Another article that caught my eye was about breaking bad news to people so that they wouldn't get a DHS. It was more or less to set the scene and let the person draw out what had happened, for example if a loved one had been killed in a car crash, to say that there had been a bad accident, and let the bereaved person say what had happened. In fact this had been practiced by police forces worldwide for decades without them knowing about GNM.

This gets better and better. I quickly glanced over the other articles, which all accorded with the German New Medicine, and found nothing about taking drugs, nothing about the latest drug discovery, nothing about gene therapy nor about a new cancer drug: absolutely nothing.

I moved on back to the main section of the paper. A full page with a number of articles about the termination of the World Health Organization. It was great news, but had it taken that long? The WHO is responsible for the deaths of more children through vaccinations than all the wars of the 20th century put together many times over. The WHO was a disaster for Africa, particularly sub-Saharan Africa. There was an article by an African president about the genocidal objectives of the WHO: white people deliberately killing black people. Another conspiracy theory, but you couldn't really blame him given all that had happened. The real truth was that all these WHO MDs had whole-heartedly believed in the Biomedical Paradigm. WHO should have been an abbreviation for the World Horror Organisation!

I read another brief article about the FAO: the UN's Food and Agricultural Organisation. They are still in existence despite everything that they had done. That sickened me. Some things never change. No such thing as a perfect exam-paper.

I moved on, flicking through the paper. There were three pages devoted to Irish matters. There was a one-page opinion-piece on the ramifications of Irish unification. There had been a referendum in early 2016 and by a small majority in Northern Ireland there had been a vote in favour of the unity of Northern Ireland and the Republic of Ireland.

That was tremendous news for me personally. At last the dreams of the great patriots that Ireland could be united under the Tricolour, the Irish flag, the green representing Catholic Nationalist Ireland, the orange representing Protestant Unionist Ireland and the white representing the unity of the two major Christian traditions living on this one small island. We had so much more in common than what divided us.

After the plebiscite there had been serious rioting and disturbances in the Protestant areas but they had gradually petered out over the last few years. This reluctant acceptance of unification by the Protestant Unionist community had been made possible by a charismatic evangelical Protestant minister. He had managed to persuade all the elected politicians from the protestant unionist tradition to enter Dáil Éireann (the Irish Parliament) in October 2020. We could now look forward to a genuinely united Ireland.

There were a lot more articles on the same vein of the realignment of Irish politics because of unification. It was fantastic. I have always wanted a united Ireland, and now that it has finally happened, well it's great, it is fantastic, but it only concerns Ireland, and that is of course important because I am Irish and I live here and I love my country. However there are no worldwide ramifications as a result of Irish unification, not like with the German New Medicine.

I flicked on through the paper. There was a picture of a former MD, a former cancer MD (oncologist), who had retrained to be a priest and had just been ordained. Many former MDs had reverted to drugs and alcohol. Some had a religious conversion. Others committed suicide: Obviously they couldn't survive their massive territorial shocks, their loss of jobs, money, status, power and prestige. The solutions to these DHSs were well known, to talk about it and reduce the isolative aspect and to move on with your life, but it is difficult if you are trapped in the past. It was very sad and depressing.

I quickly skipped over the last few pages without looking at them; I closed my eyes and had the paper arranged with the front page showing.

I looked at it and was stunned. The main story was that they were building an enormous museum to the Horror and the last days of the Biomedical Paradigm in Galway, Ireland. A museum! It had video-testimony from thousands of people (in many different languages) who had been through chemotherapy, radiotherapy and radical surgery and the devastating effect it had on them and the subsequent shocks or DHS caused by these medical interventions. A museum to the Horror and the demise of the Biomedical Paradigm! It was all over. The Horror had ended.

But there was more...

There was another article at the bottom of the front page about the number of countries with Hamer Day as a public holiday. The 7th of December was the day that Dirk Hamer died; It was also the day that Dr Ryke Geerd Hamer got a biological shock that caused testicular cancer. The 7th of December is becoming a worldwide public holiday in Israel, and in Muslim and Christian countries. It is a sombre day, remembering the people who had died because of the Horror caused by Modern Medicine and their criminal belief in the Biomedical Paradigm; It is also a joyful day, a day for public celebration because the Horror is over and we are now individually responsible for our own health. We are now free from fear. Dr Hamer is now honoured worldwide as the greatest scientist of our generation and the greatest physician of all-time for his tremendous discoveries. Dr Lanka and Klein-Klein-Aktion are honoured for their part in uncovering the Germ Theory of Disease medical myth: the central myth of the Biomedical Paradigm.

We had passed the Turning Point. The Germ Theory of Disease medical myth had finally ended in scientific circles. Dr Hamer's GNM was being finally implemented worldwide.

I would now visit my father's grave and tell him that my crusade for GNM was over. His unnecessary and premature death was the motivation for my crusade. I would never forget him: As long as I live, he lives on in me. But I no longer had anything to achieve by the time of his next anniversary. All was well with me and the world.

I laughed inwardly and glowed. It was the same feeling that you get after reading an exam script and you are certain that you will do well. In fact you will do brilliantly and you know it. However it was much better than that. You prepare at most a year for an exam. I had been working along with thousands of others for this for almost fifteen-years. I knew my father would be happy and proud. Yes, we had made the future. I felt fantastic and because I was in my own kitchen and not in an exam hall, I sang loudly:

And I think to myself.....what a wonderful world
Yes, I think to myself.....what a wonderful world

James, James! What are you doing? I woke up. It was my wife, Donna. I looked at the clock. 5 am. I remembered my dream and briefly explained it. She scolded me and told me to go back to sleep.

Donna dozed off. I lay back down in bed and I thought about the saying that my teacher and friend in the German New Medicine Harald Baumann used:

"The consciousness is the goal-setter; the subconscious is the goal-getter".

What Harald meant by this is that we set our goals, we firm them up in our conscious mind, keep them there constantly in-mind and subconsciously we achieve them. That's what we all have to do if we are going to overcome the Biomedical Paradigm.

It's like the parable from the Bible where Jesus said that if we had the faith of a mustard seed then we could move mountains. With the faith of a tiny mustard seed, nothing is impossible. If we collectively have the faith, we can move the mountain that is the Biomedical Paradigm. With faith, nothing is impossible for us.

We can expose the Ultimate Conspiracy. We can overcome the Biomedical Paradigm. We can make the future free from fear.

CHAPTER 50

Making the Future[383]

Who makes the future? Do governments, bureaucracies, organisations, companies, trade unions or the UN make the future? Or is it ordinary people that make the future?

Once we create a bureaucracy, a government, a trade-union, organisations such as the WHO, we create entities that are self-serving and it is very difficult, if not impossible, to get rid of these entities once they have been created.

Governments in the free world depend on an electoral mandate: At least we can vote them out. Their objective is to get voted in and stay in power for as long as possible. Elected governments will continue to promote the existing Biomedical Paradigm because they are being told to do so by the experts, by the white-coats, by the MDs, by the pharmaceutical industry, or by the World Health Organization.

However, governments do eventually respond to pressure from their electorate. These political machines will respond if enough of us make our voices heard. This is our only hope.

When the health ministers in our governments hear about the German New Medicine and the complete absence of proof, photographic evidence or otherwise of the existence of disease-inducing viruses like HIV, bird flu, measles, mumps and rubella, what will they do? They will defer to their chief scientific officer, their chief medical office, the medical profession, the pharmaceutical industry (that probably donates substantial sums of money to their political party) and what will their response be?

All these experts will rubbish Dr Lanka and Dr Hamer. They will attempt to persuade us with a plethora of facts about science and imply that they are the experts, they are the high priests of the Biomedical Paradigm and as experts they can assure us that all is well with the world of medicine.

These scientists and MDs (white-coats all) will claim that science is best left to the scientists. Our health is of course much too important to be delegated to the white-coats, the MDs and the pseudo-scientists.

All truth passes through three stages: firstly it is ridiculed, secondly it is violently opposed, and thirdly, it is accepted as self-evident.[384]

German New Medicine has been through the ridicule stage and survived. Dr Hamer has been jailed twice and I believe they will continue to jail him in order to suppress him and the scientific truth of his German New Medicine.

We are now at the second stage of truth where the GNM is being violently opposed by the so-called experts. They will be supported by a compliant and dutiful and supine media who will turn on the advocates for German New Medicine with all the ferocity and certainty of purpose of a pack of starving rats. However the advocates for GNM are battle-hardened and will survive the onslaught.

The procedures for the verification of German New Medicine are tried and tested: GNM has been verified before a number of times most infamously by the University of Trnva in Bratislava, Slovakia. However this time it must be tested in an open and transparent manner with a number of reputable scientists (such as engineers, physicists and mathematicians) who are unconnected with the Biomedical Paradigm and the verification should be transparent to members of the general public.

I personally believe the best way to make this transparent is to use a reality TV format with a number of patients with agreed specific medical conditions and have them cured using the therapeutic approach of German New Medicine. A second group of patients would be treated according to Modern Medicine and a third group would not be treated at all. This would all be done in accordance with the wishes of the patients. This therapeutic approach of GNM would then be compared with the approach of Modern Medicine, and with the control group who have no therapy whatsoever. It is possible that some of the patients cannot solve their conflict, but this will not invalidate the truth of German New Medicine: that all diseases and cancers follow the five Biological Laws of Nature.

Our greatest difficulties in life aren't caused by what we don't know but by our illusions, the things we hold to be true but aren't so.[385] The greatest illusion facing mankind is our collective belief in the Germ Theory of Disease medical myth, the major dogma of the Biomedical Paradigm. Once we question this central dogma of Modern Medicine, we can then question other dogmas like metastasis (cancer spreading), lung cancer and smoking. Once we understand the medical myths being propagated daily by the mass media we will have shown that we have the ability to think for ourselves. Once we understand these medical myths, we can truly comprehend the Horror that is the Biomedical Paradigm.

To make a real future for us all, we have firstly to ask ourselves are we part of the Biomedical Paradigm? If you say yes, don't cry out when the MDs, wearing their white coats and stethoscopes come looking for you, and they will. These MDs with their white coats and stethoscopes are wearing the current disguise greatly preferred by the Grim Reaper.

If you are unsure about the Biomedical Paradigm but do nothing, then you are still part of it. All that is necessary for evil to occur is for good men to do nothing.[386] If you do nothing then you are allowing the Biomedical Paradigm to continue onto its logical conclusion. God will ultimately judge us, not just by what we did but also by what we did not do.[387]

If humanity is to see through the Biomedical Paradigm, it will only be because a majority of us have started to think for ourselves.

If you realise that there is something to these discoveries of Dr Hamer and Dr Lanka and decide that they must be openly verified, what exactly can you do? What can ordinary people do? What we can do is this; we can all of us make the future, a future free from fear.

If enough of us make our voices heard, and persuade our neighbours, friends and family; the ensuing widespread public interest will become the Tipping Point that will force governments of a number of countries in the free world to accede to the following demands:

1. Clear evidence is demanded from the relevant MDs, pseudo-virologists and other white-coats about the existence of disease-inducing viruses like measles, mumps, rubella, hepatitis, HIV and bird flu.
2. German New Medicine is openly tested.

There is of course no such evidence for any disease-inducing or pathogenic virus. Once the Germ Theory of Disease is publicly accepted to be a moral and scientific fraud the era of Modern Medicine will be over. True understanding of this medical, scientific and criminal fraud will mark the beginning of a hopefully quick end to the pharmaceutical industry.

The great debate with the white-coats must also involve lawyers and judges. The legal people will demand the evidence from the white-coats that is necessary to form the burden of proof for the existence of these allegedly pathogenic viruses. A key part of this judicial and scientific debate will involve the white-coats who promote the Biomedical Paradigm accepting Dr Lanka's scientific papers about the existence of the sea algae virus that he discovered. They will be forced to admit that Dr Lanka has scientifically proven this virus to exist because it has been 1) isolated, 2) photographed and 3) biochemically characterised.

They will be requested for similar scientific papers that prove the existence of the major alleged pathogenic viruses like the HIV virus, the bird flu virus, measles, mumps and rubella viruses. When they cannot prove the existence of these viruses they will be asked by the judge why they cannot provide this evidence. Most white-coats will prevaricate at this stage. One must always bear in mind that they are brain-washed adherents of the Biomedical Paradigm. They will be pressed again and again for the scientific evidence. Eventually one-by-one they will admit that there is no evidence for the existence of any pathogenic virus. They will then be pressed about the Germ Theory of Disease in relation to so-called bacterial infections. They will be eventually forced to agree that there is no scientific evidence that proves the Germ Theory of Disease. In fact the opposite is true: The scientific evidence currently available proves that the Germ Theory of Disease is a scientific fraud.

This great scientific debate needs to occur in a very compressed time-scale. I believe a three-month judicial-scientific process would be ample time to prove or disprove the Germ Theory of Disease and the existence of viruses. This great debate cannot drag on for years. Too many lives are at risk particularly in relation to HIV-AIDS and vaccinations, but also in relation to a potential bird flu catastrophe.

There will be eventual reluctant acceptance by the white-coats that pathogenic viruses do not exist. This great debate and its determinations will mark the beginning of the end of the Biomedical Paradigm. It will also mark the beginning of the Turning Point at which the Germ Theory of Disease is rejected and eventually all the other dogmas that comprise the entire Biomedical Paradigm of Modern Medicine. The German New Medicine can now be openly verified.

The open verification and acceptance by a number of real scientific organisations worldwide of the truth of German New Medicine and the moral and scientific fraud that is the Biomedical Paradigm and more importantly, genuine acceptance by most of the general public, will complete the Turning Point, that will usher in the third stage of truth, when German New Medicine is universally accepted as being self-evident.

Once these demands are met, and once the truth of German New Medicine is finally recognised, there will be a painful introspection. Hopefully we won't allow it to become a lawyers' paradise, but a real examination of how the Biomedical Paradigm was allowed to afflict our society, and a determination to ensure that the full implications of German New Medicine are implemented.

There will be enormous public anger. There will be demands for a worldwide trial of the key players involved in promoting the Biomedical Paradigm, the WHO, the pharmaceutical companies, the MDs, the virologists and other white-coats and the mass media. I do believe that we need to bring the key players to account. But I believe that the fundamental problem is not with the key players (the MDs and the other white-coats) but with us, the ordinary citizens. We have ceded control of our own lives to these pseudo-experts, to the white-coats. We must reassert control over our own lives and especially over our own health. True freedom is when we do not blame others for our predicament but understand that we are individually culpable and responsible. We must firstly change ourselves, and be angry with ourselves, because it took us such a long time to become fully aware of the true horror of the Biomedical Paradigm.

True acceptance of GNM will mean that our society will have to change dramatically. These changes will be extremely painful for many individuals and for the many vested interests. These changes will be nothing short of revolutionary and will bring about a fundamental rethink in the way we live our lives. The world will become a much better place in which to live.

This future will be one in which we are not made afraid of so-called disease-inducing viruses like measles, mumps, rubella, HIV and bird flu. We will have no fear of WMD (Weapons of Mass Destruction) because pathogenic viruses do not exist. Pregnancy and child birth will not be treated like a disease. There will be no more vaccinations. There will be no more iatrogenic diseases like autism, dyslexia, sudden infant death syndrome (SIDS), attention deficit disorders, all caused by vaccinations. There will be no more scare stories in the media about French fries causing breast cancer or the possibility of a bird flu pandemic and all that absolute nonsense that is prevalent in the early part of the 21st century.

We have nothing to fear. We will still get biological shocks and therefore the resulting cancers and other diseases, but we now have German New Medicine to help us cure ourselves. The GNM therapists will accompany us in our return to full health, but we will be finally personally responsible for our own well-being.

A good understanding of the German New Medicine and its five Biological Laws of Nature is the ultimate preventative medicine. German New Medicine is the ultimate health insurance. You are now responsible for your own health.

My motivation for writing this book was the unnecessary death of my father from liver cancer. If the knowledge of the five Biological Laws of Nature had been universally known in 2002, he would have had an excellent chance of overcoming his liver cancer.

My objectives for this book are three-fold: Firstly, to reveal the five Biological Laws of Nature and the scientific truth of the German New Medicine; secondly, to reveal that pathogenic viruses do not exist and that the Germ Theory of Disease is a moral, scientific and criminal fraud; and thirdly, to reveal the truth behind Modern Medicine:– the Biomedical Paradigm, which is the Ultimate Conspiracy.

When your children and grandchildren ask you what you did to overcome the Biomedical Paradigm; tell them with pride how you played your part in uncovering the Ultimate Conspiracy; tell them how you helped make the future free from fear.

You know what to do.

Be not afraid.[388]

Acknowledgements

I thank my sister for introducing me to the New Medicine. I thank Ilsedora Laker for answering my initial queries and introducing me to my teacher and friend in the German New Medicine, Harald Baumann. I thank Maria and Joan who organised the course I attended in Limerick, Ireland in 2004 on the German New Medicine given by Harald Baumann. I thank Harald Bauman for his inspiring course, his patient help in nurturing my knowledge of the German New Medicine and his subsequent critical support to me particularly with the case studies and with several thorough reviews of the book. I thank Harald and Arlette Büchel for their generous hospitality at their beautiful home in Switzerland for five exhilarating days while we examined the case studies. This book would not have happened without their tremendous help and support. I cannot thank them enough. I thank Susanne Brix for all her help in enabling me to understand the mystery of the missing viruses. I thank Lauren Colby for his help with my understanding of the lung-cancer/smoking myth, which was the most difficult of all medical myths for me to personally overcome. I thank Ian Sinclair for his help in my understanding of certain vaccination related issues. I thank my friends and acquaintances who gave me comments about and help with this book. I thank Phil Roche for the seemingly never-ending task of reviewing this book, his useful suggestions and comments, and for the interesting articles he found on the internet.

I cannot repay my mother for the unconditional and total love given me by her especially as a child growing up. I have known a number of mature adults who are very insecure because they never received unconditional love from their mother in particular, but also from their father. I was lucky and received it in abundance from both my parents, and am grateful to them and am happy, secure and content in myself.

I thank my wife, Donna, for her fortitude, and for affording me the opportunity to pursue this project. Without her support and true love I could not have completed this book: For this I am most grateful.

I have a number of relations who work in the medical world. To them in particular, and to all other acquaintances of mine involved in Modern Medicine, this book should not be taken as a personal attack. It is simply a revelation of the Biomedical Paradigm and of the German New Medicine.

I found my publisher, Andy Hey of Literally Publishing, after a two-year quest using an excellent web-site for first-time writers: www.firstwriter.com. I learned from firstwriter that the big publishing houses would only consider a first-time author if they had an agent. I tried for more than a year to get an agent. Finally, after many rejections, I realised that my work did not fit in with a particular genre, and with no medical qualification whatsoever, no agent would consider me. I would have to get a publisher myself. One big publisher asked if my book had been "peer-reviewed"! I knew then that I had to find a small publisher myself. I struck gold when Andy Hey agreed to publish the book. He calmly dealt with all my queries and constant e-mails and phone-calls, and made it happen: Andy does indeed literally publish.

I gave a specific brief for the front-cover to the artists James and Laurie McAdams (a husband and wife team). They took my brief, discarded my proposal for the front-cover, but captured its message, and came up with a brilliant design: It captures the essence of this book, which is what a great front-cover should do.

I would also like to thank Ole for his proof-reading work and for some useful suggestions which were incorporated into the text.

Finally and most importantly of all, I publicly acknowledge the Holy Spirit who guided me in this endeavour. I prayed constantly about this project and received all the inspiration and help I needed from the Holy Spirit, who is God's continuing presence in this world.

Dedication

This book is dedicated to seven heroic people and to all the members of two fantastic organisations.

It is dedicated to Dr Ryke Geerd Hamer for his truly wonderful German New Medicine. It is dedicated to four individuals from Klein-Klein-Aktion: Dr Stefan Lanka, Karl Krafeld, Susanne Brix and Veronika Widmer. It is dedicated to Harald Baumann and Arlette Büchel, who both have devoted their lives to spreading the good news of the German New Medicine, and who both generously helped me with this book. With the exception of Harald and Arlette, both Swiss nationals, the others are all German: But they are all native German-speakers. They are all saving humanity from the Horror that is Modern Medicine.

This book is also dedicated to two organisations and all their respective members: Klein-Klein-Aktion and Amici di Dirk. Klein-Klein-Aktion members are dedicated to overcoming the Germ Theory of Disease medical myth and the associated viral fraud, which is the Achilles' heel of the Biomedical Paradigm. The members of Amici di Dirk are dedicated to spreading the word about the five Biological Laws of Nature. The members of both these organisations by their individual actions are helping to overcome the Biomedical Paradigm and create a world free from fear.

I have tried to accurately portray the ground-breaking work of both Dr Lanka and Dr Hamer in this book, and how they have obtained the scientific evidence necessary, for the enormous momentum required to overcome Modern Medicine and its Biomedical Paradigm. I have done my utmost to verify all the facts contained in this book. Ultimately any factual errors in this book are my responsibility, and should not reflect badly on these two scientific geniuses, nor on the empirical truth of their life work.

Viva la medicina sagrada![389]

Terminology and abbreviations used by the author

MD: is an abbreviation for medical doctor. These letters are currently used with pride by doctors worldwide particularly in the United States.

The Biomedical Paradigm: describes the philosophy and pattern of thinking employed by MDs. They believe that all disease and cancers are caused externally and not from within: They believe there is little or no mind–body connection in relation to the causes of cancers and other diseases.

The Ultimate Conspiracy: The MDs all believe in and promote the Biomedical Paradigm. Most of us (99% plus of the population) currently believe that the Biomedical Paradigm is scientific and true. This is what is meant by the Ultimate Conspiracy.

The Iatrogenic Effect: describes the tragic outcome of treatment by the MDs. It describes the effects of the treatment itself or even words used by the MD, such as "You have terminal cancer", which can cause further biological shocks providing proof of the Iatrogenic Effect.

The Tipping Point: will occur when public demand eventually forces a Government somewhere in the free world to demand scientific proof from the white-coats for the existence of any pathogenic virus.

The Turning Point: will occur when the Germ Theory of Disease medical myth is accepted by the scientific elites to be wrong. The Turning Point will be complete when the five Biological Laws of GNM are accepted by the scientific elites to be 100% correct.

The Semmelweis Reflex: the automatic summary dismissal or rejection out of hand of any new information without thought, inspection or experiment by the medical profession even though it will save many lives.

The Horror: is another name for the Iatrogenic Effect. The Horror describes the deaths and other injuries inflicted on us by Modern Medicine because of their belief in the Biomedical Paradigm and the Germ Theory of Disease medical myth. The largest components of The Horror currently are vaccinations, chemotherapy and medical treatment of the fictitious disease HIV-AIDS. Unless enough of us wake up, there could be a medically induced bird-flu pandemic that will potentially kill tens of millions of people.

White-coat: is a term used sarcastically to collectively designate most MDs, all oncologists, all pseudo-scientists and pseudo-virologists who all invariably wear white-coats.

Medical Myths: describes the dogmas that the MDs believe in even though there is no scientific basis for these myths, the dogmas such as metastasis, Germ Theory of Disease, viruses such as HIV-AIDS, measles, mumps and rubella. These myths have now acquired the status of dogmas: They are the sacred scripture of the Biomedical Paradigm and all MDs are required to believe in them.

KKA: Klein-Klein-Aktion is a German anti-vaccine, anti-Germ Theory of Disease, pro-life (in its broadest sense) and pro-GNM organisation led by Dr Stefan Lanka and Karl Krafeld. KKA strongly encourage individual citizens to ask the authorities for the scientific proof for the existence of any virus: measles, mumps, rubella, H5N1–bird flu and HIV-AIDS.

AIDS: Acquired Immune Deficiency Syndrome – a fictitious disease, which in reality is a collection of separate diseases allegedly caused by the fictitious HIV virus.

H5N1: Technical name for the putative bird flu virus. The H is an abbreviation for Haemagglutinin; The 5 is for type 5 of an alleged 15 or 16 Haemagglutin proteins which somehow has only been indirectly proven; N is an abbreviation for Neuraminidase; the 1 is for the first of nine types of the Neuraminidase enzyme that are said to exist by the white-coats.

Anamnesis: means the medical history of a patient. The patient tells his story and the GNM therapist understands the patient as a human being and how the particular event that occurred was a DHS for them causing their symptoms or "disease".

Dr: Doctor, usually an MD, possibly a PhD.

MBP: Meaningful Biological Program of Nature.

UN: United Nations.

WHO: World Health Organization, an agency of the UN.

FAO: Food and Agricultural Organization, an agency of the UN.

MMR: Measles, Mumps and Rubella fictitious viruses.

HIV: Human Immunodeficiency Virus, a fictitious virus invented and believed in by white-coats.

IQ: Intelligence Quotient.

UFO: Unidentified Flying Object.

MS: Multiple Sclerosis.

Terminology of the German New Medicine

Certain terms used in this book have been created by and are copyrighted by Dr Ryke Geerd Hamer.

GNM®: German New Medicine®. This is the body of work as discovered by Dr RG Hamer. The most important scientific facts discovered by Dr RG Hamer are the five Biological Laws of Nature.

DHS® – Dirk Hamer Syndrome – This is the biological shock that triggers the Meaningful Biological Program of Nature.

IRC® – The Iron Rule of Cancer. This is the First Biological Law of Nature.

Five Biological Laws of Nature®: These laws were discovered by Dr RG Hamer. They work 100% of the time for each and every cancer and disease.

First Biological Law: The Iron Rule of Cancer®. All cancers and other diseases (cancer-equivalent diseases) are caused by a DHS, a biological shock.

Second Biological Law: The law of two-phases®. All "diseases" or MBPs have two phases – the conflict-active phase caused by a DHS and the reparation phase caused when the conflict is resolved.

Third Biological Law: The ontogenetic system of cancers and cancer-equivalents® describes the symptoms of the MBP in the conflict-active phase and in the reparation phase.

Fourth Biological Law: The ontogenetic system of microbes® describes the nature of the microbes that operate in the reparation phase. These microbes are entirely dependent on the germ layer the organ is made up from.

Fifth Biological Law: The Quintessence®. There is a biological benefit and biological purpose behind every cancer/disease. Cancer/disease is not meaningless: It is a Meaningful Biological Program of Nature.

Conflict mass® – This is a product of the conflict duration and its intensity.

PCL® – Post ConflictoLysis.

CL® – Conflictolysis.

PCL-A® – First half of the reparation phase.

PCL-B® – Second half of the reparation phase.

EC Epileptoid / Epileptic Crisis® – midpoint of the reparation phase between PCL-A and PCL-B.

CA® – Conflict-active phase.

HH® – Hamerscher Herd or Hamer relay/Hamer focus literally in English which is viewable on a CT scan in the CA phase and in the reparation phase. It is not viewable when there is no ongoing conflict.

Tracks® – When a person experiences a DHS, he picks up on the surrounding circumstances. These surrounding circumstances are called tracks. In the case of allergies the tracks are the items such as nuts, eggs, sound, smell, taste, heat, cold, or materials that were present when the person experienced a DHS. There is no allergy without a previous DHS.

Sinnvolles Biologisches Sonderprogramm der Natur® – German New Medicine does not use the term "disease". Disease is a term used by Modern Medicine to describe the symptoms that occur in both the reparation phase and in the conflict-active phase of a Meaningful Biological Program of Nature. The original German term for this biological program is Sinnvolles Biologisches Sonderprogramm der Natur® – The abbreviation used by Dr Hamer is SBS®. This would be literally translated into English as a Meaningful Biological Special Program of Nature. In order to create a three-letter-abbreviation I have translated this term into English as a Meaningful Biological Program of Nature – and abbreviated it as an MBP.

Schizophrenic Constellation® – When a patient has two active territorial conflicts on both brain hemispheres, they are said to be in schizophrenic constellation.

Sources

Books

- Summary of the New Medicine, Dr RG Hamer.
- Krebs und alle sog. Krankheiten, (Cancer and all so-called diseases), Dr RG Hamer.
- Krebs: Krankheit der Seele, (Cancer: Disease of the Soul), Dr RG Hamer.
- Einer gegen alle, (One against all), Dr RG Hamer.
- Impfen: Völkermord im dritten Jahrtausend (Vaccination: Genocide in the Third Millenium) – Stefan Lanka and Karl Krafeld.
- Impfen – eine Entscheidung, die Eltern treffen (Vacccination: a decision parents make) Veronika Widmer.
- Guide to Natural Healing, Geddes and Grosset.
- The Turning Point, Fritjof Capra.
- The Dream and Lie of Louis Pasteur, RB Pearson.
- Béchamp or Pasteur: A Lost Chapter in the History of Biology, Ethel Douglas Hume.
- The Private Science of Louis Pasteur, Gerard Geison.
- Vaccination – The "Hidden" Facts, Ian Sinclair.
- Vaccination: A Business Based on Fear, Dr Gerhard Buchwald MD.
- The Role of Medicine, Thomas McKeown.
- In Defense of Smokers, Lauren A Colby.
- Swine Flu Expose, Eleanora McBean.
- Der Masern Betrug, (The Measles Fraud), Dr Stefan Lanka.

Articles

- Irish Times 19th October 2005.
- Medical Supplement of Irish Times every single Tuesday for way too many years.

- German New Medicine® (GNM). An Introduction to Dr. Hamer's Medical Paradigm, Caroline Markolin.
- Letter of confirmation of German New Medicine by the University of Trnva, hosted by www.newmedicine.ca & www.germannewmedicine.ca.
- The New Medicine, a new Natural Science, Dr Hans Ulrich Niemitz.
- Science and Whole Person Medicine: Enormous Potential in a New Relationship, Dr Rustum Roy.
- Modern Medicine: The New World Religion, Olivier Clerc.
- Biological Terrain vs The Germ Theory, the health advantage.
- Macht Impfen Sinn, (Does vaccination make sense), Dr Stefan Lanka.
- HIV; Reality or Artefact? Dr Stefan Lanka, Continuum, April/May 1995.
- The media campaign for AIDS tests, Liam Scheff.
- Avian Flu casts shadow over future of China's bird Lake, Jonathan Watts, Guardian newspaper Monday August 1 2005.
- Fowl play: The poultry industry's central role in the bird flu crisis, Grain Briefings, February 2006, hosted by www.grain.org.
- Second-hand Smokescreen, Steven Milloy, hosted by www.junkscience.com.
- Lord Nimmo-Smith Judgment on the relationship between smoking and lung cancer, hosted by http://www.scotcourts.gov.uk.
- NICE bowel cancer decision 'a scandal', hosted by www.menshealthforum.org.uk.
- Medical Guesswork, Business week magazine, May 29 2006.
- Is Heart Surgery Worth It, John Carey with Amy Barrett, Business Week magazine, July 2005.
- Death by Medicine, Gary Null and Associates, 2003.
- Doctors' strike in Israel may be good for health, Judy Siegel-Itzkovich, BMJ 10th June 2000.
- Doctor-Caused Disease, Monte Kline, hosted by www.pacifichealthcare.com.
- Medical Error Death Risk 1 in 300, by Sarah Hall, health correspondent, Guardian newspaper, Tuesday November 7 2006.
- There's more to vaccinations than the shot, Sharon Kimmelmann.
- Vaccination -Your child's best shot –, HPSC (Irish vaccine authority).

- Immunisation fact-file launched to promote 5-in-1 jab, Wednesday, October 13, 2004, www.pharmafocus.com.
- Deadly Immunity, Robert F Kennedy Jnr, June 2005.
- Adverse Effects of Adjuvants in Vaccines, Vera Scheibner, hosted on http://www.whale.to.
- Alert over new 5-in-1 Baby Jabs, Sunday Express, May 14 2006, Lucy Johnston.
- US scientists back autism link to MMR, Daily Telegraph 29th May 2006, Beezy Marsh and Sally Beck.
- The age of Autism, The Amish Anomaly, April 2005, Dan Olmstead, UPI reporter, hosted by http://www.whale.to.
- The age of Autism, A pretty big secret, December 2005, Dan Olmstead, UPI reporter, hosted by http://www.whale.to.
- Slaughter of the innocent, Jenny Marsh, June 2004, hosted by energygrid.
- Toxic Treatment without effect, Der Spiegel, 4th October 2004, Joerg Bleck.
- Chemotherapy of advanced epithelial cancer, a critical review, Ulrich Abel.
- Chemo's "Berlin Wall" crumbles, The Moss Reports, Ralph Moss.
- CDC Director, AIDS statement 01/12/2006, World AIDS day.
- Gibt es Beweise für die Existenz von krankmachenden Viren? (Is there any evidence for the existence of pathogenic viruses?),Dr Stefan Lanka, March 2002.
- Viruses, Dr Patrick Quanten MD.
- Die Publikation von Dr Lanka, (The Publications of Dr Lanka), Susanne Brix.
- Laws needed to target unvaccinated kids, Deborah Condon.
- From frozen Alaska to the lab: a virus 39,000 times more virulent than flu, Ian Sample, science correspondent, Guardian, October 6th 2005.
- Personal statement by Dr Patrick Quanten MD, November 1st 2001, hosted on Active Health website.
- Leben mit Zukunft (Life with a future): The bi-monthly brochure of Klein-Klein Aktion always contains many interesting articles.
- Germ Theory of Disease Causation, hosted by http://tuberose.com.

Websites

- www.dictionary.com Online English dictionary.
- www.newmedicine.ca Website maintained by Ilsedora Laker.
- www.germannewmedicine.ca Website maintained by Caroline Markolin.
- http://www.iee.et.tu-dresden.de Online English-German dictionary.
- www.klein-klein-verlag.de Website of Klein-Klein-Aktion's publishing house.
- www.klein-klein-aktion.de Website advocating action by individuals concerning the non-existence of any virus.
- www.wikipedia.org Wikipedia, the online encyclopaedia.
- www.theperthgroup.com The Perth Group also state emphatically that the HIV virus does not exist because there is no proof for its existence.
- http://www.whale.to This is mostly an anti-vaccination website.
- www.wddty.com What Doctors Don't Tell You website.
- www.virusmyth.net HIV and AIDS virus myths website.
- www.chrisreevehomepage.com Website about the actor Chris Reeve.
- www.neue-medizin.de German New Medicine website.
- www.bible.com All bible quotes were verified here.
- www.vaclib.org This is an anti-vaccination website.
- www.SickofDoctors.com
- www.yahoo.com
- www.google.com
- www.bbc.co.uk Website of the BBC – British Broadcasting Corporation.

TV

- Pandemic, the Horizon science show on the BBC, November 25th 2006. This show purporting to represent the truth that the H5N1 virus exists was a masterful piece of propaganda for the Biomedical Paradigm.

Interviews

- Interview by Christopher Ray from FAKTuell Redaktion with Dr Stefan Lanka on the 27th October 2005 called:- No Panic. The Truth about Bird Flu, H5N1, Vaccines and AIDS.
- Dr Buchwald's testimony before the Quebec College of Physicians Medical Board.
- Interview with President Mbeki, Joan Shenton, Carte Blanche, 16 April 2000.
- Interview with Shane Ellison, medicinal chemist, Jon Rappoport.

Notes

[1]This sentence is based on a quote from Dr RG Hamer.
[2]This sentence is a quote from Marcel Proust, a French writer.
[3]In this context I mean "Have a great read!"
[4]Morning News, Radio Ulster, Tuesday 19th October 2005.
[5]Stephen Nolan Show, Radio Ulster, Tuesday 19th October 2005.
[6]The term MD will be used throughout the book as an abbreviation for Medical Doctor, a practitioner of modern/orthodox/conventional medicine. Medicine is currently the ultimate professional qualification and the ultimate letters after your name in the US and increasingly in the Western world are MD.
[7]This is standard medical terminology to describe the increase in size of the liver.
[8]This is called metastasis by the MDs. Metastasis can be defined as: "a secondary cancerous growth formed by transmission of cancerous cells from a primary growth located elsewhere in the body"; www.dictionary.com.
[9]Drinking carrot juice, or eating just fruit and vegetables does not prevent any cancer/tumour from growing, because all cancers are caused by biological shocks. What is important about the food we eat is that it is wholesome and nutritious. This would exclude all processed foods–pretty much everything that is advertised on TV.
[10]www.newmedicine.ca; maintained by Ilsedora Laker.
[11]Anamnesis means the medical history of a patient; sourced from www.dictionary.com.
[12]It is common practice in the Catholic Church to have a mass offered up for the souls of the dead on or around the anniversary of their death.
[13]Summary of the New Medicine.
[14]Ilsedora Laker who maintains www.newmedicine.ca.
[15]Vermächtnis einer Neuen Medizin.
[16]This belief is from John 3:7 You must be born again.
[17]Mostly sourced from Summary of the New Medicine, Dr RG Hamer, page 175.
[18]Mostly sourced from Summary of the New Medicine, Dr RG Hamer, page 175.

[19]Mostly sourced from Summary of the New Medicine, Dr RG Hamer, page 175.
[20]Einer gegen alle, (One against all), Dr RG Hamer, page 39.
[21]The shock causing testicular/ovarian cancer is a shock caused by the loss or disappearance of a loved one.
[22]Krebs und alle sog. Krankheiten, (Cancer and all so-called Diseases), Dr RG Hamer, pages 13-17, the story of the shooting of Dirk Hamer.
[23]Krebs und alle sog. Krankheiten, (Cancer and all so-called Diseases), Dr RG Hamer, page 18.
[24]Krebs und alle sog. Krankheiten, (Cancer and all so-called Diseases), Dr RG Hamer, page 20.
[25]Krebs und alle sog. Krankheiten, (Cancer and all so-called Diseases), Dr RG Hamer, page 20–21.
[26]Krebs und alle sog. Krankheiten, (Cancer and all so-called Diseases), Dr RG Hamer, page 21.
[27]Krebs und alle sog. Krankheiten, (Cancer and all so-called Diseases), Dr RG Hamer, page 21.
[28]Krebs und alle sog. Krankheiten, (Cancer and all so-called Diseases), Dr RG Hamer, page 21.
[29]Krebs und alle sog. Krankheiten, (Cancer and all so-called Diseases), Dr RG Hamer, page 22.
[30]Krebs und alle sog. Krankheiten, (Cancer and all so-called Diseases), Dr RG Hamer, pages 22–23.
[31]German New Medicine® (GNM). An Introduction to Dr Hamer's Medical Paradigm, Caroline Markolin, www.germannewmedicine.ca.
[32]Ovarian cancer examples obtained from Harald Baumann's course in Limerick, Ireland, April 2005.
[33]Apart from diseases caused by malnutrition, bad water, poisoning, or trauma, all other diseases are classified as cancers or cancer-equivalent diseases by German New Medicine.
[34]Summary of the New Medicine, Dr RG Hamer, pages 24–26.
[35]German New Medicine® (GNM). An Introduction to Dr Hamer's Medical Paradigm, Caroline Markolin, www.germannewmedicine.ca.
[36]Reparation can be defined as "restoration to good condition", www.dictionary.com. The body restores itself back to full health in this reparation phase. One can still die in the reparation phase because of the conflict mass, because the preceding conflict has lasted too long or has been too intense.
[37]Ontogenesis can be defined as "The origin and development of an individual organism from embryo to adult, www.dictionary.com.
[38]Krebs und alle sog. Krankheiten, (Cancer and all so-called Diseases), Dr RG Hamer, page 77. The mortality rate after 5 years of chemotherapy is 95% and after 7 years of chemotherapy is 98%.
[39]The brain diagram is based on an original diagram created and copy-righted by Dr RG Hamer.

[40]Meaningful Biological Program of Nature, abbreviated to MBP, is my translation of the German term Sinnvolles Biologisches Sonderprogram der Natur, which is abbreviated to SBS.

[41]I used the term "healing phase" for the phase after a conflict has been solved up to May 2007. Following a conversation with Harald Baumann I changed the name of this phase to the "reparation phase" because the body is recuperating and restoring itself from the conflict-active phase. The term healing phase mistakenly gives the idea that everything should be fine, but in fact the healing phase can be deadly for a patient and in many MBPs it is the most deadly phase. Therefore I believe the term "reparation phase" to be a more appropriate term than "healing phase".

[42]The two-phase diagram was originally created and copy-righted to Dr RG Hamer.

[43]Summary of the New Medicine, Dr RG Hamer, page 175.

[44]Summary of the New Medicine, Dr RG Hamer, page 175.

[45]The English translation of the affidavit is on www.newmedicine.ca and www.germannewmedicine.ca.

[46]The phrase "white-coat" is used in a derogatory manner to describe all oncologists, most MDs, all pseudo-scientists and pseudo-virologists who all invariably wear white-coats. I first came across this term in an interview by Christopher Ray from FAKTuell Redaktion with Dr Stefan Lanka on the 27th October 2005 called No Panic. The Truth about Bird Flu, H5N1, Vaccines and AIDS.

[47]The Trnva verification/non-verification story was discussed with the author in June 2007.

[48]The "appalling vista" phrase originally was coined by Lord Denning in an infamous judgment concerning the Birmingham Six.

[49]Job was a rich person from the Old Testament who despite losing his children and all his possessions did not blame God, continued his belief in God, and was ultimately redeemed by God.

[50]This figure of 95% is an estimate based on the current medical procedures that are scientifically valid. This was discussed in a conversation with Harald Baumann in May 2007.

[51]http://www.iee.et.tu-dresden.de; Online English-German dictionary.

[52]www.klein-klein-verlag.de.

[53]Impfen: Völkermord im dritten Jahrtausend, (Vaccination: Genocide in the Third Millennium). Mein Weg zum Thema Impfen (My Way to the Vaccination question), Dr Stefan Lanka.

[54]No Panic. The truth about Bird flu, H5N1, vaccines and AIDS, an Interview by Christopher Ray with Dr Stefan Lanka from FAKTuell Redaktion 27.10.2005.

[55]Definition of "Paradigm" from www.dictionary.com.

[56]Hippocrates information sourced from Wikipedia, (the online encyclopedia).

[57]Hippocrates information sourced from Wikipedia, (the online encyclopedia).
[58]Hippocrates information sourced from Wikipedia, (the online encyclopedia).
[59]The Turning Point, Fritjof Capra, page 41 – 146.
[60]Guide to Natural Healing, Geddes and Grosset, page 235.
[61]The Turning Point, Fritjof Capra, page 47.
[62]The Turning Point, Fritjof Capra, page 118, Quote from George Engel.
[63]The Turning Point, Fritjof Capra, page 138.
[64]DHS or Dirk Hamer Syndrome is the GNM term for a biological shock.
[65]The phrase "It is a truth universally acknowledged" is from the first sentence of Pride and Prejudice by Jane Austen.
[66]The New Medicine, a new Natural Science, Dr Hans Ulrich Niemitz, hosted on www.germannewmedicine.ca.
[67]Quotations from: The New Medicine, a new Natural Science, Dr Hans Ulrich Niemitz.
[68]Quotations from: The New Medicine, a new Natural Science, Dr Hans Ulrich Niemitz.
[69]Science and Whole Person Medicine: Enormous Potential in a New Relationship, Dr Rustum Roy.
[70]Science and Whole Person Medicine: Enormous Potential in a New Relationship, Dr Rustum Roy.
[71]Science and Whole Person Medicine: Enormous Potential in a New Relationship, Dr Rustum Roy.
[72]Science and Whole Person Medicine: Enormous Potential in a New Relationship, Dr Rustum Roy.
[73]This information is mostly sourced from an article on the internet called Modern Medicine: The New World Religion, Olivier Clerc, based on a book of the same name.
[74]Hippocrates is the father of orthodox medicine and Pasteur is the father of the current version of orthodox medicine, so-called scientific medicine or Modern Medicine.
[75]Definition of religion obtained from www.dictionary.com.
[76]Definition of dogma obtained from www.dictionary.com.
[77]I first came across the 5000 dogmas in Modern Medicine from a course given by Harald Baumann in Limerick in April 2005 on GNM. Dr Hamer repeatedly states in his book Einer gegen alle (One against all) that there are about 5000 dogmas in Modern Medicine.
[78]Germ Theory of Disease definition, sourced from Wikipedia (the online encyclopedia).
[79]Yellow fever in Philadelphia, sourced from Wikipedia (the online encyclopedia).
[80]The Dream and Lie of Pasteur, RB Pearson, Chapter 1 Prior History of the "Germ Theory".

[81]Mostly sourced from The Dream and Lie of Pasteur, RB Pearson, Chapter 2 Bechamp, Pasteur, and Fermentation.
[82]Definition of Fermentation, sourced from Wikipedia (the online encyclopedia).
[83]Béchamp or Pasteur: A Lost Chapter in the History of Biology, Ethel Douglas Hume, page 81.
[84]Mostly sourced from The Dream and Lie of Pasteur, RB Pearson, Chapter 4 Bechamp's Microzymas or 'Little Bodies'.
[85]Béchamp or Pasteur: A Lost Chapter in the History of Biology, Ethel Douglas Hume, page 88.
[86]Béchamp or Pasteur: A Lost Chapter in the History of Biology, Ethel Douglas Hume, page 90.
[87]Béchamp or Pasteur: A Lost Chapter in the History of Biology, Ethel Douglas Hume, page 91.
[88]Mostly sourced from The Dream and Lie of Pasteur, RB Pearson, Chapter 4 Bechamp's Microzymas or 'Little Bodies'.
[89]Biological Terrain vs The Germ Theory, hosted by http://thehealthadvantage.com.
[90]Biological Terrain vs The Germ Theory, hosted by http://thehealthadvantage.com.
[91]Mostly sourced from The Private Science of Louis Pasteur, Gerald L Geison, page 18.
[92]The Private Science of Louis Pasteur, Gerald L Geison, page 18.
[93]Pasteur's deathbed saying is quoted in many articles on the internet. I do not know the original source.
[94]This sentence is based on the title of the book by Ethel Douglas Hume, A Lost Chapter in the History of Biology.
[95]Vaccination definition, sourced from Wikipedia, (the online encyclopedia).
[96]Béchamp or Pasteur: A Lost Chapter in the History of Biology, Ethel Douglas Hume, page 195.
[97]The mumps story was from a conversation with Harald Baumann in March 2007.
[98]Smallpox reference sourced from Wikipedia, (the online encyclopedia).
[99]Variolation definition, sourced from Wikipedia (the online encyclopedia).
[100]Variolation story, sourced from Wikipedia (the online encyclopedia).
[101]Impfen eine Entscheidung die Eltern treffen, (Vaccination a Decision Parents Make), Veronika Widmer, pages 18–19.
[102]Mostly sourced from Impfen eine Entscheidung die Eltern treffen, (Vaccination a Decision Parents Make), Veronika Widmer, page 20.
[103]Vaccination The "Hidden" Facts, Ian Sinclair, foreword.
[104]Vaccination The "Hidden" Facts, Ian Sinclair, page 34–37.
[105]Impfen eine Entscheidung die Eltern treffen, (Vaccination a Decision Parents Make), Veronika Widmer, page 44.
[106]Vaccination – The "Hidden" Facts, Ian Sinclair, page 60.

[107]Béchamp or Pasteur: A lost Chapter in the History of Biology, Ethel Douglas Hume, page 174. I am paraphrasing what Florence Nightingale the famous English nurse said.
[108]This is a quote from Professor Antoine Béchamp.
[109]Macht Impfen sinn? (Does Vaccination Make Sense?), Dr Stefan Lanka, March 2002.
[110]Vaccination – The "Hidden" Facts, Ian Sinclair, page 87.
[111]Vaccination – The "Hidden" Facts, Ian Sinclair, page 87.
[112]Vaccination – The "Hidden" Facts, Ian Sinclair, page 3.
[113]Vaccination – The "Hidden" Facts, Ian Sinclair, page 3.
[114]Vaccination – The "Hidden" Facts, Ian Sinclair, page 30.
[115]Vaccination – The "Hidden" Facts, Ian Sinclair, page 4.
[116]Vaccination – The "Hidden" Facts, Ian Sinclair, page 4.
[117]Vaccination – The "Hidden" Facts, Ian Sinclair, page 5.
[118]Vaccination – The "Hidden" Facts, Ian Sinclair, page 5–6.
[119]Vaccination – The "Hidden" Facts, Ian Sinclair, page 6.
[120]Vaccination – The "Hidden" Facts, Ian Sinclair, page 58.
[121]Vaccination – The "Hidden" Facts, Ian Sinclair, page 58.
[122]Vaccination – The "Hidden" Facts, Ian Sinclair, page 14.
[123]Vaccination – The "Hidden" Facts, Ian Sinclair, page 13.
[124]Vaccination: A Business Based on Fear, Dr Gerhard Buchwald MD, page 161.
[125]The Role of Medicine, Chapter 4 Infectious diseases, Thomas McKeown.
[126]Vaccination – The "Hidden" Facts, Ian Sinclair, page 34.
[127]Vaccination – The "Hidden" Facts, Ian Sinclair, page 35.
[128]Krebs und alle sog. Krankheiten, (Cancer and all so-called diseases), Dr RG Hamer, page 126.
[129]HIV; Reality or Artefact? Dr Stefan Lanka, Continuum, April/May 1995.
[130]Definition of Viruses sourced from HIV; Reality or Artefact?, Dr Stefan Lanka, Continuum, April/May 1995.
[131]Definition of a retrovirus sourced from Wikipedia (the online encyclopedia).
[132]Origins of AIDS sourced from Wikipedia (the online encyclopedia).
[133]Luc Montagnier story sourced from HIV; Reality or Artefact, Dr Stefan Lanka.
[134]AIDS definition sourced from www.stopaids.org.
[135]HIV theory of AIDS sourced from www.theperthgroup.com.
[136]HIV; Reality or Artefact? Dr Stefan Lanka, Continuum, April/May 1995.
[137]The media campaign for AIDS tests, Liam Scheff, 12/03/2005, hosted by www.aim.org.
[138]The media campaign for AIDS tests, Liam Scheff, 12/03/2005, hosted by www.aim.org.
[139]The two key AIDS diseases for Homosexuals are Kaposi's sarcoma and pneumonia.

[140]HIV-positive information sourced from The Perth Group www.theperth-group.com.
[141]HIV; Reality or Artefact, Dr Stefan Lanka Stefan Lanka, Continuum, April/ May 1995.
[142]The formation of the Perth Group sourced from www.theperthgroup.com.
[143]Klein-Klein-Aktion literally means Small-Small-Actions.
[144]The whole point of Klein-Klein-Aktion is that the white-coats must provide evidence for the existence of any virus; HIV, measles, mumps or rubella.
[145]The Martian argument is sourced from the Perth group: www.theperth-group.com.
[146]Definition of flu is sourced from Wikipedia (the online encyclopedia).
[147]The Irish vaccine authority is the HPSC - Health Protection Surveillance Centre.
[148]No Panic. The truth about Bird Flu, H5N1, vaccines and AIDS Interview by Christopher Ray with Dr Stefan Lanka, FAKTuell Redaktion 27/10/2005.
[149]No Panic. The truth about Bird flu, H5N1, vaccines and AIDS Interview by Christopher Ray with Dr Stefan Lanka, FAKTuell Redaktion 27/10/2005.
[150]Sourced from Fowl play: The poultry industry's central role in the bird flu crisis, Grain Briefings, February 2006, hosted by www.grain.org.
[151]Avian Flu casts shadow over future of China's bird Lake, Jonathan Watts, Guardian newspaper Monday August 1 2005.
[152]BirdLife International is a global alliance of conservation organisations working together for the world's birds and people.
[153]Fowl play: The poultry industry's central role in the bird flu crisis, Grain Briefings, February 2006, hosted by www.grain.org.
[154]Fowl play: The poultry industry's central role in the bird flu crisis, Grain Briefings, February 2006, hosted by www.grain.org.
[155]Avian Flu casts shadow over future of China's bird Lake, Jonathan Watts, Guardian newspaper Monday August 1 2005.
[156]Avian Flu casts shadow over future of China's bird Lake, Jonathan Watts, Guardian newspaper Monday August 1 2005.
[157]Fowl play: The poultry industry's central role in the bird flu crisis, Grain Briefings, February 2006, hosted by www.grain.org.
[158]No Panic. The truth about Bird Flu, H5N1, vaccines and AIDS Interview by Christopher Ray with Dr Stefan Lanka, FAKTuell Redaktion 27.10.2005.
[159]No Panic. The truth about Bird Flu, H5N1, vaccines and AIDS Interview by Christopher Ray with Dr Stefan Lanka, FAKTuell Redaktion 27.10.2005.
[160]From frozen Alaska to the lab: a virus 39,000 times more virulent than flu, Ian Sample, science correspondent, Guardian, October 6th 2005.
[161]No Panic. The truth about Bird Flu, H5N1, vaccines and AIDS. Interview by Christopher Ray with Dr Stefan Lanka, FAKTuell Redaktion 27.10.2005.
[162]Tamiflu information was sourced from Wikipedia (the online encyclopedia).
[163]Fowl play: The poultry industry's central role in the bird flu crisis, Grain briefings, February 2006, hosted by www.grain.org.

[164]Passive smoking is called ETS or Environmental Tobacco Smoking by the white-coats.
[165]Unlike President Bill Clinton who claims that when he was a young man that he smoked a joint but did not inhale.
[166]Alveolar lung cancer is caused by a "Fear of Death" biological shock.
[167]This section is mostly sourced from In Defense of Smokers by Lauren A Colby.
[168]In Defense of Smokers, Lauren A Colby, Chapter 2: The Burden of Proof.
[169]In Defense of Smokers, Lauren A Colby, Chapter 8: Smoking Myths and the Role of Detection Bias. Burch's paper was called Smoking and lung cancer: the problem of inferring cause (1978) J. Royal Statistical Society A 141:437–477.
[170]In Defense of Smokers, Lauren A Colby, Chapter 7: The Surgeon General's Reports. Brownlee's paper was called A Review of Smoking and Health (1965) J. Amer. Statist. Ass. 60, 722–739.
[171]In Defense of Smokers, Lauren A Colby, Chapter 6: The Propaganda machine.
[172]Second-hand Smokescreen, Steven Milloy, hosted by www.junkscience.com.
[173]In Defense of Smokers, Lauren A Colby, Chapter 8: Smoking Myths and the Role of Detection Bias.
[174]Summary of the New Medicine, Dr RG Hamer, Page 153.
[175]Lord Nimmo Smith judgment, http://www.scotcourts.gov.uk/opinions/2005CSOH69.html.
[176]Lord Nimmo Smith judgment, http://www.scotcourts.gov.uk/opinions/2005CSOH69.html.
[177]The real effects of smoking were discussed in a conversation with Harald Baumann in March 2007.
[178]French fries are called chips in Ireland and Britain.
[179]Definition of Metastasis from www.dictionary.com.
[180]The New Medicine, a new Natural Science, Dr Hans Ulrich Niemitz, hosted on www.germannewmedicine.ca.
[181]Krebs und alle sog. Krankheiten, (Cancer and all so-called Diseases), Dr RG Hamer, page 88.
[182]Krebs und alle sog. Krankheiten, (Cancer and all so-called Diseases), Dr RG Hamer, page 144.
[183]The phrase "disease is born in us and from us" is a quote from Professor Antoine Béchamp.
[184]Summary of the New Medicine, Dr RG Hamer, Page 157.
[185]Placebo definition from www.dictionary.com.
[186]Irish Times 19th October 2005.
[187]NICE bowel cancer decision 'a scandal', www.menshealthforum.org.uk.
[188]NICE bowel cancer decision 'a scandal', www.menshealthforum.org.uk.
[189]This section is mostly sourced from Medical Guesswork, Business Week magazine, May 29 2006.

[190]This section is mostly sourced from Is Heart Surgery Worth It, John Carey with Amy Barrett, Business Week magazine, July 2005.
[191]Death by Medicine, Gary Null and Associates, 2003.
[192]Doctors' strike in Israel may be good for health, Judy Siegel-Itzkovich, BMJ 10th June 2000.
[193]Doctor-Caused Disease, Monte Kline, www.pacifichealth care.com.
[194]Doctors' strike in Israel may be good for health, Judy Siegel-Itzkovich, BMJ 10th June 2000.
[195]Medical Error Death Risk 1 in 300, by Sarah Hall, health correspondent, Guardian newspaper, Tuesday November 7 2006.
[196]The acronym PFLS is contained in the article: There's more to vaccinations than the shot, Sharon Kimmelmann.
[197]Vaccination schedule obtained from Irish Government website www.citizensinformation.ie.
[198]Immunisation fact-file launched to promote 5-in-1 jab, Wednesday, October 13, 2004, www.pharmafocus.com.
[199]This section is mostly sourced from Deadly Immunity, Robert F Kennedy Jnr. All quotations are from this article.
[200]This suspicion is according to the article Deadly Immunity, Robert F Kennedy Jnr.
[201]Adverse Effects of Adjuvants in Vaccines, Vera Scheibner, hosted on http://www.whale.to.
[202]Mostly sourced from: Alert over new 5-in-1 Baby Jabs, Sunday Express, May 14 2006, Lucy Johnston.
[203]This document was publicised by What Doctors Don't Tell You (www.wddty.com) who produce a monthly newsletter that questions conventional medicine.
[204]Alert over new 5-in-1 Baby Jabs, Sunday Express May 14 2006, Lucy Johnston.
[205]US scientists back autism link to MMR, Daily Telegraph 29th May 2006, Beezy Marsh and Sally Beck.
[206]A cot is the word used in Ireland and Britain for a crib in the US.
[207]Dr Buchwald's testimony before the Quebec College of Physicians Medical Board, hosted on http://www.whale.to.
[208]Vaccination a Business based on Fear, Dr Gerhard Buchwald MD, 1995, page 247–248.
[209]Vaccination a Business based on Fear, Dr Gerhard Buchwald MD, 1995, back page.
[210]Vaccination a Business based on Fear, Dr Gerhard Buchwald MD, 1995, page 297.
[211]The age of Autism, The Amish Anomaly, April 2005, Dan Olmstead, UPI reporter, hosted by http://www.whale.to.
[212]The age of Autism, A pretty big secret, December 2005, Dan Olmstead, UPI reporter, hosted by http://www.whale.to.

[213]Krebs und alle sog. Krankheiten, (Cancer and all so-called Diseases), Dr RG Hamer, page 77.
[214]Slaughter of the innocent, Jenny Marsh, June 2004, hosted by energygrid.
[215]Toxic Treatment without effect, Der Spiegel, 4th October 2004, Joerg Bleck.
[216]Toxic Treatment without effect, Der Spiegel, 4th October 2004, Jörg Blech.
[217]Chemo's "Berlin Wall" crumbles, The Moss Reports, Ralph Moss.
[218]Chemo's "Berlin Wall" crumbles, The Moss Reports, Ralph Moss.
[219]Chemotherapy of advanced epithelial cancer, a critical review, Ulrich Abel.
[220]Toxic Treatment without effect, Der Spiegel, 4th October 2004, Joerg Bleck.
[221]Future radiation therapy treatment confirmed in a conversation with Harald Baumann in June 2007.
[222]Krebs und alle sog. Krankheiten, (Cancer and all so-called diseases), Dr RG Hamer, page 129.
[223]Krebs und alle sog. Krankheiten, (Cancer and all so-called diseases), Dr RG Hamer, page 129.
[224]Krebs und alle sog. Krankheiten, (Cancer and all so-called diseases), Dr RG Hamer, page 129 and 130.
[225]The German for "Cancer is curable" is "Krebs ist heilbar": I think it sounds poetic in the German language.
[226]With the exception of bloodletting all the others medical horrors were inflicted on us by Modern Medicine the current form of orthodox medicine.
[227]The information about bloodletting was sourced from Wikipedia (the online encyclopedia).
[228]The information about Semmelweis was sourced from Wikipedia (the online encyclopedia).
[229]Gibt es Beweise für die Existenz von krankmachenden Viren? (Is there any evidence for the existence of pathogenic viruses?),Dr Stefan Lanka, March 2002.
[230]Semmelweiss's book was called Die Ätiologie, der Begriff und die Prophylaxis des Kindbettfiebers.
[231]The term "Semmelweis Reflex" was sourced from Wikipedia (the online encyclopedia).
[232]General information about the Spanish flu was sourced from Wikipedia (the online encyclopedia).
[233]This paragraph explaining other possible reasons for the deaths of young soldiers was inserted based on a conversation with Harald Baumann in June 2007.
[234]Swine Flu Expose, Eleanora McBean, Chapter 3 Anti-Typhoid Vaccine Causes a worse disease which the Doctors name Paratyphoid, hosted by http://www.whale.to.

[235]Swine Flu Expose, Eleanora McBean, Chapter 2 The Spanish Influenza Epidemic of 1918 was caused by vaccinations, Hosted by http://www.whale.to.
[236]Swine Flu Expose, Eleanora McBean, Chapter 1 Swine Flu another medically-made epidemic, Hosted by http://www.whale.to.
[237]Mbeki AIDS story sourced from Wikipedia (the online encyclopedia).
[238]Interview President Mbeki, Joan Shenton for Carte Blanch, 16 April 2000, hosted by www.virusmyth.com.
[239]CDC Director, AIDS statement 01/12/2006, World AIDS day.
[240]The possible bird flu catastrophe section was inspired by a masterful piece of propaganda for the Biomedical Paradigm, Pandemic, a Horizon science show on the BBC, November 25th 2006.
[241]Mostly sourced from Viruses, Patrick Quanten MD.
[242]No Panic. The truth about Bird flu, H5N1, vaccines and AIDS, Interview by Christopher Ray from FAKTuell Redaktion with Dr Stefan Lanka 27.10.2005
[243]The UFO analogy has been used in various writings by Karl Krafeld and Stefan Lanka from Klein-Klein-Aktion.
[244]Mostly sourced from Gibt es Beweise für die Existenz von krankmachenden Viren? (Is there any evidence for the existence of pathogenic viruses?), Dr Stefan Lanka, March 2002.
[245]Die Publikation von Dr Lanka, (The Publications of Dr Lanka), Suzanne Brix.
[246]Gibt es Beweise für die Existenz von krankmachenden Viren?, (Is there any evidence for the existence of pathogenic viruses?), Dr Stefan Lanka, March 2002.
[247]Emperors New Clothes story sourced from Wikipedia (the online encyclopedia).
[248]This is an invented story to give an example of the type of conflict that could cause mumps. It is sourced from Lisa and the Mumps, The Strong family and their medical adventures, Volume 3, Harald Baumann and Daniela Amstutz.
[249]Mammy is the term used in Ireland for Mummy or Mum in England or Mom in the US.
[250]Cidona is an Irish apple-based soft-drink that I really like.
[251]This is an invented story to give an example of the type of conflict that could cause measles or rubella. It is sourced from Lisa and the red spots, The Strong Family and their medical adventures, Volume 1, by Harald Baumann and Daniela Amstutz.
[252]Sourced from Page 17 of Sammy has a rash, The Strong family and their medical adventures, Volume 5, by Harald Baumann and Daniela Amstutz.
[253]Der Masern Betrug, (The Measles Fraud), Dr Stefan Lanka, page 150.
[254]Der Masern Betrug, (The Measles Fraud), Dr Stefan Lanka, page 150 .
[255]Sourced from the World Health Organization's website www.who.int.

[256]Possible causes of measles were suggested by Harald Baumann in a phone conversation in May 2007.
[257]This sentence is based on the title of a book by Dr Gerhard Buchwald–Vaccination: A business based on Fear.
[258]Origin of cause of liver cancer and all cancers/diseases obtained from the Psyche-Brain-Organ disease chart created by Dr RG Hamer.
[259]Summary of the New Medicine, Dr RG Hamer, page 155.
[260]Prevalence of liver cancer in starving children discussed in a conversation with Harald Baumann in March 2007.
[261]Great Expectations is a novel by Charles Dickens.
[262]Case study with Harald Baumann, discussed with author in March and June 2007.
[263]Case study with Harald Baumann, discussed with author in March and June 2007.
[264]Case study with Harald Baumann, discussed with author in March and June 2007.
[265]Case study with Harald Baumann, discussed with author in March and June 2007.
[266]Case study with Harald Baumann, discussed with author in March and June 2007.
[267]Case study with Harald Baumann, discussed with author in March and June 2007.
[268]Case study with Harald Baumann, discussed with author in March and June 2007.
[269]Brain tumour definition sourced from Wikipedia (the online encyclopedia).
[270]Brain tumour statistics sourced from Wikipedia (the online encyclopedia).
[271]Summary of the New Medicine, Dr RG Hamer, Page 90–91.
[272]German New Medicine® (GNM). An Introduction to Dr Hamer's Medical Paradigm, Caroline Markolin, www.germannewmedicine.ca.
[273]German New Medicine® (GNM). An Introduction to Dr Hamer's Medical Paradigm, Caroline Markolin, www.germannewmedicine.ca.
[274]Case study with Harald Baumann, discussed with author in March and June 2007.
[275]Case study with Harald Baumann, discussed with author in March and June 2007.
[276]Summary of the New Medicine, Dr RG Hamer, page 157.
[277]Summary of the New Medicine, Dr RG Hamer, page 157–160. 6,000 Syrian hamsters were exposed to a life-time of cigarette smoke and not one hamster developed bronchial cancer nor alveolar lung cancer.
[278]Case study with Harald Baumann, discussed with author in March and June 2007.
[279]Case study with Harald Baumann, discussed with author in March and June 2007.

[280]Case study with Harald Baumann, discussed with author in March and June 2007.

[281]Dana Reeve case study was suggested by Harald Baumann in March 2007. The factual accounts of her cancer were sourced from www.chrisreevehomepage.com.

[282]Poison – Chemotherapy, Slash – Surgery, Burn – Radiotherapy.

[283]The experiment to prove the cause of lung cancer and tuberculosis was suggested by Harald Baumann in March 2007.

[284]Detection of breast cancer, sourced from the BBC website: www.bbc.co.uk.

[285]This is an invented story to give an example of the type of conflict that could cause glandular breast cancer. It is sourced from Mummy Strong has a Lump in her Breast, The Strong Family and their medical adventures, Volume 6, Harald Baumann and Daniela Amstutz.

[286]Case study with Harald Baumann, discussed with author in July 2007.

[287]Case study with Harald Baumann, discussed with author in July 2007.

[288]Based on a picture and story on page 105 of Krebs und alle sog. Krankheiten (Cancer and all so-called Diseases), Dr RG Hamer.

[289]Based on a picture and story on page 97 of Krebs und alle sog. Krankheiten (Cancer and all so-called Diseases), Dr RG Hamer.

[290]Case study with Harald Baumann, discussed with author in March and June 2007.

[291]Symptoms of prostate cancer, sourced from the BBC website: www.bbc.co.uk.

[292]Detection of prostate cancer, sourced from the BBC website: www.bbc.co.uk.

[293]Case study with Harald Baumann, discussed with author in March 2007.

[294]Case study with Harald Baumann, discussed with author in March and June 2007.

[295]Symptoms of colon cancer, sourced from the BBC website: www.bbc.co.uk.

[296]Detection of colon cancer, sourced from the BBC website: www.bbc.co.uk.

[297]Case study with Harald Baumann, discussed with author in March and June 2007.

[298]Case study with Harald Baumann, discussed with author in March and June 2007.

[299]Case study with Harald Baumann, discussed with author in March and June 2007.

[300]Case study with Harald Baumann, discussed with author in April 2005 and March 2007.

[301]Case study with Harald Baumann, discussed with author in March and June 2007.

[302]Case study with Harald Baumann, discussed with author in March and June 2007.

[303]Definition of allergy, sourced from Allergy UK http://www.allergyuk.org.

[304]Case study with Harald Baumann, discussed with author in June 2007.
[305]Nut allergy case study sourced from a German-language GNM website www.neue-medizin.de.
[306]Case study with Harald Baumann, discussed with author in March and June 2007.
[307]This is called a tiger robbery because of the predatory stalking that precedes it.
[308]Definition of diabetes sourced from Wikipedia (the online encyclopedia).
[309]Diabetes information sourced from the GNM website, www.neue-medizin.de.
[310]Mellitus is the Latin word for sweet. Yes, some MDs must have tasted the urine to discover that it is sweet when the patient has diabetes mellitus (beta cells).
[311]Any of these conditions cause the right-handed woman to react to a biological shock like a right-handed male.
[312]Case study with Harald Baumann, discussed with author in March and June 2007.
[313]Case study with Harald Baumann, discussed with author in March and June 2007.
[314]Even with an excellent German language understanding, Swiss-German can still be almost incomprehensible. Certainly the author (with basic German) on a trip to Switzerland visiting Harald Baumann, could understand the written language but had no idea of what the Swiss were saying. They might as well have been speaking Swahili.
[315]Case study with Harald Baumann, discussed with author in March and June 2007.
[316]Case study with Harald Baumann, discussed with author in March and June 2007.
[317]Case study with Harald Baumann, discussed with author in March and June 2007.
[318]Case study with Harald Baumann, discussed with author in April 2005 and March 2007.
[319]An Achilles' heel is a fatal weakness in spite of overall strength, actually or potentially leading to downfall, sourced from Wikipedia (the online encyclopedia).
[320]The Sunday Business Post is an Irish Newspaper.
[321]Laws needed to target unvaccinated kids, Deborah Condon, January 2003. Hosted on www.irishhealth.com.
[322]There were some typographical errors in the original e-mail that was sent. The content is the exact same.
[323]There were some typographical errors in the original e-mail that was sent. I also gave the internet links for these two books and for Dr Lanka's scientific publication rather than their titles. Apart from that the content is the exact same.
[324]There were some typographical errors in the original e-mail that was sent. The content is the exact same.

[325]I also gave the internet links for these two books rather than their titles in the original e-mail. Apart from that the content is the exact same.
[326]There were some typographical errors in the original e-mail that was sent. Apart from that the content is the exact same.
[327]There were some typographical errors in the original e-mail that was sent. Apart from that the content is the exact same.
[328]There were some typographical errors in the original e-mail that was sent. Apart from that the content is the exact same.
[329]There were some typographical errors in the original e-mail that was sent. Apart from that the content is the exact same.
[330]There were some typographical errors in the original e-mail that was sent. Apart from that the content is the exact same.
[331]Taoiseach is the Irish/Gaelic for Prime Minister. Taoiseach is pronounced phonetically Tee-shock.
[332]There were some typographical errors in the original e-mail that was sent. Apart from that the content is the exact same.
[333]Tánaiste is pronounced phonetically Tawn-ash-te.
[334]There were some typographical errors in the original e-mail that was sent. Apart from that the content is the exact same.
[335]"The Troubles" describes the low-intensity war mostly in Northern Ireland (6-counties of Ireland) from 1968–1994.
[336]An Tánaiste is the Irish/Gaelic for the Deputy Prime Minister.
[337]I also gave the internet links for these two books rather than their titles in the original e-mail. Apart from that the content is the exact same.
[338]There were some typographical errors in the original e-mail that was sent. Apart from that the content is the exact same.
[339]The link to Dr Lanka's scientific publication is given in the original e-mail. Apart from that the content is the exact same.
[340]The link to the text book is given in the original e-mail. Apart from that the content is the exact same.
[341]Impfen – Völkermord im dritten Jahrtausend? (Vaccination – Genocide in the Third Millennium?) Was ist Wissenschaft (What is science) chapter, Karl Krafeld.
[342]The link to the text book is given in the original e-mail. There were some typographical errors in the original e-mail that was sent. Apart from that the content is the exact same.
[343]There were some typographical errors in the original e-mail that was sent. Links were used in the original e-mail. Apart from that the content is the exact same.
[344]Links were used in the original e-mail rather than the titles. Apart from that the content is the exact same.
[345]There were some typographical errors in the original e-mail that was sent. Links were used in the original e-mail rather than the titles. Apart from that the content is the exact same.

[346]In the original e-mail I got the proper name of the recipient Kalpana Chauhan completely wrong. This is because I had never come across a name like that before. I wrote back to her and apologised for misspelling her name and re-sent the original e-mail with my queries.
[347]There were some typographical errors in the original e-mail that was sent. Apart from that the content is the exact same.
[348]I used the term "healing-phase" up to May 2007. I now believe that the term "reparation phase" is more appropriate.
[349]The rejection of empirical medical evidence without testing it is called the Semmelweis Reflex in honour of the way Semmelweis himself was treated by the medical establishment of his day.
[350]In the original e-mail the title of the fourth Biological Law was the same as the third Biological Law. Glandular breast cancer was mistakenly said to occur in the reparation phase instead of the conflict-active phase. Apart from these errors, the content of the printed e-mail is the same as the original e-mail that was sent.
[351]There were some typographical errors in the original e-mail that was sent. Apart from that the content is the exact same.
[352]www.germannewmdicine.ca.
[353]There were some typographical errors in the original e-mail published on www.germannewmedicine.ca. Apart from that the content is the exact same.
[354]For example Profesor Duesberg states that the HIV virus exists but that it is harmless.
[355]There were some typographical errors in the original e-mail that was sent. Apart from that the content is the exact same.
[356]Jon Rappoport interview with a former vaccine researcher, hosted by http://www.whale.to.
[357]Radio Telefís Éireann, RTÉ, Ireland's Public Service Broadcaster.
[358]There were some typographical errors in the original e-mail that was sent. Apart from that the content is the exact same.
[359]BBC – British Broadcasting Corporation.
[360]Sourced from Fowl play: The poultry industry's central role in the bird flu crisis, Grain Briefings February 2006, hosted by www.grain.org.
[361]Sourced from Fowl play: The poultry industry's central role in the bird flu crisis, Grain Briefings February 2006, hosted by www.grain.org.
[362]Encephalitis Lethargica information sourced from Wikipedia (the online encyclopedia).
[363]There were some typographical errors in the original e-mail that was sent. Apart from that the content is the exact same.
[364]The Irish newspapers were The Irish Times, The Irish News, The Examiner and The Belfast Telegraph. The English Newspapers were the Guardian and The Independent.
[365]There were some typographical errors in the original e-mail that was sent. Apart from that the content is the exact same.

[366]The phrase "The Turning Point" comes from a brilliant book of the same name by Fritjof Capra.
[367]Interview with Shane Ellison, former medicinal chemist, hosted by http://www.whale.to.
[368]Interview with Shane Ellison, former medicinal chemist, hosted by http://www.whale.to.
[369]This sentence is based on a quotation from St Bernard of Clairvaux.
[370]Dr Buchwald's testimony before the Quebec College of Physicians Medical Board, hosted on http://www.whale.to.
[371]Personal statement by Dr Patrick Quanten, MD November 1st 2001, hosted on Active Health website.
[372]Surgeon story sourced from two conversations with Harald Baumann April 2005 and March 2007.
[373]Psychiatrist story sourced from two conversations with Harald Baumann April 2005 and March 2007.
[374]This sentence is paraphrased from a quote by Martin Luther King jnr.
[375]John 8:7 "Let him who is without sin, cast the first stone".
[376]This sentence came from the article: No Panic. The truth about Bird flu, H5N1, vaccines and AIDS, an Interview by Christopher Ray with Dr Stefan Lanka from FAKTuell Redaktion 27.10.2005.
[377]The back cover and spine of the book depict the staff of Asclepius. This symbol is used by many medical and pharmaceutical organisations worldwide. The staff of Asclepius is used by the author as a symbol for Modern Medicine.
[378]The Role of Medicine, Thomas McKeown, Page 3.
[379]The Role of Medicine, Thomas McKeown, Page 3.
[380]20-20 vision describes perfect eye-sight. Hopefully by the year 2020 most of us will be able to see clearly with new eyes and understand the Horror that is Modern Medicine. This chapter has been inspired by the "Aisling"/ Dream poems from Irish literature.
[381]Louis Armstrong was a famous Jazz musician. His version of "What a wonderful life" is both definitive and memorable.
[382]Diabetes is caused by a fear-disgust/revulsion conflict. Every Tuesday I read the Irish Times medical supplement and was revolted and disgusted by it. I never got a DHS because I was mentally prepared for it, knowing that most medical stories were absolute fiction. Despite my continuing disgust there was no shock involved and hence no DHS.
[383]The chapter heading was inspired by the bi-monthly magazine of Klein-Klein-Aktion, called Leben mit Zukunft (Life with a Future)
[384]This sentence is a quote from the German philosopher Schopenhauer.
[385]This sentence has been reworded from a quotation from the contents section of Vaccinations the "Hidden" Facts, Ian Sinclair.
[386]This sentence is a quote from Edmund Burke Irish/British Statesman.

[387]Based on Catholic/Christian teaching – The sin of Omission.
[388]One of the last statements by Pope John Paul 2.
[389]Viva La Medicina sagrada, Long live the sacred medicine, in Spanish. La Medicina sagrada is a Spanish term for the New Medicine or German New Medicine.

Made in United States
North Haven, CT
10 November 2026

22081994R00241